CCRN®

CERTIFICATION FOR ADULT, PEDIATRIC, AND NEONATAL CRITICAL CARE NURSES

2009 EDITION

OTHER KAPLAN TITLES FOR WORKING NURSES

Your Career in Nursing

First-Year Nurse

Kaplan Legal Nurse Consultant

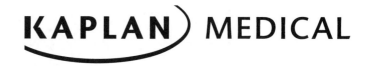

CCRN®

CERTIFICATION FOR ADULT, PEDIATRIC, AND NEONATAL CRITICAL CARE NURSES

2009 EDITION

PROVEN, PRACTICAL TOOLS TO HELP YOU PASS THE TEST

© 2009 Kaplan, Inc.

Published by Kaplan Publishing, a division of Kaplan, Inc.
1 Liberty Plaza, 24th Floor
New York, NY 10006

Printed in the United States of America

10 9 8 7 6 5 4 3 2 1

ISBN-13: 978-1-4277-9772-8

Kaplan Publishing books are available at special quantity discounts to use for sales promotions, employee premiums, or educational purposes. Please email our Special Sales Department to order or for more information at *kaplanpublishing@kaplan.com*, or write to Kaplan Publishing, 1 Liberty Plaza, 24th Floor, New York, NY 10006.

CONTRIBUTING EDITOR

Sailesh C. Harwani, MD, PhD

Contributing Authors

Nancy Baumhover, RN, MSN, CCRN
The Cardiovascular System

Cynthia Gurdak Berry, RN, MSN
Multiorgan System

Doris Denison, MSN, ACNP-BC, CCRN
The Endocrine System
The Neurologic System
Professional Caring and Ethical Practice Using the Synergy Model

Sailesh C. Harwani, MD, PhD
The Pulmonary System

Terry J. Landgraff, MSN, CCRN
The Cardiovascular System
The Hematologic & Immunological Systems
The Renal System

Darlene Mathis, DNP, RN, FNP-BC, NP-C, CNE, CRNP
The Gastrointestinal System

AVAILABLE ONLINE

Free Additional Practice

kaptest.com/booksonline

As owner of this guide, you are entitled to get more practice and help online. Log on to *kaptest.com/booksonline* to access additional CCRN practice questions.

Access to this selection of online CCRN practice material is free of charge to purchasers of this book. You'll be asked for a specific password derived from the text in this book, so have your book handy when you log on.

For Any Test Changes or Late-Breaking Developments

kaptest.com/publishing

The material in this book is up-to-date at the time of publication. However, the AACN may have instituted changes in the test after this book was published. Be sure to carefully read the materials you receive when you register for the test. If there are any important late-breaking developments—or any changes or corrections to the Kaplan test preparation materials in this book—we will post that information online at *kaptest.com/publishing*.

Feedback and Comments

kaplansurveys.com/books

We'd love to hear your comments and suggestions about this book. We invite you to fill out our online survey form at *kaplansurveys.com/books*. Your feedback is extremely helpful as we continue to develop high-quality resources to meet your needs.

Contents

Contents

PART I

The CCRN: Information and Strategies

Introduction

ABOUT THE CCRN

If you have picked up this book, then you have probably decided that you are ready to take a step toward obtaining your CCRN (Critical Care Registered Nurse) certification. Congratulations! This is an exciting step and this book will be instrumental in helping you succeed.

The CCRN certification exam is intended to gauge how well you can apply your medical knowledge, concepts, and principles to care for the complex needs of critically ill patients. By achieving certification, you will demonstrate to both patients and employers that you have the advanced knowledge and skills necessary to care for the acutely and/or critically ill, as well as demonstrate that you are competent in a specialized area of care.

CCRN certification is administered by the American Association of Critical-Care Nurses (AACN) Certification Corporation, although membership in AACN is not a requirement to take the exam. Currently, there are over 40,000 certified CCRNs. The certification was first introduced in 1976 and it includes CCRN exams for adult, pediatric, and neonatal patients. Although the exam was introduced over 30 years ago, it is updated to keep pace with the changes in the health care world. It reflects the environment in which nurses care for acutely and critically ill patients—whether in an intensive care unit, trauma unit, or any other clinical arena. It is interesting to note that approximately 40 percent of certified CCRNs work in areas outside of the intensive or cardiac care unit settings. This shows that acutely and critically ill patients are cared for in a variety of clinical settings.

WHAT IS CCRN CERTIFICATION?

The CCRN is a specialty certification, the goal of which is to validate the knowledge of the nurses who provide care to acutely and critically ill patients in areas such as intensive care units, cardiac care units, combined intensive care and cardiac care units, medical/surgical intensive care units, trauma units, and critical care transport and flight. In a sense, the certification provides hospitals, health care agencies and health care consumers with a standard way of measuring qualifications.

Using CCRN Credentials

Once you pass the CCRN exam, you can—and should—list CCRN after your licensing title. Thus, Mary Jones, RN would become Mary Jones, RN, CCRN after passing the CCRN exam. Note that there are no periods in CCRN. You will receive a wallet card signifying that you are CCRN certified. Carry this with you in case you need to validate your credentials at any time.

REGISTERING FOR THE EXAM

To register for the CCRN certification exam, the AACN must deem that you are eligible to take the exam, which it does by reviewing an application. In this section, we'll outline the application and scheduling process for the CCRN exam.

CCRN Exam Eligibility Requirements

In order to be eligible to sit for the CCRN exam, you must meet certain requirements. To start, you must have unencumbered licensure as an RN or APRN in the United States. Not sure if your license is unencumbered? To be considered unencumbered, your license cannot have any provisions or conditions that limit your practice in any way. If you meet the licensure requirement, you can look at the requirement for practice hours. The AACN states that CCRN candidates must have 1,750 hours in direct bedside care of acutely or critically ill patients (in the patient population of the exam for which you are applying: neonatal, pediatric, or adult) during the previous two years. Of those hours, 875 must have taken place in the year immediately preceding your application. In addition, only hours that take place in a U.S.- or Canada-based (or comparable) facility will count.

The Application Process

While the application process is not overly complicated, there are a few keys steps that you will need to take to ensure that you are properly registered for the exam.

First, request an application (available from the AACN Certification Corporation at *aacn. org*) or print out the online version. To access the online CCRN registration, enter the following URL into your web browser:

http://web.aacn.org/DM/Certifications/CertificationCenter.aspx

You will need to set up an online registration in order to use the website. This process is straightforward and requires basic information, such as your name and address. You will choose a member name and a password to use for when you return to the site. Once you have registered to use the AACN website, you can apply for the exam. Note that the online registration can only be used to apply to take the computer-based CCRN exam. If you know that you need to take the paper and pencil exam, you will need to apply the old fashioned way—using a paper form available from AACN.

You will need to submit your application, along with a one-page honor statement, listing your verifier information and RN or APRN license information, and your application fee to the AACN Certification Corporation. AACN accepts applications via fax at (949) 362-2020 or via mail at:

AACN Certification Corporation
101 Columbia
Aliso Viejo, CA 92656

Peace of Mind

You can buy yourself some peace of mind by sending your application via certified mail or by requesting a return receipt. These options will inform you when your application has been received by the AACN Certification Corporation. You can purchase these mailing upgrades at your local post office for a nominal fee.

AACN takes approximately six to eight weeks to process the applications. Once the application has been processed, the AACN will notify Applied Measurement Professionals, Inc. (AMP), the company that administers the exam for AACN, of all the eligible exam candidates. If you are deemed eligible to take the exam, AMP will send you a postcard and an email informing you that your application has been approved. If, for some reason, AACN finds that you are not eligible to take the exam or if it has questions about any part of your application, you will be contacted in writing. You should respond to any requests from AACN quickly and thoroughly.

CCRN Certification Application Honor Statement

The Honor Statement is a form that you fill out, certifying that you have met the minimum requirements for taking the CCRN exam. You do not need to write the statement yourself; you will use the preprinted form from the AACN Certification Corporation, which is available in its text booklet and online. You will fill in your name, AACN number, and contact information for a professional associate who can verify that you have actually met all of the eligibility requirements. It doesn't matter whether your verifier is an RN colleague or a clinical supervisor (RN or physician); the person you choose must be able to accurately and truthfully verify that you are eligible to take the exam.

If you are aware that you are not fully eligible for the exam, you should not apply for it. All applications are subject to a random audit of eligibility. If you are selected, you will be notified in writing and have 60 days to respond. Your verification contact will be asked to confirm your eligibility in writing, and you will be asked to submit a copy of your RN or APRN license.

Application Fees

The application fees are the same, whether you take the neonatal, pediatric or the adult CCRN exam. The CCRN computer-based exam fee is $220 for AACN members and $325 for nonmembers. The retest fee and the current CCRN renewal fee are both $170 for members and $275 for nonmembers.

For the paper and pencil exam, however, the fees are significantly higher. The fees depend on the number of people taking the exam simultaneously at one location. If you need to take the paper and pencil exam, you should inquire about pricing when applying.

Scheduling Your Exam

Once you have received notification that you are eligible to take the CCRN exam, you need to schedule a time to do so. As with most things, however, it is wise to stay flexible and plan ahead. Before scheduling your exam date, visit the AMP website to see what exam locations are near you. There are over 160 testing centers in the United States where you can take the computer-based exam, most of which are H&R Block offices. To find exam locations and schedule your exam online, type the following URL into your web browser:

www.goamp.com

Make a note of one of two specific locations so that you'll have this information handy when you schedule your test date. Be advised that although you can sometimes schedule your exam almost immediately, in other cases dates may not be available for several weeks. It all depends on the availability of slots at the location you choose, as well as how popular that exam location and time period are with other examinees.

Exams are given by appointment only, which must be made *at least* four days before your chosen testing date. It is important to note that your exam eligibility only lasts for 90 days, so you should schedule your exam immediately after receiving your postcard and email. Both the postcard and the email will clearly note the expiration date of your eligibility period. Since the exam is offered twice a day, five days a week throughout the year, you should not have a problem scheduling your exam within your eligibility period.

That said, if you are unable to schedule your exam during the 90-day eligibility period, you should call AACN to request a new 90-day period. You are allowed to do this only once and you must pay a $100 change fee for the new eligibility period.

In addition to listing the exam locations, the AMP website has a user-friendly interface for scheduling and even rescheduling your exam. If you prefer to schedule your exam by phone rather than online, call 888-519-9901. Before calling or going online, make sure you have your confirmation postcard handy. You will need your AACN customer number (which will be printed on your postcard) in order to schedule your exam.

If the testing center closest to you is more than a three-hour drive one way, you can apply to take a paper and pencil exam. To do so, you need to apply for authorization *at least three months* in advance of the test date by calling 800-899-2226. This is true for people who live outside of the United States as well.

GENERAL CCRN EXAM CONTENT

Whether you take the neonatal, pediatric or adult CCRN exam, the general format will be the same. You will have three hours to complete 150 multiple choice questions, 125 of which will be scored. The remaining 25 unscored questions are used by the AACN to plan for future exams.

CCRN at a Glance

Examination Length: 3 hours
Number of Questions: 150 total (125 scored, 25 unscored)
Question Types: Multiple choice

Which CCRN Exam Should I Take?

The exam that you take should correlate with your experience. You should take the adult exam if you have experience in direct bedside care of acutely or critically ill adult patients, and likewise, for the pediatric and neonatal exams. Do not register for an exam for which you do not have adequate experience.

Each of the CCRN exams consist of two sections: Clinical Judgment, which is 80 percent of the exam questions, and Professional Caring and Ethical Practice, which is the remaining 20 percent of the exam questions. The questions in the Clinical Judgment section are specific to the population (adult, pediatrics, neonatal) of the exam that you are taking. The questions in the Professional Caring and Ethical Practice section, however, can be about patients of any age.

CCRN Adult Exam

The following is a brief overview of the content of the CCRN Adult Exam, along with the percentage of questions that are in each category.

Clinical Judgment (80% of the exam)

Cardiovascular	32%
Pulmonary	17%
Endocrine	4%
Hematology/Immunology	3%
Neurology	5%
Gastrointestinal	6%
Renal	5%
Multisystem	8%

Professional Caring and Ethical Practice (20% of the exam)

Advocacy/Moral Agency	2%
Caring Practices	4%
Collaboration	4%
Systems Thinking	2%
Response to Diversity	2%
Clinical Inquiry	2%
Facilitation of Learning	4%

CCRN Pediatric Exam

The following is a brief overview of the content of the CCRN Pediatric Exam, along with the percentage of questions that are in each category.

Clinical Judgment (80% of the exam)

Cardiovascular	19%
Pulmonary	22%
Endocrine	5%
Hematology/Immunology	6%
Neurology	10%
Gastrointestinal	5%
Renal	4%
Multisystem	9%

Professional Caring and Ethical Practice (20% of the exam)

Advocacy/Moral Agency	2%
Caring Practices	4%
Collaboration	4%
Systems Thinking	2%
Response to Diversity	2%
Clinical Inquiry	2%
Facilitation of Learning	4%

CCRN Neonatal Exam

The following is a brief overview of the content of the CCRN Neonatal Exam, along with the percentage of questions that are in each category.

Clinical Judgment (80% of the exam)

Cardiovascular	10%
Pulmonary	36%
Endocrine	4%
Hematology/Immunology	4%
Neurology	6%
Gastrointestinal	7%
Renal	2%
Multisystem	11%

Professional Caring and Ethical Practice (20% of the exam)

Advocacy/Moral Agency	2%
Caring Practices	4%
Collaboration	4%
Systems Thinking	2%
Response to Diversity	2%
Clinical Inquiry	2%
Facilitation of Learning	4%

YOUR CCRN SCORE

At the end of the day, what you really want to know is whether or not you passed the exam. Luckily, if you take the computer-based exam, you will receive your score report immediately upon completion. Those who take the paper and pencil exam will have to wait six to eight weeks for their results to be sent in the mail.

Duplicate score reports are available for both the computer-based and the paper and pencil exams. You may request a duplicate report from AMP, within 12 months of sitting for your exam. Your request should be made in writing and should include the following;

- Your name
- AACN customer ID number
  (preceded by the letter C, as listed on your initial eligibility confirmation postcard)
- Your address
- Your telephone number
- The date and type of exam that you took
- Check or money order for $25, made payable to AMP

Be sure to sign your request and mail it to:

Applied Measurement Professionals, Inc.
18000 W. 105th Street
Olathe, KS 66061

You should receive your duplicate report in approximately two weeks.

Passing Score

If you pass the CCRN exam, you will receive a wallet card and wall certificate stating that you are certified within six to eight weeks. Your certification is good for three years, starting the first day of the month in which you passed the exam. So, if you take the exam in April 2009 and you pass, your certification will last from April 1, 2009 through March 31, 2012.

What to Do If You Fail

The first thing to do if you fail the exam is keep your chin up! Don't be discouraged; you can take the CCRN exam up to four times in a 12-month period. So, if you don't pass on your first try, spend a little more time preparing and then register to take the exam again.

If you do fail the exam, you won't be allowed to appeal your score. You can apply for a retest and receive discounted retest fees.

Renewing Your CCRN Credential

Your CCRN certification is good for three years. When the time comes to renew your certification, you have several options to choose from. Briefly, you will be able to choose:

1. *CCRN renewal by Synergy CERPs* (Continuing Education Recognition Point), which involves meeting eligibility requirements for CCRN recertification and completing the Synergy CERP Program.

2. *CCRN renewal by CERPs* will be phased out starting January 1, 2010.

3. *CCRN renewal by exam,* which involves meeting the eligibility requirements for CCRN recertification and successfully completing the CCRN certification exam.

You can also choose these non-renewal options:

1. *Inactive CCRN status,* which is available to those nurses who do not meet the CCRN recertification eligibility requirements and who wish to keep their CCRN certification status.

2. *Alumnus CCRN status,* which is available to nurses who no longer provide bedside care to critically ill patients.

3. *Retired CCRN status,* which is available to current CCRN nurses who are retiring or retired from nursing.

You should plan to review the renewal criteria from AACN throughout your three-year certification period to keep abreast of any changes to the requirements.

HOW THIS BOOK CAN HELP YOU

This book is designed to make your dream of CCRN certification a reality. In chapter 2, we'll cover the ins and outs of the exam's computer interface so you can enter the testing environment feeling comfortable with computer-based testing. Chapter 3 will provide you with specific exam strategies and advice for test day. Chapters 4 through 12 are content-based and each of these chapters covers a particular category of the exam, from the cardiovascular system to multiorgan, providing you with in-depth content to study for the exam.

The CCRN Computer Interface

2

In recent years, most medical licensure and other professional certification organizations have switched from paper test booklets to computer-based testing (CBT). From the testing organization's viewpoint, CBT offers many advantages. First, it takes place year-round in hundreds of sites throughout the United States and the world. Every test site offers standard testing conditions in terms of the computer equipment used and the rules governing the behavior and monitoring of examinees. There is also increased security as compared with paper tests because completed exams do not need to be physically shipped back to testing agencies for scoring. Instead, examinee data are sent electronically to the testing agency, thus reducing the chance that grid sheets and exam booklets could be lost during shipping. Additionally, examinees often receive their scores immediately, as compared with the six to eight week waiting period for paper tests. In the case of the CCRN, as stated in chapter 1, the scores are available immediately after taking the computer-based CCRN exam.

The future holds even more opportunities that make CBT attractive. Paper test booklets must be assembled and printed many months before testing dates; therefore, typographic corrections or other changes are difficult to make or must await a new test-creation cycle. With electronically based testing, test developers have quicker and more numerous options for making changes, such as adding fresh photographic material, replacing poor items, or simply correcting typographic mistakes.

Because most medical licensing organizations now require not only initial certification by examination, but also periodic recertification testing to maintain professional certification on a regular basis, there is good reason to become comfortable with these types of tests and with effective ways to review for and deal with multiple-choice questions. After all, if you can't avoid it, you may as well take steps to become good at it!

The CCRN exam is given in a CBT environment, except in special situations when candidates request and are authorized to take a paper and pencil version of the exam. The paper and pencil version is an option for those candidates who live more than three hours (one way) from a testing center. Unless you meet this criterion, you should be prepared to take the computer-based exam.

This chapter will explain what you can expect from the testing environment and what to look out for on the day of the exam.

THE CCRN TESTING ENVIRONMENT

As we mentioned earlier, the CCRN certification exam is administered by AMP and is typically given at H&R Block offices. The exam locations are set up to be conducive to test-taking but there are a few things that are worth noting to make your exam experience as stress-free as possible.

Know Where You're Going

When you register for the exam, you will select an exam location. You will want to keep the address of the exam location and the directions to it handy. If you misplace either piece of information, you can look up the address and find directions on the AMP website at *www. goamp.com*. This information is very important because you need to know exactly where you are going on the day of the exam. Ideally, you should be familiar with the area so you will know how long it will take you to get to the exam location. If you are not familiar with the area, you should attempt to cover the route to the location prior to the day of the exam, whether by car or mass transit, so you will know what to look out for, where to park, what the travel time will be, and the possible alternate routes to get to the testing location (in case there is a traffic emergency, roadblock, or detour). It is critical that you know how long the trip will take you because you do not want to be late reporting to the exam. In fact, if you arrive more than 15 minutes late, you will not be allowed to take the exam.

Arriving at the Exam

At the exam location, you will be asked to *show two forms of identification,* one of which must be a photo ID. The forms that you choose must be current, show your signature, and the name on the identification must be the same as the one that you registered with. So, for example, if you recently were married and changed your name, and then you registered for the exam with your new name, both forms of identification would need to show your new name. If you had not yet gotten around to changing your name on your driver's license, however, you would not be able to show that card as a form of identification. Make sure that you have your IDs in order well in advance of test day.

ID Savvy

You must bring two forms of identification with you to the CCRN exam. One of the IDs has to be a photo ID. The AACN accepts the following as photo IDs:

- Driver's license

- State identification card

- Passport

- Military identification card

For your non-photo ID, you can show a credit card or any other card that has your current name and signature.

Inside the Testing Area

We suggest that you dress in layers on test day so that you can adjust accordingly if the center feels either too warm or too cool for you. Except for the identification needed when you check in, all other personal items should be left in your car or at home. You will be allowed to carry only your identification with you into the examination room.

Food and beverages are not allowed in the testing rooms. You can choose to leave exam location to get a drink, take medication, or use the restroom, but the amount of time allowed for the exam is not stopped when you are away from your computer. Because your computer is still running, inadvertent data entry from your keyboard can also occur, so it is recommended that you try not to take a break unless you absolutely must.

You are not allowed to bring any scratch paper, or any other materials, into the testing room. Instead, you will be provided with scratch paper for making notes. This paper must be turned into the proctor after you complete the exam in order to receive your score report.

Once you are brought to the testing cubicle designated for your use, center staff will start your testing software. In the unlikely event that there is a hardware or software problem during your exam, center staff should be notified immediately so that they can correct the problem and so that you will not lose valuable test response data or testing time.

Although center policies are designed to provide all examinees with a comfortable test area equipped with functioning equipment and a reasonably quiet environment, don't expect a soundproof cubicle. Other examinees are taking exams or may be taking breaks and so you should expect some background noise.

Don't Be Dismissed!

After all of your preparation for the exam, you don't want to run the risk of being dismissed from the exam and having your exam score rendered null and void. According to the AACN, exam candidates can be dismissed from the exam for any of the following:

- Entering the exam without authorized admission
- Taking the exam for someone else
- Recording test questions or making notes
- Bringing notes, unauthorized electronic devices (PDAs, hand-held computers, cell phones, pagers, etc.), or other resources into the exam location
- Creating any sort of disturbance, including being abusive or uncooperative
- Leaving the exam location without notifying the proctor

Cancellations

Should an emergency or illness prevent you from keeping your exam appointment, you will be allowed to reapply to take the exam in the future. If you reapply for the CCRN exam within one year of your original application, you reactivate your application by simply paying the initial exam fee. However, if you reapply more than one year after your original application, you will need to resubmit a full application and pay the initial exam fee again.

What about cancellations of the exam itself? If inclement weather or an emergency on the day of the exam warrants cancellation of the exam, it will be rescheduled. AMP offers a 24-hour weather hotline available by calling 913-495-4418. If you think that there is a chance the exam may be cancelled, call the hotline to check. It is only in rare circumstances that the exam actually has to be cancelled but if it happens to you, you will be notified of the rescheduled date or how to reapply for the exam.

THE BASICS OF THE COMPUTER-BASED CCRN EXAM FORMAT

Once you have checked in at the exam location, you will have to log in at the computer terminal assigned to you for the exam. You will be directed to enter your AACN customer identification number, preceded by the letter C. This is the number that was printed on your eligibility confirmation postcard. If you failed to bring the postcard with you and you do not remember your AACN number, the exam proctor should be able to give it to you. But, you should plan to bring the postcard with you to the exam location on test day.

After you enter your AACN number, your photograph will be taken by the computer. This photo will stay on-screen during your exam and will be included on your score report. This helps ensure that you are not taking the test for someone else or that someone else is not taking the exam for you.

Test Items

The CCRN exam is comprised of 150 multiple-choice questions. Test items may contain a variety of information sources. Some items include colored photographs, diagrams or other reference material that may be useful in answering the item. Only one item will be shown at a time. The question number will appear in the lower right-hand corner of the screen. The entire test item, including the question and four answers labeled A, B, C, and D, should appear on the screen. To answer a question, use the mouse to click on the answer or use the keyboard to input the letter (A, B, C or D) of your answer. After doing so, you will see your answer in the lower left-hand corner of the screen.

Changing your answer is simple. To do so, click on a different answer or enter a different letter as many times as you want. Before second-guessing yourself (or third- or fourth-guessing!), review our thoughts about it in chapter 3 on page 27.

When you have answered a question, you can move on to the next item by clicking on the forward arrow (>) in the lower right-hand corner of the screen or by clicking on the "NEXT" key. This will move you ahead one item. If you change your mind and need to go back to a previous item, click on the backward arrow (<) in the lower right-hand corner of the screen. As with moving forward, this will move you backward by one item. Repeat either action if you need to move forward or backward by more than one item.

Timed Exam

As you know, the CCRN exam is a timed exam. The computer that you are using will monitor the time and will automatically end the exam if you run out of time. So, you will need to work quickly and efficiently.

If you have not taken a computer-based exam before or you are not comfortable with computers, you may be worried that your lack of familiarity with the computer-based testing process will put you at a disadvantage. Don't worry. At the start of the exam, you will be given a practice test so you can gain comfort with the computer-based testing process before you start the actual exam. Further, by practicing at home prior to arriving at the exam you can increase your familiarity with the computer-based testing format and help decrease your anxiety even more. The time that you spend on the practice test does not count as part of the timed exam. So, relax and practice using the computer interface until you feel comfortable with it. All of the instructions that you need for the exam will be available on-screen once you finish the practice test and begin the actual exam.

At any point during the exam, you can display a digital clock showing the time remaining by clicking the "TIME" button in the lower right-hand corner of the screen or selecting the "TIME" key. This will allow you to watch your pace so you can keep on track. If you decide that you no longer want to have the clock displayed, you can turn it off by clicking the "TIME" button or key again at any time.

DURING THE EXAM

After making sure you have adequate experience, studying hard for months, and gearing yourself up to take the CCRN certification exam, the last thing you want to do is jeopardize your score by making a silly error at the testing site. Here is a quick look at some of the things you are allowed and, perhaps more important, not allowed to do during the exam:

During the exam you CAN . . .	During the exam you CANNOT . . .
Dress in layers. Dressing in layers is a good idea so you can make adjustments if the room is hot or cold.	**Take purses, briefcases or jackets into the testing room.** You are not allowed to bring any personal items into the test area. Leave all such items either at home or in your car.
Use a calculator. This comes with some stipulations. Your calculator must be non-programmable, silent, hand-held, either solar or battery operated, and it must not have printing capabilities or an alphabetic keypad.	**Take books, papers or any reference books or materials into the testing room.** The CCRN is definitely not an "open book" test. Leave all study aids and other books and materials at home.
Comment on any item on the exam. Click on the exclamation point to the left of the TIME button to open a dialogue box to leave your comments.	**Ask questions about content.** You may not ask the proctor any questions about the exam content during the exam.
Make notes. The proctor will give you scratch paper to use for notes during the exam. This is the only paper that you may use and it must be returned to the proctor at the end of the exam in order to receive your score.	**Take notes or other material home with you.** You cannot take any material related to the exam, including the scratch paper provided to you for making notes, out of the testing site.

During the exam you CAN . . .	During the exam you CANNOT . . .
Take a break. If you need to take a break, you must request authorization to do so. However, it is important that you understand that breaks count toward your total exam time. If you take a break, you will not be allowed any extra time on the exam.	**Leave the exam location without permission.** If you take a break or leave the testing site for any reason without authorization, your score will automatically be rendered null and void.
End the exam early. If you are a quick test-taker and you finish before the allotted time, you may opt to end the exam early. To do so, click on the COVER button on the computer screen.	

AFTER THE EXAM

When you have completed the exam, you will undoubtedly be anxious to receive your score report. You will need to be patient and take one additional step before seeing your score; you will need to complete an evaluation of your testing experience. The evaluation is brief and should not take you too much time.

When you are done with the evaluation, the proctor will give you your official score report, showing the percent of correct answers for each major category.

FINAL THOUGHTS

Now that you know what to expect from the exam location, the computer-based testing environment, and the CCRN certification exam itself—we're ready to review some exam strategies. In chapter 3, we'll show you some tips and techniques to ensure that you pass the CCRN.

CCRN Exam Strategies 3

To get to where you are in your career, you have had to be prepared for and pass hundreds of examinations over the years. You probably have an established method for test preparation that has worked well in the past, so you may feel little need to create a specific plan of study for the CCRN, but each exam may differ in regard to the focus on content, style of questions, format, time limits, etc. Hence, it is important to realize that while you may be able to rely on your previous test taking skills, you should adapt them to the CCRN.

SPECIFIC STRATEGIES FOR THE CCRN

The CCRN assesses your knowledge of the skills and abilities necessary to practice in acute and critical care settings. The questions will require more from you than simple recall of isolated facts. The questions are designed to elicit *critical thinking* to assess your ability to apply knowledge in a wide variety of contexts and patient-care situations.

To be able to walk into the exam location on test day with confidence that you will do well, you need a plan. This chapter will help you to develop a study plan and manage where you most need to invest your review time so that all of your efforts result in a score that truly reflects the knowledge, skills and abilities that you have worked so hard to acquire.

Develop a Study Plan

An effective study plan involves the following key factors:

- Determining how much time you need for each area
- Setting a sequence of topics
- Establishing a good study process
- Minimizing forgetting
- Monitoring your performance
- Determining when you are ready to take the exam

The first step in creating your plan is to figure out how much time you need for reviewing each area. To do this, you need a current assessment of your strengths and weaknesses by using practice questions to measure your current level of knowledge. Take 10 questions per subject area and score the items. Calculate your percent correct for each area. This initial performance profile will help you determine where you are weaker and need to put more time, and where you are stronger and need less time to review.

Weight Your Review

Studying everything equally wastes limited review time by investing the same amount in every subject. As we showed in chapter 1, not every subject appears on the exam in equal proportion. You should weight your review time more heavily toward the subject areas that are emphasized on the exam.

In chapter 1, we outlined the percentage of questions in each subject area that are on the CCRN exams. Using that list, along with your personal performance profile, will be useful in determining how much time you will need to spend reviewing each subject area. By thinking carefully about what needs more time and what needs less, you will derive the maximum benefit from your review.

Familiarize Yourself with Exam Content

A key strategy for the CCRN certification exam is to become familiar with the exam content. This will help you to sequence the subjects in your study plan. Because the AACN outlines the percentage of questions from each subject area that will appear on the exam (see page 8), you can use that as your guideline. In this book, each system is covered in a chapter, allowing you to progress from the cardiovascular system to pulmonary to endocrine and so on. Follow the systems as we've included them in this book as you study for the exam, spending more time on the systems that have a higher percentage of questions on the exam and less time on the systems that have a lower percentage of questions.

In the past, nurses were required to have accomplished a specific set of technical skills before they were allowed to take the CCRN exam. This is no longer the case. However, having experience with certain skills and technologies will most likely improve your score on the exam. The AACN has a list of experiences that it suggests that CCRN certification exam candidates have. The lists for adult, pediatric and neonatal are available on the AACN website at *www.certcorp.org*. Navigate to the CCRN Eligibility Requirements to review the list of suggested experiences. If you do not have experience in these areas, it may be to your benefit to seek them out prior to taking the exam.

No standardized licensing examination is 100 percent predictable and question writers work hard to create questions that require understanding and integration of the material. The best overall goal in reviewing, therefore, is to aim for genuine understanding of major concepts, key definitions, and integration of the knowledge across subject areas.

Establish an Effective Study Process

One of the most common myths about studying and test performance is the belief that merely going through the material results in being able to successfully apply the learned material to test items. If this were true, then doing well would require only that you reviewed good notes or a good review book. This myth assumes that reviewing equals the ability to apply, which is not the case.

Nearly everyone has had some experience with individuals who seem to be able to do well on examinations even when they study less than many others. Are they simply geniuses or do they possess photographic memories? Usually neither. Most of these individuals have discovered that the key to doing well on exams lies in the study process itself.

A good study process involves using your time strategically and systematically working to address your weak areas. The other component of a good study process is using practice questions (like those included in this book) to test how well you can apply what you are studying. In this way, you will not be simply studying in isolation from the application. You will engage the material, which will help you learn and remember it so that you can be one of those test-takers who achieves a top score on the CCRN exam!

Actively Engage with the Material

So, you understand that you need to engage with the material that you are studying. But what does that mean? This means you *should not* simply run your eyes along the words you are reading and, in effect, merely following what is being said. Simply reading your review material will do you little good. You have to *do* something with what you are reading. Here are some methods:

- Transform the material be extracting key aspects into a briefer, personally meaningful version.

- Use arrows and boxes to diagram a process.

- Stop after reviewing a topic and summarize outloud.

- Do practice questions that relate to what you just read and clarify any misunderstandings or forgotten elements by searching your notes or the review book.

- Make quiz cards with a topic or item on one side and key features on the other. Looking at the item side of the card, try to recite the features.

Any other study methods that call for you to make judgments about the material, express it in your own words, show linkages between things, or mimic the demands of actual test items are all effective techniques to use. You may find that one method works better for you than others. Or, you may find that you need variety so you'll try all the methods listed. Do whatever makes you comfortable.

Beware of Passivity

Passive study methods are deceptive because you tend to assume that you know the material well when, in reality, you only followed along and recognized the material as familiar. If what you do when you study results in frequent nodding off or mind wandering, then you need to change your methods. Perk it up so you can ensure you are really learning, and retaining, the material. Oftentimes this has to do with what time of day you study. Some people are more effective if they study in the evening or night and others are more effective if they study in the morning or afternoon. You need to decide this for yourself if you have not already figured it out.

Methods of Remembering

Everyone must deal with forgetting because there is so much information to review that whatever you study first is going to fade away to some degree by the time you finish studying everything else. To combat this problem, you must create a *greatly condensed* summary of notes that you can use later on to refresh your memory during the final days before the exam. Tackling practice questions on a regular basis that cover all previously reviewed material is another method of keeping material fresh in your memory. If you don't address the problem of forgetting information, your performance will reflect how recently you studied each area, with earlier topics yielding a lower performance than the topics you studied closer to the day of the exam.

Practice What You Learn

If you are serious about doing well on the CCRN exam, then we strongly suggest that you do practice questions from the beginning and continue this through the entirety of your studying. We refer to this as the "practice all along" approach. One way to look at practicing with questions is to realize that self-testing is analogous to medical diagnosis. You want to discover the problem while you still have time to treat it. Waiting until the end of your studying to do questions is not recommended because you will be finding out what you still don't know right before the actual examination, when there is no time left for "treatment." Further, the "practice all along" approach will help you review material that you may have recently studied and prevent you from forgetting key points. Finally, it is a way to keep your study interesting.

Know When You're Ready

The final aspect of a solid study plan is determining if you are ready for the exam. The most reliable way to do this is to take a longer practice test in a manner that is as similar as possible to the testing conditions you will face on exam day; in other words, you should take a full-length "mock test." This means that if you have three hours to complete 150 questions on the day of the exam, then your simulation test should also be taken at the same pace. And, obviously, the items in the simulation must be as similar as possible to those you will see on test day (how well you do on the simulation will be a pretty good indicator of how well you might score on the actual examination).

Don't wait until a day or two before the exam to take your "mock test." You will want to make sure that you have enough time to analyze your errors and clarify any misunderstandings or forgotten elements.

Answer All the Questions

Your CCRN exam score is based on the number of questions answered correctly. Therefore, you will want to answer all of the questions on the exam, but that doesn't mean you have to answer a question the first time you see it. You can leave items unanswered as you progress through the exam and return to them later. This will allow you to skip difficult questions and move on to the questions to which you know the answers. Then, if you have time at the end of the exam, you can return to the difficult questions that you left unanswered.

By clicking on the blank square to the right of the TIME button, you can bookmark an item so you'll know to return to it at the end of the exam. If you do have time to review your unanswered items, click on the hand icon or select the NEXT key. Doing so will show you your first unanswered item. Continue to click on the NEXT key or the hand icon to progress through all of your unanswered items. You will need to practice this before you get to the test, so you are familiar with the software!

At the end of the exam, you will receive a report of the number of items that you have answered. If there is still time remaining, you can go back and answer any unanswered questions. Even if you do not know the answer to a question, if you have time to answer it, you should. Remember, your score is based on the number of *correct* answers you select. There is *no penalty for guessing* so take a chance and answer every question that you can. You never know, you may even guess correctly!

GENERAL TEST-TAKING STRATEGIES

Test-taking is a performing art. To perform well, you must practice the skills, get feedback, and try again until the whole thing becomes internalized and finely tuned, and every aspect of the piece has been rehearsed in advance. The following general test-taking strategies are designed to help you do just that!

Identify and Correct Your Error Patterns

As you progress with your practice questions and studying, you should routinely analyze your errors. Overall performance tells you just that—how you did on a mixture of items covering various aspects of the material. Take some time to sort out where your mistakes were made. Did errors load up on a particular aspect? Did you do much better on the Clinical Judgment section than on the Professional Caring and Ethical Practice one, or vice versa? Are you a whiz with questions related to the cardiovascular system but not as good with questions on neurology? If so, you may have discovered what material you tend to understudy or avoid, which, in turn, shows you what material you need to spend more time studying.

Continue looking for patterns among the items that you missed. Some possible error patterns might include the following:

Test Anxiety

If many of your errors occurred on items early in the exam, this may be an indicator of test anxiety, which is often most strongly felt during the early stages of taking an exam. Alternatively, it may simply reflect the fact that difficult content happened to be asked early in the test. However, most often the answer is test anxiety.

Pace Yourself and Avoid Mental Fatigue

If many of your errors occurred on the final pages of the exam, and you answered the items in numerical order instead of jumping around, then mental fatigue may be a problem for you. Are you getting enough sleep at night? Are you finding that you run short of time near the end of the exam, causing you to rush through answering the final items? Did you feel that the most difficult material was covered mainly in the final portion of the exam? Try finding a better pace to ensure that you have enough time to answer all of the questions without having to rush. If fatigue is an issue for you, practice more to raise your testing endurance, or plan to get more sleep in the weeks leading up to the exam.

Misreading

Reading mistakes are more common during exams than most people think. After all, people feel nervous, rushed, or simply tired toward the end and may easily misread a word or key phrase—or even answer the question they *expected* to be asked, rather than the one *actually* asked. How can you tell if an error was made because of a reading mistake? Read the item and note the correct answer, as well as the answer you selected. If your choice makes no sense, given what was asked, then it is highly likely that you misread the question at the time.

Beware of misreading. Only a few letters in a prefix or suffix can change the entire meaning of a question (i.e., hyper versus hypo). Negatively phrased items (i.e., "What is the least likely diagnosis?") can trip people up, too. Read the questions carefully to avoid this common mistake.

Frustration

Were there any items on the exam that at the time made you upset or frustrated? Test-takers often describe such questions as picky, tricky or unfair. The reason you should identify these anger-triggering items is that test-takers frequently make silly mistakes on items following the ones that made them upset. So the test-takers pay the price for the tricky, unfair or frustrating item because their strong emotions interfered with their concentration on subsequent items.

Second-Guessing Yourself

Most test-takers second-guess themselves at some point. Unfortunately, most second-guessing does not lead to more correct answers. Instead, when people change answers they often change a wrong answer to another wrong answer and sometimes a correct answer to a wrong answer. Here is a way for you to identify what happens when you second-guess yourself.

When you take a practice test, make a mark (such as a triangle in the margin) so that you will be able to spot all items where you changed your initial answer. Now tally the three possibilities:

- Wrong to wrong
- Wrong to right
- Right to wrong

Don't be surprised if you discover that most changed answers end as the first option. These reflect knowledge gaps, not a problem with whether you do or do not change answers. Next, if the sum of those that fit the second possibility is greater than those that fit the third possibility, then you are using good judgment and don't have a problem with answer changing. If the sum of those that fit the third possibility is greater than those that fit the second possibility, however, then you have an answer-changing problem. The solution? Simple: Adopt a rule, based on the data you've collected and analyzed, that you will never change an answer.

Knowledge Gaps

Are many of the errors you make referring to a common topic or similar kind of material? For example, you might notice that test after test, you tend to answer questions on the renal system incorrectly. This pattern clearly signals its own solution—you must spend more time studying the renal system if you want to improve. Adjust your study strategy accordingly and put more time into practicing the problematic areas identified in your error analysis.

Other Obstacles

The potential patterns identified in error analyses can't all be described here. Not every test error will fall into a pattern. But the process of scanning your performance for patterns is extremely worthwhile if you have adopted active, sound study strategies, you try to anticipate what might be asked, and yet your test performance is still not improving.

Master the Multiple-Choice Format

The CCRN certification exam consists solely of multiple-choice questions so you will want to deal with that format in your study plan. Let's look at the approach to questions used by many test-takers and focus on why it works.

The Basic Steps

1. Read the question stem carefully to locate important clues.

2. Make sure you fully understand what is being asked.

3. Before looking at any answer choices, put the clues together with what you are being asked and allow your mind to form some kind of answer.

4. Look at the choices offered, and if one of them fits your anticipated answer, mark it.

5. If no choice is a good fit, use general knowledge, larger concepts, and logic to eliminate as many choices as you can.

6. Select an answer from the remaining choices.

Interestingly, not all of these steps will necessarily be used in every question. However, in most standardized exams, many questions will ask you to assess specifics that you won't be able to recall. It is in dealing with these that good test-takers have a real advantage over those who aren't as adept. So, just what methods are used to get more correct answers?

The Methods

Unconfident test-takers are prone to an "either/or" mindset when they encounter questions. If, after reading the question, they aren't sure of an answer based on what they recall, they quickly give up and guess. Good test-takers don't admit defeat that quickly. Instead, they use information presented in the question itself or more of their general knowledge to chip away at the question. By persevering and exploiting whatever they can to eliminate choices, they more frequently end up with correct answers. Here are some methods for you to follow to get more correct answers on the CCRN exam:

- *Recognize a question in disguise*
  It is crucial that you fully understand what is being asked in every question. Take your time to read and re-read the questions, if you need to. Ask yourself, "What is really being asked?" Once you are confident that you know what the question is, then you can move on to find the answer.

- *Eliminate distracters*
  Distracters are designed to do just what their name implies—to distract you from the correct answer. For most questions, you can eliminate at least one or two of the distracters by applying your basic knowledge of the subject area.

- *Visualize the correct situation*
  As you read through a question, visualize the information that is being presented. Imagine what a patient looks like in the situation being described; visualize any injuries or symptom. Then, follow up by visualizing the proper response to the question that is being asked. If you can see the situation in your mind, you will often be able to see the answer, too.

- *Be wary of suspicion*
  People who have struggled on multiple choice exams often carry around strong negative emotions about having to take these kinds of tests. Sometimes they feel that the items are designed to trick them into choosing wrong answers. In fact, it is often those feelings that cause them to choose the wrong answer. A suspicious test-taker will read a clue in the question stem and immediately reason that it was put there to lure them into making a mistake. So, instead of using the clue to select the right answer, the suspicious test-taker will choose another answer, the wrong one.

- *Don't let sharp turns confuse you*
  While we don't want you to be too suspicious, we do want you to look out for what is often referred to as a "bait-and-switch" question. In such questions, the focus in the point of view changes, usually sharply and sometimes slyly. These types of changes require you to read the question very closely to ensure that you really do understand what is being asked. In these types of questions, one or more of the answers

will relate to the focus *prior* to the sharp turn. If you don't notice that a change has occurred, you may choose the wrong answer. So, read carefully and follow all the twists and turns of the question.

ADVICE FOR TEST DAY

As the CCRN exam day approaches, many test-takers become increasingly anxious. This is a natural reaction, but it is wise to recognize the symptoms of pre-exam anxiety and to take steps to manage it. You don't want your nervous feelings to lead to counterproductive behaviors that can decrease your exam performance.

Mental Turmoil

One of the most common symptoms of test anxiety is a tendency to lose focus and concentration. Rather than thinking about the material they are studying, people find their minds racing with thoughts about the material they still haven't mastered, questioning whether they should stop studying this topic and review another topic instead, or worrying about what they will do if they fail the examination. Their regimen of studying, taking breaks, and practice testing also tends to become harder to adhere to, so many people abandon their study plans and begin to flit from one thing to another. Others may decide to do only practice questions from dawn to dusk, believing that the more items they see in the final days, the more likely it is that they will encounter similar items on the actual exam. Still others engage in polling their colleagues, feeling that whatever their friends are doing in these final days must be the right thing for them to do as well. All of these behaviors are symptomatic of test anxiety and often result in feeling less and less in control at the worst of times. *Remember that your goal is to adhere firmly to your study plan and to allow the structure it provides to help you rein in the pre-exam jitters.*

Nutrition

Eating habits affect everyone's ability to deal with life's challenges, whether they involve sports, taking a test, avoiding fatigue and moodiness, or becoming more vulnerable to illness. Diabetics must monitor their food intake closely to prevent dangerous fluctuations in their blood glucose levels, but all of us are affected by the ups and downs of our blood sugar levels and excessive intake of junk foods. Caffeine, alcohol, too much sugar, and not enough variety in your diet can all disrupt your metabolism and leave you feeling short on energy or, in some cases, overstimulated.

Taking a long exam like the CCRN burns many calories, so it's a good idea to think ahead about fueling up properly before the exam. Since you will not be allowed to bring any food or drinks into the testing site, make sure that you eat enough before you arrive. Avoid heavy foods or eating a large meal before the exam, both of which can leave you suffering from postprandial droop, resulting in grogginess or abdominal discomfort. Finally, be sure to drink enough fluids; dehydration is another potential cause of fatigue, headache and general listlessness.

Insomnia

People's personalities vary greatly, with some reacting to increased stress by seeking out favorite activities that help them mentally regroup and feel physically tired, allowing them to fall asleep and regain their equanimity. Other people turn to drugs or alcohol, self-medicating to bring on sleep. Nearly everyone occasionally finds sleep elusive when they are worried about something they must deal with soon, such as a certification exam. Although most adults can function on six hours of sleep, some individuals require eight or nine to feel fully rested and alert. Tune into your own sleep requirements and make sure that in the weeks and days leading up to the CCRN exam, you are allowing yourself ample rest.

Prescribed medications can alter sleep requirements, making it difficult to fall asleep or to wake without grogginess. Perhaps the best advice that can be given to test-takers who fear they will not be able to fall or stay asleep the night before the exam is to avoid foods or beverages containing caffeine later than mid-afternoon the day before the exam.

The day before the exam, take some extra steps to ensure that you wake well-rested. First, avoid strenuous exercise too close to bedtime. While exercise may help tire you out, therefore helping you sleep, if it is done too close to retiring, vigorous exercise can actually overstimulate you, making it even harder for you to fall asleep. The most important thing to avoid doing late on the day before your exam is studying. Whatever material you madly race through that evening is not going to settle into your long-term memory. Instead, bits and pieces of it will still be spinning around in your working memory the following morning, and this can directly interfere with recall of the far larger body of information that you spent the last few months and weeks working with. In addition, cramming the night before the exam may also overstimulate your mind so that you have trouble relaxing and falling asleep.

Your best bet for a good night's sleep the night before the CCRN exam? Have a relaxing evening that doesn't veer too far from your normal routine, but that doesn't include any last-minute cramming.

Five Tips for Concentration, Pacing and Test Anxiety

Tip One: Reflect on Your Strengths

Several weeks before the exam, use an index card to list several of your greatest personal strengths and attributes, such as, "I'm an intelligent person who reacts well under pressure," or, "I am an excellent nurse and I have the experience and knowledge required for CCRN certification." Keep this card handy so that whenever negative thoughts intrude while you are studying, you can pull the card out, read each statement, and reflect on their truth. Luxuriate in the calm, positive feelings you associate with each of the statements. Fairly soon, you won't even need the card because you will know all the statements by heart and will be able to mentally review them as an antidote to negative thoughts and self-doubt.

Tip Two: Become Aware of Mind-Wandering

Keep a master tally sheet nearby each time you sit down to study. Make a check or a hash mark each time you find yourself engaging in negative thinking, daydreaming, or otherwise mentally escaping from the study situation. For many people, the very act of counting the frequency of mind-wandering actually reduces the frequency of those behaviors. This is a mild form of behavior modification that you can apply to your own study behavior. Although simple, it works well for many people.

Tip Three: Relive Your "Hero" Moments

As you prepare for the exam, spend some quiet time thinking back over your life experiences to find one event in which you were the "hero" of the situation. Perhaps you walked in on a serious fight between two friends and were able to bring about a peaceful resolution. Perhaps you'll recall the first time you successfully intubated a patient with respiratory failure or the time you successfully led a fund-raiser for your favorite charity. Whatever life event you select, it must be a situation in which your abilities and actions solved a problem or redeemed a bad situation.

Spend 10 minutes each day in a quiet place reliving this event, trying to bring back the memory in as much detail as possible. What time of year or day was it? What were you wearing? What was the setting like? As you practice this, it will take less and less time for you to retrieve the memory in graphic detail. The purpose of this exercise is to allow you to mentally revisit the event quickly because stored with this remembered event are all of the associated psychological feelings of being in control, a successful problem solver, confident, and in general, winning over adversity. When you retrieve this memory as part of a time-out taken during the exam when anxious feelings arise, positive emotions serve to counteract the negative emotions associated with the test-taking process.

Tip Four: Go At Your Optimal Pace

To find your optimal pace, be sure to work through several practice tests during your preparation. This book is filled with sample questions; use them not only to test yourself but also to learn how long it takes you to answer the questions as well. With practice, you will sense the right pace and will be able to walk into the exam location on test day confident that you can handle it because you have already done so in practice mode.

During the actual exam, use the same pacing plan that you used in practice over the final week or two of studying. Worrying about running out of time contributes to anxiety and often leads to time-wasting behaviors, such as checking the clock every few minutes. This nervous habit continually interrupts your thought process and often results in the need to re-read once you return to the question.

Tip Five: Take Time Out

If you feel anxiety during the exam that is interfering with your ability to concentrate on the questions, take a brief mental time out. Shut your eyes, lean back, and slowly rotate your neck and roll your shoulders to relax them. Take several slow, cleansing, deep breaths and exhale each breath slowly. Recall your "hero" moment if you think it will help re-invigorate you. This time out helps break the cycle of anxiety and will usually help you return to the task at hand with a greater sense of calm and improved concentration.

Signs of Anxiety That May Require Professional Help

There are some anxiety symptoms, such as muscle twitching, chronic insomnia, nausea, hyperventilation episodes, or chest tightness, for which self-help tactics may not be enough. If you experience several of these symptoms and they are severe, seek professional help from a psychiatrist or a cognitive psychologist who is experienced in helping people overcome situational anxiety. Therapies may include anti-anxiety medications, self-hypnosis instruction, behavioral retraining, or a variety of other interventions. But don't delay making an appointment—each of these treatment modalities requires time before they become effective. In seeking a professional, don't see just anyone. The professional you choose should have experience in treating this type of problem.

Managing Time during the Examination

Don't skip around frantically searching for easier items to answer. Doing this can result in missing items and will leave you feeling out of control in the test situation—something you definitely want to avoid. Also, because you won't easily be able to estimate how many items you have left to answer at any given point, skipping around makes following any pacing plan very difficult.

Decision Rules

Use decision rules to make the most of your testing time. Everyone needs at least two deciding rules. *Rule One* is used when you have thought about the question and are able to narrow the possible answers to two options. At this point, self-honesty is paramount. If you have already used recall and any strategies appropriate to such a question, it's time to choose and move on. Rule One gives you a way to decide, preventing you from reading and re-reading the item, hoping that something else will occur to you that will help you decide between the final two choices. To apply Rule One, mark the *upper* of the final two choices and move on to the next question. Then, the very next time that you are faced with the same final two choices dilemma, you should mark the *lower* of the final two choices. This is actually a time-management rule, designed to prevent you from endlessly obsessing between the final two choices.

Rule Two pertains to questions about material that you've never come across before. Fortunately, you are unlikely to encounter very many of these "clueless" items (especially since you are using this book!). Most test-takers report that on standardized examinations, they encounter only a handful of items that they truly have no idea how to answer. If you encounter a question dealing with totally unknown content, then have a favorite among A through D in mind, mark the answer that corresponds to your favored letter and move on. There is little to be gained from reading and re-reading the question multiple times in hopes that lightning will strike your synapses and make the correct answer apparent. Cut your losses (time loss in this case), so that subsequent items that you have a far stronger chance of answering correctly can be answered without rushing through them.

FINAL THOUGHTS

In this chapter, we covered the importance of developing a solid study plan and following a good study process as well. We outlined several test-taking skills that you can employ to enhance your chances of acing the CCRN certification exam. We also looked at how to improve your concentration, find your optimal pacing and reduce your anxiety on test day. All of these issues are important for you to consider as you prepare for the CCRN exam. Now that you are aware of them and understand what and how you need to study, we'll move on to the exam content, starting with the cardiovascular system.

Remember: Engage with the material, do the practice questions and you will do well. Good luck!

PART II

CCRN
Subject Review

The Cardiovascular System

4

Knowledge and the ability to apply information regarding the cardiovascular system is extremely important for the CCRN. Approximately 33 percent of the total number of scored questions on the CCRN examination involve the cardiovascular system. You will need to master a basic understanding of cardiovascular anatomy and physiology, ECG interpretation, and advanced cardiac life support (ACLS), as well as more complex physiology and disease management to do well on the CCRN.

Understanding major concepts such as preload and afterload, diagnostic and clinical complications associated with myocardial infarction in particular anatomical areas of the heart, pharmacological effects and shock states based on hemodynamic parameters, and differences between right and left heart failure are also important. It is also imperative to know that when terms such as pulsus alternans, pulsus paradoxus, narrowed pulse pressure, and Lewis lead appear on the exam—they relate to specific cardiovascular conditions. Knowing the particular conditions that these terms apply to is paramount in mastering cardiology for the CCRN; for example, pulsus paradoxus is an indication of pericardial effusion.

ANATOMY OF THE CARDIOVASCULAR SYSTEM

The position of the heart is slightly left of the midline, above the diaphragm, and within the anterior thoracic cavity behind the sternum. With this positioning, the right atrium and ventricle are primarily inferior and anterior, while the left atrium and ventricle are posterior and anterolateral. This will be important when the location of myocardial ischemia or damage is identified. To locate the point of maximal impulse (PMI), the health care provider places his fingers over the apex of the heart which is located at the left fifth intercostal space in the midclavicular line. This provides information as to the possible dilation of the left ventricle. As the left ventricle dilates, the PMI will be located more laterally and inferiorly. When describing the size of a normal adult heart, the clenched fist can be used as a guide for approximate size. Weight varies based on whether there are conditions that enlarge the heart such as heart failure or cardiomyopathy. In general, a male heart weighs slightly more than the female heart. There are four layers of the heart with different functions and attributes:

Pericardium

The pericardium is composed of two layers and forms a pericardial sac. The two layers of the pericardium are the fibrous and serous pericardium. The serous pericardium is further broken down into two layers: the parietal (outer) and visceral (inner, sometimes referred to as the epicardium) pericardium. Since the parietal layer is fused to the fibrous pericardium, you can think of the heart as essentially having two membrane layers: the parietal/fibrous pericardium and the visceral pericardium. The area between these two layers forms the pericardial sac, which holds approximately 10 cc of viscous fluid. Not only do the layers of the pericardium provide protection, but the fluid between the parietal and visceral layers allows the chambers of the heart to fill with blood and contract smoothly, and prevent the heart from overexpanding. However, when there is a pericardial effusion, fluid or blood accumulates between these two membranes and may impede cardiac function by not allowing the chambers of the heart to fill normally. As a result, the heart cannot effectively fill and contract, resulting in tamponade (a critical emergency). Typically, once diagnosed, a directed needle pericardiocentesis will be done to aspirate the fluid temporarily and allow normal contraction of the heart.

Inflammation may also occur between the two layers of the pericardium and can be painful. This is referred to as pericarditis. Pericarditis causes muffled heart sounds and a friction rub is often present over the precordium (the anterior chest wall).

Myocardium

This is the muscle layer of the heart. The contractile muscle fibers are located in this layer and arranged in multiple, interlacing levels. These are effective in pushing the blood flow through the chambers and into the lungs for reoxygenation and to the critical organs and extremities for oxygenation. This is the layer which is damaged in acute myocardial infarction. A blockage in coronary blood flow is the most common cause of this damage.

Endocardium

The innermost lining layers of the heart are called the endocardium. This lining forms a continuous layer with the vessels and intracardiac structures such as the papillary muscles and heart valves.

The anatomical structures within the heart include heart chambers, cardiac valves, nervous conduction system, and coronary vessels. There are two upper chambers of the heart which are considered low pressure chambers. The right atrium receives deoxygenated venous blood from the superior/inferior vena cava and coronary sinus, while the left atrium receives oxygenated blood from the pulmonary veins. The right atrium and ventricle are separated by the tricuspid valve, while the left atrium and ventricle are separated by the mitral valve. These valves initially open during ventricular diastole (relaxation) and close during ventricular systole (contraction). Approximately 80–85 percent of the blood is received passively from the atria. The contraction of the atria is responsible for "pushing" the remaining 15 percent of the blood from the atria into the ventricles; this is often referred to as the "atrial kick." The loss of this "kick" due to heart irregularities such as atrial fibrillation or flutter may cause a significant drop in cardiac output which causes the patient to become symptomatic. The valves which separate the outflow tracts of the right and left ventricles are the pulmonic and aortic valves respectively. These are referred to as semilunar valves. Chordae tendineae and papillary muscles join the valves to the wall of the ventricles.

The muscular wall of the left ventricle is three times thicker than that of the right ventricle. The right ventricle forms the greatest majority of the anterior surface of the heart. There are three types of cardiac muscle: atrial muscle, ventricular muscle, and excitatory and conductive muscle fibers. The atrial and ventricular muscle contracts similarly to skeletal muscle, except that the duration of the contraction is longer. The excitatory and conductive muscle exhibits autonomic electrical discharge which controls the rhythmical beating of the heart.

Coronary Vasculature

The arterial system that supplies the heart branches off the base of the aorta. There are four major vessels: right coronary artery (RCA), left coronary artery (LCD), left anterior descending artery (LAD), and the left circumflex artery (LCA). There are also collateral arteries which support circulation and may enlarge when there is damage to the other major vessels. During myocardial ischemia or infarction, it is possible to tell where the symptoms are originating from by changes on the EKG related to the location of the symptoms. For example, anterior changes on the EKG in "V" leads or a right bundle branch block may indicate blockage in the LAD. The RCA feeds the posterior wall of the myocardium, the AV node, and the SA node in approximately 55 percent of adults. The LCA branches into the LAD and the circumflex arteries. The LAD supplies the anterior septum, anterior wall of the left ventricle, right bundle branch and the anterosuperior left bundle branch.

The coronary veins serve to return the deoxygenated blood from the heart to the right atrium. The major vessels in this system include the great cardiac vein, small and middle cardiac veins, and the thebesian veins. These veins join to form the coronary sinus.

The important fact to remember about the coronary blood flow system is that there is a reserve which, when necessary, *can increase* the circulation to the heart by as much as six times normal. Myocardial oxygen demand may *increase* during hyperdynamic states such as strenuous exercise and conditions such as sepsis (elevated fevers). Coronary blood flow may *decrease* during states such as decreased tissue perfusion (hypotension), decreased left ventricular diastolic pressure, increased myocardial mass (heart failure), or mechanical obstruction (valvular disease).

FIGURE 4.1 *Arterial Supply to the Heart*

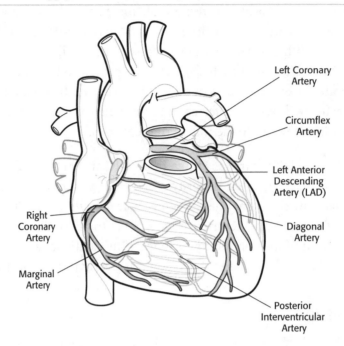

PHYSIOLOGY OF THE CARDIOVASCULAR SYSTEM

Conduction System

The cardiac cycle is initiated in the healthy heart by the **sinoatrial** (SA) **node**, which is located in the mouth of the vena cava on the posterior aspect of the right atrium. The SA node is considered the heart's natural pacemaker due to its characteristics of high automaticity and/or intrinsic heart rate. Typically, this heart rate is 60 to 100 beats per minute (BPM). The SA node contains two very specialized types of cells: **specialized pacemaker cells** and **border zone cells.**

Once the SA node cells are depolarized, the impulse generated is conducted down through the border of the atrium to four specialized pathways: Bachmann's bundle toward the left atrium and three internodal pathways directed to the atrioventricular (AV) node. The AV node is located posteriorly on the interatrial septum. Between the atria and ventricle are non-conducting tissues and therefore, the impulse travels to ventricle via the AV node. The AV node also contains pacemaker cells, but their intrinsic rate is lower than the SA node. The AV node is technically reset by the functioning SA node to prevent it from initiating its own impulse. However, in the event the SA node is non-functional or dysfunctional, the AV node will stimulate the impulse to the ventricles at a rate between 40 to 60 BPM. There is a slight delay in the conduction as the impulse travels through the AV node. The effect of this delay is to allow time for optimum ventricular filling and in turn, ventricular ejection during contraction.

FIGURE 4.2 *Cardiac Conduction System*

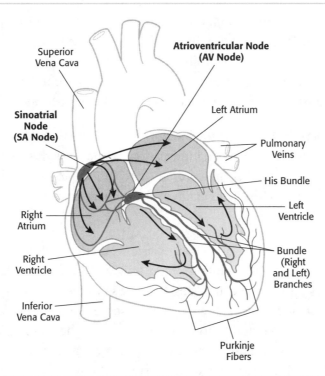

The normal AV node contains only one pathway to the ventricle for conduction. If there is an additional abnormal pathway, it is considered to be an accessory pathway. These circular pathways can allow the impulse to reenter the atrial circuit and cause rapid dysrhythmias which would then override SA node function. An atypical situation may develop where the pathway travels between the atria and ventricles, but outside the AV node. This dysrhythmia is called Wolfe-Parkinson-White (WPW) syndrome which can cause premature impulses in the atria or ventricle causing tachydysrthymias. An EKG of a person with WPW will demonstrate the presence of delta waves just immediately preceding the QRS complex.

The final conduction pathway is through the Bundle of His, bundle branches, and Purkinje fibers. This pathway runs through the subendocardium down the right side of the intraventricular septum. The two bundle branches follow toward the right apex and the left ventricular wall. These branches narrow into a thin anterior branch and a thick posterior branch. A serious conduction defect, called a hemiblock, can occur when the left bundle is blocked. With any blockage in the bundles, a widening of the QRS complex will occur on the 12 lead EKG, indicating a lengthening of conduction. Eventually the right and left bundles divide into the Purkinje fibers which attach to the subendocardial surface of both ventricles. The Purkinje fibers, which provide for rapid depolarization of the ventricles, have the fastest conduction velocity of all heart tissues.

Nervous Regulation

Within the regulatory nervous system there are two systems which can directly impact cardiovascular functions. These are the **sympathetic nervous system** (SNS) and the **parasympathetic nervous system** (PNS). Typically the PNS has the effect of *decreasing* most of the cardiovascular functions such as automaticity, contractility, rate, and velocity of contraction. The SNS has the opposite effect and will *increase* all of these functions.

Parasympathetic fibers are located at the level of the SA and AV node and, more specifically, the right and left vagus nerves. Sudden bradycardia can occur with stimulation of the vagus nerve. Sympathetic fibers parallel the coronary circulation before the fibers innervate the myocardium. It appears that the right chain of these fibers tends to affect rate while the left chain impacts contractility.

Within the nervous system there are also intrinsic regulatory reflexes which provide feedback to the brain and work to maintain blood flow and perfusion. The first of these are called **baroreceptors**. As the name indicates, they are sensitive to pressure and are located in the aortic arch and carotid sinuses. These receptors sense changes in volume, as a measurement of pressure, and will respond through stimulation of the autonomic nervous system. If a sudden drop in blood volume should occur such as in gastrointestinal bleeding, the baroreceptors would stimulate an increased heart rate through the vasomotor center in the medulla. The second of these reflexes are the **chemoreceptors**, located in the aortic arch and are provided by a rich blood supply and innervated by the PNS. They have the ability to detect oxygen tension and respond to a decreased oxygen tension by the stimulation of respiration. The Bainbridge reflex causes reflex tachycardia in response to increased right atrial pressure. This reflex is designed to protect right heart function.

Although not specifically a reflex, another control mechanism of the heart involves the atrial release of a hormone called atrial natriuretic factor. The response is due to an increase in atrial pressure. The effects are that sodium and water are excreted by the kidneys and vasodilation occurs. The dual effect of reducing extracellular fluid volume and improving the capacity of the venous system results in a restoration to the blood volume.

Concepts of Cardiac Output

The definition of cardiac output is fairly simple; however, the actual potential of cardiac output has many factors. **Cardiac output** (CO) is the volume of blood which is ejected by the heart over 1 minute and is reported in liters/minute. Considering this definition, the two major components of the equation are *heart rate* and *stroke volume*. A calculation can be made for cardiac index (CI), which is the CO divided by the patient's body surface in square meters (m^2). The normal range for CO is 5–6 L/min and the average CI is 2.5 to 4.5 L/min/m^2.

Additionally, there is a component of efficiency involved. Simply increasing CO does not necessarily mean increased functional capacity of the heart. Eventually, the resultant increase could lead to decompensation of the heart, resulting in clinical heart failure.

Preload

Preload was actually not recognized as a fundamental concept until the early 1900s. The researcher who wrote about his findings with relation to preload was Ernest Starling. Starling's Law is still recognized today as one of the primary concepts in cardiac function. The basis for this law is that the heart will respond to an increased volume and compensate for a period of time to improve cardiac output until a certain point, at which time the contractility actually diminishes and the heart function decreases. These changes occur on a molecular level with the actin and myosin cross-bridges in the myofilament. Therefore, preload is a combination of blood volume entering the left ventricle and the contractility of that ventricle. It is also known as left ventricular end diastolic pressure (LVEDP), and can be measured with the use of a pulmonary artery catheter and pulmonary capillary wedge pressures. Factors which affect preload are venous return, total blood volume, "atrial kick" (mentioned earlier), and compliance of the ventricles.

Afterload

Afterload of the heart is the pressure or stress which the ventricular wall faces when ejecting its blood volume. Afterload may be considered the resistance in the circulation as well. Factors which impact afterload include: increased systemic vascular resistance (SVR) or vasoconstriction, increased blood volume, aortic impedance such as with aortic valve sclerosis/stenosis, and septal hypertrophy. Along with increased afterload and work of the heart comes increased myocardial oxygen demand; therefore, the goals for reducing afterload should include decreasing SVR with the use of vasodialtors, reducing blood volume, or repairing valvular dysfunction with valve replacement.

The concepts of preload and afterload are important aspects of cardiac output and in most abnormal heart and circulation functions, one or both are severely altered from normal.

Contractility

Contractility is essentially the ability of the heart to contract and the subsequent force of contraction. The body will compensate for decreased contractility by increasing heart rate to a certain point as discussed earlier with Starling's law. This is done via stimulation of the sympathetic nervous system. In critical care patient management, pharmacologic agents which function similarly to the sympathetic nervous system stimulus may also be used to increase cardiac contractility. Pharmacologic agents that increase cardiac contractility are referred to as inotropic agents.

CARDIOVASCULAR CONDITIONS

Hypertensive Crisis/Emergency

Hyptertensive crisis, otherwise known as hypertensive emergency, is a sudden event involving a critically elevated blood pressure, and requires immediate medical attention. Hypertensive emergency is diagnosed when there is a critically elevated blood pressure associated with end-organ damage. Hypertensive crisis was once known as malignant hypertension. The presenting clinical manifestations include: altered level-of-consciousness or disorientation, seizure, vomiting, severe headache, epistaxis, visual disturbances, and diastolic blood pressure exceeding 120 mm Hg. Hypertensive encephalopathy as well as irreversible end-organ damage to the brain, kidneys, and heart or death can result if not corrected.

The primary cause of hypertensive crises is most often due to untreated or uncontrolled hypertension. Secondary causes include renal dysfunction or endocrine disorders. Risk factors associated with hypertensive crisis include: diabetes, smoking, obesity, oral contraceptive agent use, hypertension during pregnancy, and hyperlipidemia. Hypertension enhances sympathetic stimulation causing systemic vasoconstriction. which decreases blood flow to vital organs. Complications of hypertensive crisis include: cerebrovascular accident (CVA), increased intracranial pressure (IICP), myocardial infarction (MI), decreased mesenteric blood flow, and renal failure. The goals of treatment are to: (a) determine the cause, either primary or secondary, (b) immediately detect and prevent clinical sequelae, (c) reduce the blood pressure no more than 25 percent in the first one to two hours of presentation, (d) provide patient teaching to decrease risk factors and promote compliance with prescribed medial regimen.

The "gold standard" treatment for hypertensive crisis is the administration of a potent vasodilator such as *Nitroprusside (Nipride), Hydralazine,* or *Fenoldopam Mesylate (Corlopam).* Other agents than can be used in the treatment of hypertensive crisis include nitroglycerin (produces more venodilation than arteriolar dilation), Nicardipine, Labetalol, Esmolol, Enalaprilat, and Phenolamine. However, Nitroprusside can cause fetal renal impairment and should not be used in pregnancy for this reason. Nipride also causes cyanide toxicity (confusion, seizure activity, visual disturbances, and tinnitus) and requires thiosulfate as an additive to prevent cyanide toxicity. Fenoldopam isn't always preferred due to its longer half-life (5 to 10 minutes) and hypokalemic effects. Other effects of Fenoldopam are headaches and reflex tachycardia. Hypotension caused by Fenoldopam can be treated with IV fluids and Trendelenburg position. *Nicardipine Hydrochloride (Cardene)* a calcium channel blocker/antihypertensive is gaining popularity as a choice infusion for the treatment of hypertensive crisis, due to gentler effects and lack of toxicity. Other useful agents include: *Nitroglycerin (Tridil), ACE inhibitors (Lisinopril, Captopril, Enalapril, Enalaprilat), β-blockers (Labetalol, Esmolol, and Metoprolol), calcium channel blockers (Nicardipine and Amlodipine), and diuretics (Furosemide and Bumetanide).*

Chronic Stable Angina Pectoris

Chronic stable angina pectoris is chest discomfort that does not increase in severity or frequency over time. This type of angina is predictable and typically follows some type of exertion (physical activity, stress, anxiety, extreme emotions or a meal). This type of chest pain is easily relieved with *nitrates (nitroglycerin)* and rest. During the episode of chest pain, the patient's ECG may reflect the following changes: T wave inversion or ST segment depression in ECG leads correlating with decreased coronary blood flow and oxygen delivery (myocardial ischemia).

Myocardial ischemia causes the symptom known as angina or chest discomfort. Most victims of chronic stable angina pectoris describe this discomfort as a pressure, indigestion, heaviness, or achy feeling across the chest lasting anywhere from 5 to 20 minutes. Others describe the discomfort by location: chest, jaw, arms, substernal, back, or epigastric region. Accompanying symptoms include: nausea, diaphoresis, shortness-of-breath, and dizziness. Angina occurs as a result of the myocardium lack of blood supply due to coronary artery disease (CAD), namely, atherosclerosis. It may also occur as a result of an embolus and/or vasopasms of the coronary arteries. Atherosclerosis results in the loss of elasticity of the vessel and progresses as we age. The culprit of this type of angina is that myocardial oxygen demand exceeds supply. Coronary artery disease (CAD) is the most prominent risk factor associated with chronic stable angina pectoris. Most importantly, serum cardiac biomarkers (CK and CK-MB isoenzymes, myoglobin, and T/I troponins) are not elevated with episodes of stable angina.

The goal of treatment for this type of angina is to increase myocardial oxygen supply (nitrates) and decrease demand (nitrates, calcium channel blockers, and β-blockers). This can also be accomplished by lifestyle modification teaching, such as; smoking cessation, diabetic education, weight control, stress or anxiety reduction, promotion of a non-sedimentary lifestyle, proper diet, blood pressure and cholesterol control. Illicit drug use is often associated with this condition; therefore, a thorough patient history is necessary. Prinzmetal's angina (coronary vasospasm) is primarily seen with illicit drug use. Oftentimes, an *anti-platelet (Aspirin 81 mg daily) or antithrombotic (Clopidogrel 75 mg daily)* may be prescribed. Adequate Nitroglycerin instruction is needed for patients with chronic stable angina pectoris. Angiography and percutaneous coronary interventions (PCI) such as percutaneous transluminal coronary angioplasty (PTCA), laser angioplasty, cutting balloon angioplasty, bare-metal stent placement, drug-eluding stent placement, brachytherapy, directional and rotational atherectomy can be the treatment for this condition as well as coronary artery bypass grafting (CABG).

Acute Coronary Syndromes

Acute coronary syndrome (ACS) includes the following medical conditions: unstable angina pectoris, non-ST segment elevation myocardial infarction (NSTEMI), and ST-segment elevation myocardial infarction (STEMI). Acute coronary syndromes result from coronary artery disease, thrombosis, atherosclerotic plaque, vasoconstriction, and occlusion. All three of these syndromes are similar in initial presentation and medical management. However, unstable angina pectoris does not cause elevations in cardiac biomarkers (CK and CK-MB isoenzymes, myoglobin, and T/I troponins). The following criteria conclude the diagnosis of STEMI or NSTEMI acute myocardial infarction: (a) a change on the electrocardiogram indicating myocardial ischemia or injury (ST elevation, ST depression, presence of a Q wave), (b) elevated cardiac biomarkers, **and** (c) symptoms of acute coronary syndrome lasting longer than 20 minutes, or chest discomfort that occurs at rest. Other related symptoms include dyspnea, nausea, vomiting, chest pain, diaphoresis, syncope, and referred pain. Pain may be referred to arms, jaw, neck, shoulder, and between the scapula of the back. The pain associated with ACS is typically reported as chest "pressure" and feel as if someone is "sitting on their chest."

Differentiation of a transmural (endocardium to epicardium) from a nontransmural (subendocardial) myocardial infarction is dependent upon the extent of the necrosis. In the past, the medical terms "transmural and subendocardial" were used to be synonymous with "Q wave and non-Q wave" respectively based upon the presence or absence of Q waves. Currently, Q-wave detection is pathologic and mainly associated with larger infarctions. If Q waves become apparent, then they appear within hours of myocardial infarction. Abnormal Q waves greater than 0.04 seconds in duration and 25 percent of the height of the R wave develop within the first 24 hours.

Unstable Angina Pectoris

Unstable angina pectoris is often referred to as "crescendo or preinfarction angina" since this type of chest discomfort becomes more difficult to relieve and lasts longer. Often, this is the result of multi-coronary artery disease. Unstable angina pectoris neither causes elevations in cardiac biomarkers (CK and CK-MB isoenzymes, myoglobin, and T/I troponins) nor causes myocardial cell death (necrosis). Patients present with the same symptoms as STEMI and NSTEMI. However, clinical presentation is unstable compared to chronic stable angina pectoris.

Non-ST Segment Elevation Myocardial Infarction (NSTEMI)

The major difference between unstable angina pectoris and NSTEMI and STEMI is the myocardial cell death or necrosis associated with these two types of myocardial infarctions. The danger associated with this type of myocardial infarction is that the ECG may or may not show evidence of myocardial injury or ischemia. Troponin T and I levels are more than 0.1ng/ml in NSTEMI. These elevations are present for 8 to 12 hours after the onset of symptoms and are generally trended to determine the peak. Elevated troponin values are difficult to interpret in the context of acute renal insufficiency, as they will artificially be elevated because the kidneys excrete troponin from the bloodstream. ST segment changes sometimes occur with chest pain and ST segment depression or inverted T waves may be present.

ST-Segment Elevation Myocardial Infarction (STEMI)

ECG changes correlate with the location of the necrosis in STEMI. Table 4.1 demonstrates the associations between location of infarction and ECG leads. A low percentage of people with chest discomfort who seek medical attention may present with normal ECG rhythms initially. Therefore, a normal ECG does not rule out acute myocardial infarction. A combination of terms also describe the location of the myocardial infarction, such as anterolateral or anteroseptal. Patients diagnosed with acute inferior myocardial infarction should be routinely screened with a right-sided EKG due to the possibility of a right ventricular infarction.

Acute Coronary Syndrome Treatment (ACS)

The goal of treatment in ACS is to rapidly identify the cause of chest pain or symptoms, exclude non-ischemic chest pain, stratify patients with coronary ischemia, and provide immediate treatment, including interventional procedures such as percutaneous transluminal coronary angioplasty (PTCA) or coronary artery bypass graft (CABG) if necessary, to prevent further damage. Emergency medical service to coronary artery stent should be less than 90 minutes. The noteworthy acronym *MONA (morphine, oxygen, nitrates, and aspirin)* has always been associated with remembering the treatment for acute coronary syndromes. During states where myocardial oxygen is limited, supplemental oxygen will help improve the availability of oxygen. Morphine serves both to reduce pain and also as a mild vasodialator which, similarly to nitrates, reduces venous return or preload. Nitrates relax smooth muscle and cause venodilation, thus decreasing the venous return to the heart. In turn, it reduces myocardial oxygen demand and consumption. In cases of myocardial artery spasm, it may help reduce the spasm and assist in improving blood flow and oxygenation to the tissue of the myocardium. Aspirin has been demonstrated to prevent platelet aggregation and should be administered prehospital if possible.

TABLE 4.1

Area of Infarction	Indicative Changes (ST segment elevation)	Reciprocal Changes (ST segment depression)	Coronary Artery Involved
Inferior wall	II, III, aVF	I, aVL, V5 and V6	RCA or Circumflex
Septal wall	V1 and V2	II, III, aVF	LAD
Anterior wall	V2 - V4	II, III, aVF	LAD
Lateral wall	I, aVL, V5 and V6	II, III, aVF	Circumflex or Obtuse Marginal
Right ventricle	V3-4R	I, aVL	RCA

The use of *beta blockers (Atenolol, Metorprolol)* is standard in the treatment of acute MI patients. Beta blockers reduce heart rate and contractility, thus reducing myocardial oxygen demand and afterload. These drugs are contraindicated in the patient with a history of bronchial asthma, AV blocks, or hypotension.

Heart Failure

Heart failure is one of the most predominant conditions in the Medicare population. In fact, it is the most frequent diagnosis-related group (DRG) for acute care hospital admission in this population. Heart failure is a general term that describes an impaired cardiac function where either one or both of the ventricles are unable to maintain an adequate cardiac output to meet the metabolic demands for the body. Classification of heart failure is done with the use of the New York Heart Association (NYHA) Functional Classifications: Classes I–IV. The highest classification (Class IV) is when the patient remains symptomatic even at rest. Heart failure can be due to either a systolic dysfunction, such as cardiomyopathy or vavular disease, or diastolic dysfunction such as acute myocardial infarction or drug abuse (cocaine).

When educating patients about heart failure and how this impacts their future quality of life, it is best to discuss the preservation of ejection fraction. This education should focus on diet, exercise tolerance, compliance with medication, daily weight monitoring, and when to discuss changes in their weight or breathing with their primary care physician. Non-compliance with medications can play a large role in heart failure hospital admissions; hence, it is important to clearly discuss the medication and diet regimen with each patient diagnosed with heart failure.

The pathophysiology of heart failure is complex and cyclical which often leads to involvement of other organs, particularly when there is chronic fluid overload. The primary indicator of heart failure is ejection fraction. This is assessed with the use of a transthoracic echocardiogram (TTE), commonly referred to as "echo." The TTE will describe systolic and ventricular function, valvular dysfunction, chamber sizes, and may be able to estimate pulmonary artery pressure. Symptoms and clinical findings in heart failure are as follows:

Left-Sided Heart Failure–Systolic

Left-sided heart failure is demonstrated by a series of events which ultimately leads to a failure of the left ventricle. Examples of etiologies of this type of heart failure include **idiopathic dilated cardiomyopathy** and **myocardial infarction**. This type of heart failure begins with a reduction in left ventricular contractility resulting in an impairment of the cardiac output. The ejection fraction (EF) then falls to below normal (normal range = 55–70 percent). The ventricle compensates by dilating and the heart rate increases as it attempts to maintain an adequate cardiac output. As discussed earlier, based on Starling's Law, initially the contractility of the heart will increase; thereby increasing the stroke volume and cardiac output.

TABLE 4.2

LEFT-SIDED HEART FAILURE		RIGHT-SIDED HEART FAILURE
Systolic	**Diastolic**	
Fatigue, weakness, lethargy	Exercise intolerance	Easily fatigued
Orthopnea	Orthopnea	Dependent/pitting edema
Tachycardia on exertion	Tachycardia on exertion	Anorexia
Basilar rales, rhonchi, crackles, and wheezes	Basilar rales, rhonchi, and wheezes	Weight gain
Elevated PCWP, PADP	Elevated PCWP, PADP	Oliguria
Murmur of mitral insufficiency	Holosystolic murmur if evidence of tricuspid or mitral regurgitation	Venous distension
Skin cool, moist, cyanosis		Extra heart sounds—S3
Hypoxia, respiratory acidosis	Hypoxia, respiratory acidosis	Elevated CVP, right atrial and right ventricular pressures

However, if the dilation persists, the contractility will begin to decrease, further depressing the cardiac output. These responses may be satisfactory to increase the cardiac output, despite a poor EF. As stroke volume and heart rate increase, myocardial oxygen demands may increase. In addition, left atrial and pulmonary venous pressures increase as a result of myocardial dilatation and/or decreased left ventricular compliance. Pulmonary congestion and edema occur as these pressures rise and fluids leak into the pulmonary interstitial space. Subsequently the patient may demonstrate signs and symptoms of right-sided failure, as a result of fluid overload and increased pulmonary pressures.

Left-Sided Heart Failure–Diastolic

In this type of heart failure, the ventricle is considered stiff or non-compliant. Etiologies of this type of heart failure include mitral stenosis, constrictive pericarditis, hypertrophic cardiomyopathy, or restrictive cardiomyopathy. The condition results in inadequate filling pressures and rising diastolic pressures. With increasing diastolic pressures also come increased left atrial, pulmonary venous and pulmonary capillary pressures. In these cases, the systolic function may remain normal, or be hyperdynamic.

Right-Sided Heart Failure

The etiology of right-sided heart failure can be varied but commonly is caused by fluid overload such as in renal failure, cardiomyopathy, or valvular disease. In these conditions, the patient's right ventricle is unable to adequately pump blood into the pulmonary bed, which causes a drop in cardiac output. As a result the right ventricle enlarges, resulting in peripheral edema and elevated jugular venous pressure and corresponding distention. Occasionally in left ventricular myocardial infarction, the patient may show evidence of a right ventricular infarction which could also result in right-sided heart failure. Another indication of right-sided heart failure is the presence of the hepatojugular reflex. Place the patient in a 30–45 degree angle, compress the right abdomen and observe for distension of the neck veins. Positive distention of the jugular veins is indicative of heart failure.

Typically when a patient is admitted with heart failure, the first line of treatment is pharmacological. Once the causative condition is determined, the appropriate medications can be administered. For reduction of preload, *diuretics* can be ordered either orally or intravenously based on the severity of the fluid overload. Careful monitoring of electrolytes, particularly sodium, potassium, and magnesium, is necessary to assure balance. Low dose *morphine,* 3–5 mg IV, produces a mild vasodilatation and decreases venous return to the heart, decreases anxiety, and reduces pain.

DOPamine or DOBUTamine (written in tall man letters to aid in the differentiation of the drug, a JCAHO patient safety standard) is often ordered based on the expected outcomes and cause of the failure. *Dopamine* has dopaminergic, alpha- and beta-adrenergic effects based on the dosage of the drug. At low doses (1 to 2 mcg/kg/min) the effect is dopaminergic and increases blood flow to the kidneys and mesentery by acting as a vasopressor. As a result, diuresis occurs and urine output increases. At moderate doses (2–10 mcg/kg/min), the result is the beta-adrenergic effect and there is an increase in heart rate, blood pressure, cerebral and renal perfusion. Finally, at higher doses (>10 mcg/kg/min), alpha-adrenergic effects will cause peripheral vasoconstriction, increased systemic vascular resistance, and increased blood pressure. Unfortunately, the beta adrenergic effects can cause tachycardia, thereby increasing myocardial demand. If the drug should extravasate, there is a potential for tissue necrosis and sloughing. Therefore, if possible, the drug should be infused through a central line catheter which can also be used to measure central venous pressure (CVP).

Dobutamine is administered to improve myocardial contractility and has a direct inotropic effect, which can result in increased stroke volume and cardiac output. This drug is especially effective in the hypotensive patient which is caused by cardiogenic shock. Infusions are titrated based on effect at rates of 2.5–10 mcg/kg/min. At low doses it may actually potentiate excessive diuresis and decrease blood pressure.

Amrinone (milrinone) is a drug which directly relaxes smooth muscle in the vasculature and produces a reduction in both preload and afterload. It is infused at a rate of 2–20 mcg/kg/min after an initial bolus of 0.5–0.75 mcg/kg. The reduction in afterload reduces the work of the heart.

Finally, *nitroprusside* may be used to reduce afterload, especially if the patient is hypertensive. This effect occurs due to arterial dilatation and reduction of systemic and pulmonary vascular resistance. Rate of this infusion is 0.1 mcg/kg/min. Similarly to Dopamine, this drug causes tissue sloughing and necrosis with extravasation.

Nesiritide can be effective in patients with acutely decompensated heart failure who experience shortness of breath at rest. This drug is a recombinant form of the natural human peptide, hBNP. Nesiritide relaxes smooth muscle and causes both venous and arterial dilation (both which cause a reduction in systemic vascular resistance) and may be effective for patients where other therapies have not reduced the symptoms of heart failure. One of the significant side effects of nesiritide is hypotension, so it is critical that this patient be monitored closely. Immediate interventions of placing the patient in trendelenburg position and an IV bolus may be required to treat the hypotension, which may last for a period of time due to the half-life of the drug.

With all of the above intravenous medications, it is imperative for the critical care RN to closely monitor blood pressure and ECG to observe for hypotension and arrhythmias such as conduction defects. Neurological status should be monitored for decreased cerebral perfusion as well.

Cardiogenic Pulmonary Edema

As the name implies, cardiogenic pulmonary edema is the result of some type of cardiac dysfunction which occurs in late-stage heart failure. Typically this occurs suddenly after an event which causes temporary overload of the work of the heart. It then becomes a vicious circle as the patient is unable to compensate for the changes. The cycle begins as a temporary increase in the load on the heart often due to decreased pumping capacity of the heart, e.g., myocardial infarction, heavy exercise, or severe infection. The result is backing up of blood into the pulmonary bed. The increased blood in the lungs causes pulmonary capillary pressure to increase. Leaking of fluid begins to occur in the tissues and alveoli. Blood flowing through the capillary bed then cannot be oxygenated and as a result, the body tries to conserve oxygen by causing peripheral vasodilatation. To compensate, the body tries to increase venous circulation from the periphery. There is more evidence of damming of the blood within the lungs. Further leaking occurs and the cycle becomes circular. Symptoms the patient may experience include acute shortness of breath, frothy, pink-tinged sputum, and hypotension. The patient often requires immediate intubation and control of airway.

Late End Stage Heart Failure

In late stage heart failure, all reserves are exhausted and the patient becomes end stage, or if the patient is determined to be a good candidate for transplantation, more interventional procedures such as insertion of a left ventricular assist device, right ventricular assist device, or bi-ventricular assist device can be done to allow more time until an organ becomes available.

Left Ventricular Assist Device (LVAD)

The use of LVADs to bridge the period between end stage heart failure and transplant has decreased and the goal of LVAD has changed to become a standard treatment for heart failure patients and permanent definitive therapy. Despite these advances, the mortality rate for heart failure patients remains high at 70 percent. Not all heart failure patients are candidates for ventricular assist devices. Younger patients with fewer morbidities are the best candidates for LVADs.

The criteria for insertion of LVAD include a lack of response to conventional medical therapies, as discussed above. Additionally, if the purpose of this device is a bridge to transplantation, the patient must meet the transplant criteria as well. It is also important that the patient not suffer from deterioration of renal and hepatic function, as these functions will be critical in the recovery during the post-operative period and for quality of life in the long run. If the patient has suffered respiratory failure requiring ventilation prior to transplant, the mortality risk significantly increases.

The device is typically inserted via a sternotomy while patient is on cardiopulmonary bypass. The inflow cannula is inserted into the left ventricle and tunneled to the external pump, while blood is returned via an outflow tract which has been inserted subcostally into the ascending aorta. The patient must be anticoagulated to prevent clot formation either in the blood exterior to the body or in the vasculature where the devices lie. The cannulas are connected to an external pump, via a pneumatic hose, to a blood sac which pumps via alternating pressure and vacuum. The cannulas are covered with a synthetic material which encourages endothelial cell ingrowth, thus sealing the tract of the cannula to the mediatstinum. This process can take up to 10 days.

Electrical back-up is also required for the device, even though it primarily runs on a pneumatic system. The pump can be run on either a manual fixed rate that does not respond to the patient's own intrinsic heart rate or the preferred trigger, which is that when the device blood sac reaches full fill, the device then pumps the blood back to the patient. The second method reduces the chances of thrombus formation.

There are also totally implantable devices which are electrically driven pulsatile LVADs made of titanium. The patient wears an external battery pack which is connected to the system controller. These are positioned either in the left upper abdominal quadrant or intra-abdominally. The insertion of this device requires entry into two compartments (thoracic via a sternotomy and abdominal via a laparotomy) which increases the opportunity for infection. Similar positioning of the cannulas occurs during insertion of the device. In these devices, air is displaced through a pump and the air reenters through the same housing as a space is created by the ejection of the blood from the pump. The device also has the capability to be hand pumped in emergencies or be reconnected to a pneumatic device for patients who have to be rehospitalized.

Complications of the LVAD postoperatively include: multi-organ failure which is often due to preoperative conditions such as low perfusion states, right ventricular failure, especially (if there is evidence of respiratory failure requiring mechanical ventilation preoperatively), bleeding due to anticoagulation or prolonged cardiopulmonary pump time, infection, thromboembolism, and device malfunction. These are best managed with standard approaches to the patient's care in medical centers which are known for their expertise in use of these devices.

Right Ventricular Assist Device (RVAD)
Unfortunately one of the complications of LVADs is right-sided heart failure. This is often due to the fact that the failing heart, particularly the right side, does not have the capability to provide enough blood flow through the pulmonary circuit to fill the device. Occasionally, the patient can be managed with inotropes, nitrous oxide, or protaglandins to increase the cardiac output and RV function. The effect of nitrous oxide is lowering of the pulmonary vascular resistance and mean pulmonary artery pressure, thus increasing LVAD flow. The challenge with RVADs is that there is no small, biocompatible, inexpensive implantable device. The RVADs currently in use for clinical trials require external drive systems. The RVAD receives blood from the right atrium, diverting it from the right ventricle, and delivers it to the pulmonary artery for distribution by the pulmonary vasculature. The device is connected to the right atrium and the pulmonary artery via vascular grafts from one of the passageways of the RVAD and exits via either a sternotomy or parasternal incision. Similar complications may develop with the use of RVADs as with LVADs and include thrombosis, bleeding, infection, secondary organ failure, and air emboli.

Biventricular Assist Device (BiVAD)
In conditions when there is failure of both ventricles such as extensive cardiomyopathy or cardiogenic shock, biventricular assist devices can be used to bridge the period prior to transplantation or extend the period of cardiovascular support to promote recovery of the patient's own heart. Occasionally these devices are used when the patient cannot be successfully removed from the cardiopulmonary bypass devices intraoperatively. Based on the location of the cannula placement at the time of insertion, either one or both ventricles can be bypassed. The system consists of two single-use blood pumps, cannulae (which are used to secure openings into the ventricles), aorta, and pulmonary artery, and a pneumatic drive console.

Nursing Considerations with VADs

It is imperative that critical care nurses caring for the patient with VADs are familiar with the technical aspects of the device which their organization uses to provide ventricular assist. There are specialists who typically work in the cardiovascular operating arena called *cardiac perfusionists* who are specially trained with these types of devices and will serve as a resource. Additionally, device vendors typically have clinical nurse specialists who will assist with training on the devices.

Hemodynamic monitoring is continuous and the frequency is based on the patient's clinical condition but should include vital signs, cardiac output measurements, hemodynamic measurements including pulmonary artery (PA) pressures, pulmonary capillary wedge pressures (PCWP) except in RVAD use, central venous pressure (CVP), and arterial pressures, intake and output, circulatory checks, and monitoring of arrhythmias.

The patient must be able to support a reasonable cardiac output for consideration for weaning to occur, as well as a mean arterial pressure > 60 mm/Hg. Similar to ventilator weaning, the ventricular assist device flow rate is decreased gradually, to ascertain if the patient's own ventricles will be able to sustain the cardiac output.

Acute Inflammatory Disease

Inflammation of the heart can occur as a result of bacterial or viral microorganisms, chemical agents, or medications. The location of the inflammation often determines the subsequent effect on the heart and includes the myocardium, pericardium, and endocardium. There are no age limitations to these inflammations and there can be significant impact on the function of the heart if severe enough.

Myocarditis

The myocardium, as described earlier, is the muscle layer which surrounds the heart and has contractile abilities. Myocarditis refers to the inflammation of the heart muscle. Viral etiologies of mycoarditis include influenza, cytomegalovirus (CMV), human immunodeficiency virus (HIV), viral hepatitis, cocksackie, or mumps/rubella. Bacterial etiologies include, but are not limited to, streptococci, meningococci, and rickettsia. Finally, fungal infection can also lead to myocarditis and the most common is aspergilliosis.

As a result of the inflammation, myocardial fibers may become injured and then hypertrophy, causing cellular death to occur. Contractility and cardiac output decrease, and intolerance to activity occurs as the heart cannot compensate for the increased demand placed on the body. Heart failure may also ensue if left ventricular function is impaired significantly.

Treatment is focused on the cause of the inflammation and improving cardiac contractility with pharmacological agents or interventional support such as IABP (intra-aortic balloon pump) or LVAD if necessary. It is important to monitor the patient's cardiac output and/or venous oxygen saturation to assure adequate perfusion. Modification of activities may be required to preserve cardiac function.

Endocarditis

The endocardial layer contains anatomical structures such as the valves, chordae tendoneae, septum, and endothelium. Inflammation of these structures and layers will cause endocarditis.

Similar to myocarditis, microorganisms can also infect the endocardial layer, often through introduction into the bloodstream. Injury of key mechanisms of this layer can occur and cause substantial impact on cardiac function. Additionally, thrombotic lesions can form as a result of the clumping of platelets and fibrin at the location of the injury. Valvular tissue can be destroyed and the leaflets can actually rupture, become incompetent or perforate. Often the left heart valves are infected, typically as a result of IV drug abuse. The introduction of these agents can be from multiple causes including, but not limited to, open heart surgical procedures, congenital heart defects, dental procedures, prolonged IV therapies such as hyperalimentation, and immunosuppressive therapies. Treatment is targeted toward the source of the inflammation aimed at supporting cardiac function. Anticoagulants have not been found to be effective with this type of thromboembolus and in fact, may increase the likelihood of intracranial hemorrhage.

It is important to note that not all endocarditis is infectious. Endocarditis may also occur from inflammation on the endocardium that leads to the formation of a thrombus. This is often referred to as a marantic vegetation. In these cases, anticoagulation may be of benefit. To better characterize endocarditis, a TTE may be enough to reveal the vegetations; however, a transesophageal echocardiogram (TEE) is paramount in attaining detailed characterization of the endocardium and the vegetation. In most institutions, a TTE is often ordered prior to the TEE, unless clinical suspicion is extremely high.

Pericarditis

Inflammation of the pericardial layer can be more diverse and have a variety of etiologies other than infection. There are some very distinct features of pericarditis that are important for critical care nurses to be able to identify. First, pericarditis is often associated with a general syndrome. This syndrome includes fever, chest pain, the presence of a pericardial friction rub, diffuse ST elevation, and the potential for pericardial effusion causing pericardial tamponade.

Pericardial effusions may be created slowly or rapidly, based on the cause of the effusion. Rapidly accumulating effusions, particularly of blood, can lead to cardiac tamponade and is an emergent event requiring a pericardiocentesis or an operative pericardial window. Hypotension and death can ensue in minutes if not treated. Evaluation for tamponade can be done by listening for decreased heart sounds, and observing for sudden increases in CVP, jugular venous distention, and pulsus paradoxus. Pulsus paradoxus is evidenced when the pulse becomes weaker as one inhales and stronger as he exhales. Pulsus paradoxus is an inspiratory reduction in systolic pressure >10 mmHg. This is best measured using a manual cuff, although some digital electronic blood pressure cuffs are amenable to measuring pulsus paradoxus.

Constrictive pericarditis occurs as a result of more chronic scarring of the pericardium after an inflammation initially occurs. The layer becomes thickened with fibrous tissue and the heart is unable to fill as readily, causing a decrease in cardiac output and a residual increased jugular venous filling pressures. Right heart failure often develops. In these situations, a pericardiectomy is required, but it can be very risky for the patient.

Acute Myocardial Complications

Papillary Muscle Rupture

The papillary muscles extend from the chordae tendineae and are part of the structures which attach the valves to the walls of the myocardium and give stability to the leaflets of the valves, thus preventing prolapse during systole. Damage to the papillary muscles can cause an insufficiency of the valve, specifically the AV valves, and a murmur can be heard.

After an acute myocardial infarction, the papillary muscles are at increased risk for rupture due to an inadequate blood supply from the coronary circulation. Rupture of the papillary muscles on the left side of the myocardium cause an insufficiency of the mitral valve and a regurgitation murmur can be heard. Damage of this nature can also cause increased pulmonary congestion, and, in turn, lower cardiac output. Partial rupture can be treated with aggressive management using the IABP and vasodilators until surgical intervention can be performed. Complete rupture most often results in acute mitral regurgitation, shock and subsequently death.

Ventricular Aneurysm

A ventricular aneurysm is a structural defect in the wall of the ventricle which results most commonly after a transmural myocardial infarction. The myocardium bulges and the wall is thinned at the location of the aneurysm, which produces a reduction in the stroke volume of the ventricle. Common complications occurring as a result of a ventricular aneurysm include acute heart failure, thrombus formation, which can embolize systemically, and ventricular tachycardia.

Diagnosis is typically made with a TTE and physical assessment. Treatment is symptomatic and surgical intervention and repair of the aneurysm. Prognosis is often dependent upon the size of the aneurysm. Rupture of the aneurysm is not common and is caused most often by a reinfarction of the muscle surrounding the aneurysm, but is nonetheless a surgical emergency and can be life threatening.

Ventricular Septal Rupture

This condition results only in approximately 1 percent to 2 percent of the population who suffer from a transmural myocardial infarction. This event can take place up to a week following the MI. However, the mortality associated with ventricular septal rupture is significant and can occur in 5 percent to 10 percent of acute MI deaths. Initial manifestations of septal wall rupture include severe chest pain, syncope, hypotension, and acute deterioration in the hemodynamic stability of the patient. Subsequently heart failure, shock, and death become imminent. The blood from the high pressure left ventricle is suddenly shunted into the low pressure right heart causing an immediate fluid and pressure overload. Immediate stabilization and surgical intervention are required for survival.

Cardiac Tamponade

Cardiac tamponade was discussed briefly earlier. Cardiac tamponade is a result of an effusion of fluid or blood into the pericardial space and causes increased pressure on the myocardium, thus restricting the diastolic filling of the ventricles and myocardial contractility. The etiology of cardiac tamponade includes cardiac trauma, iatrogenic trauma (e.g., pacemaker wire perforation or cardiac contusion during CPR), aortic dissection, or acute MI with myocardial rupture. The treatment for cardiac tamponade with hemodynamic instability is immediate removal of the effusion either by pericardiocentesis or surgical pericardial window.

Peripheral Vascular Disease

Similar to coronary artery disease, peripheral vascular disease develops most commonly due to atherosclerotic vessel disease. As a result of the narrowing or occlusion of the vessels, decreased perfusion to the extremities will occur and damage to tissues most likely will result.

Arterial versus Venous Occlusion

Peripheral vascular disease (PVD) is divided into two categories: arterial and venous. Venous peripheral disease is chronic, evolves over time, and can be managed on an outpatient basis once diagnosis is made and the patient is adequately anticoagulated. On the other hand, arterial peripheral vascular disease may require acute intervention for a thrombotic occlusion to preserve the limb. PVD may occur in any peripheral vessel but most often occurs in the lower extremities.

Acute Arterial Occlusion

Vessels that are most commonly affected from arterial peripheral vascular disease are the superficial femoral artery, popliteal artery, distal aorta, and iliac arteries. In arterial peripheral vascular disease, blood flow is occluded either by a thrombus or narrowing of the vessel and ischemic muscle pain ensues. These symptoms appear after 75 percent of the vessel is occluded. The pain from ischemia can be extreme. If the vessel is not totally occluded, the patient may experience claudication, which is an intermittent aching pain when walking. Claudication can be relieved by rest and may remain unchanged for many years. Arterial peripheral vascular disease can be clinically assessed using doppler ultrasound to calculate ankle-brachial indices (ABI). Low ABI are diagnostic of arterial PVD.

Acute arterial occlusion is evidenced by sudden onset of severe pain, loss of pulse to the extremity, cold skin, pallor of the skin, and impaired motor and sensory function. These symptoms are also known as the three "P's": pain, pallor, pulselessness. This condition is a surgical emergency and requires immediate intervention to remove the obstruction or to stent the artery. Without rapid intervention, the patient will likely suffer the loss of the limb due to excessive tissue damage and gangrene, which can lead to sepsis.

Venous Occlusion

One of the most common forms of venous occlusion is the **deep vein thrombosis** (DVT). The etiology of DVT is often immobility when blood flow is diminished to the vessel for hours and venous stasis occurs. Clots form and can occlude lower extremity vessels even as far up as the iliac vein and the inferior vena cava. These clots can also become systemic and cause pulmonary embolus, which may be life threatening. The acute treatment for venous occlusion is anticoagulation with *heparin* or *t-PA therapy*. Prevention is the most appropriate treatment including early mobilization and prophylaxis with low molecular weight heparin and is why all bedfast critically ill patients should be on this medication unless contraindicated. Hospitals have also begun to institute the use of sequential compression devices (SCD) to intermittently inflate and compress the veins of the lower extremities, simulating muscular contraction during ambulation. For renal patients, heparin subcutaneously is the drug of choice, but low molecular weight heparin should be avoided.

Arterial Aneurysm Locations

An aneurysm is described as a weakening of a vessel wall resulting in a bulging and wall stress at the site. Within the body there are several sites where aneurysms can develop as a result of atherosclerosis. These include the following vessels: thoracic and abdominal aorta, femoral and popliteal arteries, and the circle of willis (Berry Aneurysm). There are several potential complications which can occur as a result of arterial aneurysms, including rupture, dissection, and stenosis. Location of the aneurysm and expediency in the treatment will determine the outcome for the patient if one of these complications occurs. Dissections and ruptures require immediate surgical intervention especially to prevent rapid blood loss. The mortality remains high for these situations, up to 80 percent. We will focus our discussion in this section on the complications associated with aortic dissections.

Aortic Rupture

When the wall of the vessel weakens beyond a certain point, the vessel ruptures and immediate arterial blood loss occurs. Rupture more likely occurs if the vessels are dilated beyond 5–6 cm. Immediate treatment would include fluid and blood replacement, and surgical intervention. With aortic rupture, there is a significant amount of blood loss resulting in hypoperfusion to key end organs, including the brain and kidneys. If the patient survives the initial event, end organ failure is likely to occur and is a result of lengthy hypoperfusion.

Aortic Dissection

The primary difference between aortic rupture and aortic dissection is that in aortic dissection, a tear likely occurs in the intima of the vessel, which then moves up and down the vessel causing a larger tearing and leaking of blood into the column of the intima. The patient will describe the pain from this dissection as "tearing or ripping" in which the onset is sudden and abrupt. This pain may also be described as radiating to the back between the blades of the scapula. Perfusion to key organs may still occur. However, if the bleeding extends into the valves and pericardium, ischemia may occur and end organ damage will occur as a result. The patient can be initially managed with antihypertensives and pain control, however, immediate surgical intervention is required. Even with surgical intervention, the mortality for aortic dissection remains at approximately 80 percent.

Carotid Artery Stenosis

Similar to the above-referenced peripheral vascular conditions, the carotid arteries may also develop atherosclerosis and plaque development. Symptoms that may develop as a result of carotid artery stenosis are primarily neurological since these vessels provide blood flow to the brain. With significant blockage the patient may experience transient ischemic attacks (TIAs) or stroke. Permanent brain damage can occur as a result of lengthy hypoperfusion to the brain. Often, if the occlusion or stenosis is gradual in onset, collateral circulation will develop and provide adequate circulation. Stenotic areas of more than 75 percent in the vessels are more prone to the development of thrombosis due to the sluggish blood flow and adhesion of platelets and fibrin. Diagnosis is made by carotid Doppler studies.

Carotid Stent

If the carotid artery blockage is due to stenosis, the physician may elect to implant a stent to provide a more permanent means to keep the artery open. This is a minimally invasive procedure done under local anesthetic. An incision is made in the femoral artery and a guide wire is threaded to the site of blockage. A balloon is used to dilate the artery and a stent is inserted to keep the vessel open.

Endarterectomy

Another surgical procedure to clear the blockage in the carotid artery is called an endarterectomy. The vessel is surgically opened and the atheromatous plaque substance is removed. Once hemostasis is achieved, the vessel is closed. The disadvantage of this procedure over stenting is that it typically requires general anesthesia and there is a chance that the blockage may reappear, requiring another surgical procedure.

Angioplasty

Angioplasty is used in conjunction with the stenting procedure for carotid artery occlusion. Angioplasty is dilatation of the vessel via a balloon catheter inserted via a major vessel, typically in the groin or arm. Occasionally, simply the opening of the vessel via the balloon angioplasty is enough to provide adequate blood flow through the vessel, and the vessel remain opens. More commonly, however, the stent is placed to allow for long-term recovery. These procedures are fairly new for carotid blockages, even though they have been used for some time with coronary artery occlusion.

Peripheral Stenting

As with coronary artery and carotid artery stenting, new techniques are being developed with the use of the balloon catheter, angioplasty, and insertion of stenting for peripheral vessel occlusion. The most common sites are the iliac, femoral popliteal artery, and renal arteries.

CARDIOTHORACIC SURGERY

Despite a brief period of reduction in the frequency of deaths due to cardiovascular disease during the period from 1980 to 1990, there has been an increase in deaths from cardiovascular disease in the following 10-year period. It is even more bothersome that there is an increase in deaths in women from cardiovascular disease, while deaths in men remain stable. Atherosclerosis remains the number one cause for coronary artery disease. Diet and genetic predisposition to the disease are contributing factors.

Acute coronary artery occlusion occurs as a result of the following:

1. The atherosclerotic plaque is an uneven surface where blood platelets form, and fibrin is deposited. Red blood cells are attracted to this area and a clot forms in the coronary artery. Occasionally, this clot will break away and move to a more peripheral vessel of the coronary artery. The vessel may be partially or completely occluded. The patient experiences chest pain as a result and coronary ischemia or infarction occurs from the point of the blockage and peripherally. EKG changes include ST elevation or depression in electrical leads that correspond with the ischemic tissue (see Table 4.1 earlier for area of infarction and 12 lead EKG changes).

2. Additionally, local muscular spasm of the coronary artery can occur which stimulates local nervous system reflexes and in turn, wall contraction. Theories exist that this, too, may cause secondary thrombosis in the vessel.

3. Collateral blood flow develops, which sustains the coronary tissue health. It is felt that this may occur as soon as seconds after the primary occlusion and may provide up to 50 percent of the coronary blood flow to that area. This initial development does not change significantly until approximately two to three days after the injury, when there is a significant increase in the blood flow from the collaterals.

Coronary Artery Bypass Grafting (CABG)

The first coronary artery bypass was performed in 1967. In CABG, the myocardium is revascularized using grafts to bypass the blockage in the obstructed coronary arteries. It has been accepted as a safe and effective means in relieving medically uncontrolled angina pectoris and for revasculature of left main coronary artery, triple vessel disease, double vessel disease involving the LAD, or coronary artery disease with EF < 35 percent. There are cases where additional vessels will be grafted based on quality of circulation to the myocardium; however, the outcome may not be as successful in the prevention of mortality compared to coronary artery stenting. The length of an acute hospital stay for CABG has decreased considerably over the most recent past with the length of stay now five to six days, nine for Medicare patients.

On-pump CABG

Cardiopulmonary bypass is a mechanical device used for diverting and oxygenating the patient's blood away from her heart and lungs during CABG surgery. The patient must be systematically heparinized during the period on pump. Incorporated into the pump is a means to chill the blood to approximately 28° C and then to warm it prior to discontinuance of bypass. This reduces tissue oxygen requirements during the surgical procedure.

The sites for securing the graft vessels include the saphenous veins, internal mammary arteries, gastroepiploic artery, and radial artery. At this point, long-term patency is better with the mammary arteries. In addition, using mammary arteries prevents the need for leg incisions.

Post Perfusion Syndrome

Post perfusion syndrome, or "pumphead" as it is more commonly called, is a neurocognitive syndrome that is evidenced in post on-pump CABG patients. The symptoms of this include memory impairment, stilted speech, depression, confusion, and decreased hand–eye coordination. This syndrome is considered transient and most patients resume normal cognitive function within a short period post surgery. Most functions return within 3 months and after 12 months there is negligible evidence of the syndrome. There are varying theories as to the potential causes of this syndrome. One theory is that there are microemboli which are showered during the pump time. However, regardless of the theories behind the etiology of "pumphead," surgeons have moved to try and eliminate the use of cardiopulmonary bypass altogether.

Off-pump CABG

Approximately 20 percent to 25 percent of the CABG procedures performed in the United States are done without the use of the cardiopulmonary bypass pump device. This procedure was implemented with the goal of reducing mortality and morbidity related to the on-pump procedure, particularly in the high risk groups. Thus far, studies have demonstrated that the graft patency rates are equal.

This procedure appears to be more successful in patients with focal stenosis versus diffuse disease. It also prevents the "pumphead" syndrome that develops in the post-operative period from the on-pump procedure. In contrast to the cooling of the patient's blood during the period when it is out of the patient, the off-pump procedure warms the patient with warming mattresses, warmed fluids and warmed anesthesia gases. Off-pump CABG requires very specific positioning of the patient to maximize the visibility and access to the coronary arteries which are to be bypassed, specifically displacement of the heart to the right, and the use of mechanical stabilizers by compression or suction to control the constantly moving heart. Medications such as beta blockers or calcium channel blockers are used to slow the heart to reduce movement as well. The sequence of the grafting of the vessels is from the easiest graft to the most difficult. It is felt that this will help with perfusion of tissues while the more difficult vessels are being repaired.

Long-term studies will provide additional support for this procedure over the on-pump procedure, with more data on long-term survival and graft patency.

Endoscopic Vein Harvesting

One of the most uncomfortable parts of the recovery from CABG in the past has been the healing of the wounds from where the graft vessels were harvested, particularly the legs. This process was often hampered in the diabetic patients who occasionally would have prolonged healing times and the development of infections. A new technique in harvesting graft veins using an endoscopic approach is now being used. The benefits of this approach are smaller incisions required to remove an appropriate length of the vein, decreased pain, fewer wound-healing complications, reduced scarring, and a faster recovery time.

Robotic Assisted Surgery

Another new technique in cardiovascular surgery is using a robotic surgery system, which combines the traditional approach with laparoscopic techniques. The most common cardiovascular procedure for which this device is used is mitral valve replacement (MVR).

Some of the benefits of this type of surgery are that the sternotomy and rib spreading are not required—there is a shorter recovery period, less opportunity for infection, less blood loss, and potentially better outcomes.

One of the drawbacks for this procedure is that the surgeon has to be specially trained on the device and become efficient with hand-to-eye coordination which is quite different than the traditional use of surgical instruments. Another deterrent for many organizations is the cost of the device, which exceeds one million dollars.

Valve Replacement

Insufficient, prolapsed, or stenotic valves often require replacement in order to eliminate the hemodynamic dysfunctions which are associated with these problems.

However, medical management is used as long as the patient is asymptomatic. The goal is to maintain as much left ventricular function as possible during this phase. With surgical valve replacement, there are inherent risks with the use of both prosthetic and biological tissue valves.

Valvular Defects

Not all valvular defects require surgical intervention. The most common valves replaced in a surgical intervention are the aortic and mitral valves. The nursing interventions which should be undertaken with patients who have valvular defects include the following: a thorough assessment of hemodynamic stability and adequacy of tissue perfusion, evaluation of dysrhythmias, assuring diagnostic studies are carried out in a timely and efficient manner, standardized post-operative care, education based on assessed needs, and administration of medications which are pertinent to the patient's care.

Aortic Stenosis

In aortic stenosis, the inability of the valve to function effectively is due to the obstructive narrowing of the valve. Over time, the valve becomes thickened and calcified. As a result there is impedance of blood flow to the aorta. To adapt to the increased pressure gradient, it has to push against the left ventricle hypertrophies, and so becomes stiff and non-compliant. Left atrial and pulmonary artery pressures subsequently increase as the stiffened left ventricle works to eject the blood. Pulmonary congestion and right heart failure will then develop. Currently the only effective surgical intervention for aortic valve disease is aortic valve replacement (AVR). The goal of AVR is to preserve ventricular function.

Valve replacement is done with either a mechanical valve made from a combination of metal alloys, such as pyrolite carbon, Dacron, and Teflon, or a bioprothetic valve, such as bovine, porcine, or human heart valves. This procedure requires open heart surgery and carries the

FIGURE 4.3 *Aortic Stenosis*

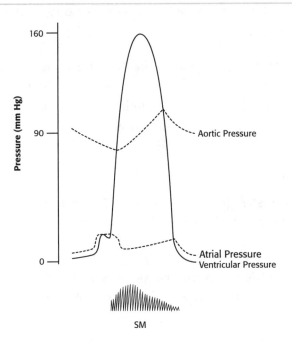

risks associated with an interventional procedure such as infection, bleeding, hemodynamic instability, etc. Post valve replacement, the patient will initially require anticoagulation with intravenous *heparin*. *Warfarin* may be used when the patient is stabilized and being prepared for discharge.

The normal International Normalization Ratio (INR), a measure of the effects of warfarin, without anticoagulation is 1.0. The expected therapeutic range for patients who have undergone valve replacement is 3.0 to 4.0. There are special diet modifications for patients who are on anticoagulants, including avoidance of foods high in vitamin K (broccoli, lettuce, spinach, and liver). Additionally, medications that can alter bleeding times should be avoided as well, e.g., aspirin, ibuprofen, birth control pills, and certain antibiotics.

Mitral Stenosis

The definition of mitral stenosis is a progressive narrowing of the mitral valve opening to less than 1.5 cm. This can be caused simply by the aging process, but may also develop as a result of inflammation and rheumatic fever. Fibrosis of one or more leaflets of the valves can cause fusion of one or both commisures. The chordae tendonae may also become thickened and shortened and decrease the mobility of the valve. As with aortic stenosis, the blood flow is impeded and chamber pressures increase. If the orifice of the valve diminishes to less than 1 cm^2, pulmonary hypertension occurs and increased pulmonary pressures cause an increase in right ventricular pressures, which could ultimately cause right-sided heart failure.

FIGURE 4.4 *Mitral Valve Stenosis*

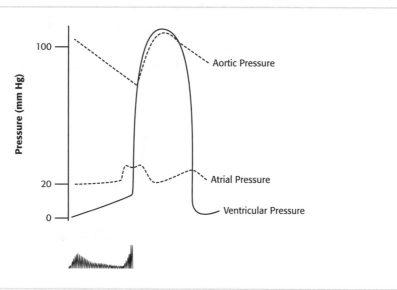

With mitral stenosis, the choices for correction are commissurotomy and valve replacement. During a commissurotomy the fused leaflets of the stenotic valve are incised and debrided to improve valve mobility. Reconstruction avoids the potential complications which come with valve replacement surgery and prosthetic valves. Commissurotomy may eliminate the need for long-term anticoagulation.

Aortic Regurgitation

Regurgitation occurs when the cardiac valve becomes incompetent or weakened by damage or degeneration of the cusps of the valves. The valves become "floppy" and blood flows backward during diastole as a result of the lack of complete closure of the valve. In turn, forward flow of blood in inhibited, peripheral vasoconstriction occurs, and aortic diastolic pressure decreases. The body attempts to compensate for the reduced blood flow by increasing heart rate and as a result, oxygen myocardial demand increases and can potentially lead to ischemia and sudden death. *Widening pulse pressures* also occur and demonstrate low aortic diastolic pressures in the presence of high systemic pressures. The etiology of aortic regurgitation can be infection, idiopathic calcifications, congenital malformations, hypertension, trauma, and aneurysms.

As stated earlier, at the present time, the only surgical intervention for aortic valve disease is open aortic valve replacement. However, a new technique using a percutaneous AVR for aortic stenosis is currently in clinical trials. The first human case of this procedure was done in 2002. A standard interventional approach is used to introduce the catheter, which removes the diseased valve and replaces the new valve. At the present time, this procedure is limited to end stage disease where the candidate has been eliminated as a candidate for

FIGURE 4.5 *Aortic Regurgitation*

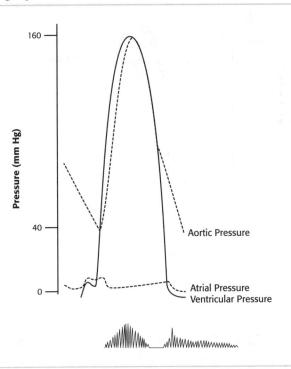

conventional surgical replacement of the valve. Medical therapy to control blood pressure, improve oxygenation, and improve stroke volume (inotropic drugs) should be instituted to preserve ventricular function until the patient is significantly decompensated and valve replacement becomes necessary.

Mitral Valve Regurgitation

Mitral valve regurgitation can occur chronically or acutely. Causes of chronic mitral valve disease of this nature can be infectious or autoimmune, congenital malformations, dilation of the left ventricle from other causes, and connective tissue diseases such as Marfan's syndrome. Acute disease can be caused by rupture of the chordae tendonae from endocarditis or rheumatic heart disease, traumatic injury, or papillary muscle dysfunction.

In mitral valve regurgitation, blood flows back into the left atrium (regurgitation) as a result of the incompetent valve. Left atrial diastolic pressures suddenly increase when this occurs acutely. As a result of the rapid onset, the left atrium cannot compensate for the change and cardiac output output falls dramatically, causing pulmonary edema and cardiogenic shock. Often the patient requires an intra-aortic balloon pump (IABP) and vasopressors for support until the patient is stabilized for surgical intervention.

FIGURE 4.6 *Mitral Valve Regurgitation*

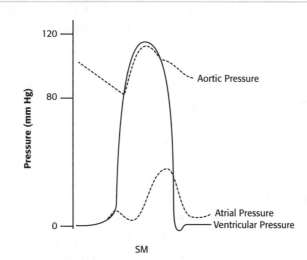

Most Common Congenital Repairs

When caring for patients with congenital or acute defects of the heart, it is imperative for the critical care nurse to be observant for hemodynamic stability and changes which occur as a result of the increase in the ventricular and atrial pressures. This includes assessing the patient for evidence of shunting and the possible direction of the shunt, monitoring for atrial and junctional rhythms and conduction blocks, pre- and post-operative care, and administration of antibiotics to prevent infection.

Septal Defects

Structural defects may occur as a result of acute myocardial infarction in adults or may be congenital in infants and children. With these defects, blood most often is shunted from the areas of high pressure to low pressure, which is typically left ventricle to right ventricle. If the shunt is severe, the patient may develop acute heart failure, shock, and death. When the left to right shunt is long standing, the right ventricular pressures may increase and surpass that of the left ventricle, causing peripheral cyanosis, referred to as Eisenmenger's syndrome (see next page).

Atrial Septal Defect

A defect may occur in the septum at the level of the atrium which allows shunting of blood to occur between left and right atria. There are typically three types of atrial septal defects; sinus venosus, ostium secundum, and ostium primum defects. These are named based on the location of the defect. A sinus venosus occurs where the right atrium and superior vena cava join. The ostium secundum occurs around the area of the foramen ovale. This type of defect is the most common of the three. The final defect, ostium primum, occurs at the lower end of the septum.

Most often the blood is shunted from the area of higher pressure to the lower pressure, in this case, left atrium to right atrium. Fluid overload subsequently occurs due to increased blood flow from the right heart. A systolic murmur is audible as blood flow increases across the pulmonic valve. Echocardiography and cardiac catheterization can assist with the diagnosis of atrial septal defect.

The exact cause of this type of defect is not known but may be related to maternal and fetal infections early in the pregnancy, medications, or genetic factors. Surgical intervention is recommended to avoid long-term pulmonary hyptertension. A pericardial or Dacron patch is used to repair the defect. With repair of septal defects, there is a chance that the patient may develop conduction blocks due to injury of the bundle of His. In these situations, the patient may require a temporary pacemaker.

Ventricular Septal Defect

The ventricular septal defect (VSD) occurs between the ventricles within some portion of the membranous or muscular septum. The VSD is the most common type of congenital defect in children and occurs along with other types of defects. In addition to the membranous or muscular types, there are three additional types: supra-cristal, AV canal type, and crista superventricularis.

Smaller defects may actually close spontaneously and do not cause significant hemodynamic instability. Larger defects will cause shunting a left to right shunt and an increase in the pulmonary venous return to the left atrium, and, subsequently, the left ventricle. As pressures increase on the left, pulmonary congestion occurs and over time can lead to pulmonary hypertension. The pulmonary hypertension may then become irreversible and systemic pressures can increase so that the shunt becomes right to left. This condition is called Eisenmenger's syndrome.

The repair of these defects requires open heart surgery with a sternotomy and cardiopulmonary bypass. A patch will be applied to the defect. Similar to the atrial septal defect, conduction arrhythmias can occur due to potential injury to the AV node or Bundle of His. Patients will also be treated prophylactically with antibitiocs to prevent infections such as endocarditis.

Patent Ductus Arteriosus

During fetal development there is a patent connection between the descending aorta and the pulmonary artery to bypass the underdeveloped lungs. On occasion this patency does not seal off as it should at the time of birth and there remains a ductus (hole) between those two vessels. Since the aorta has a higher pressure flow, oxygenated blood will flow from the aorta through the patent ductus to the pulmonary artery and subsequently to the lungs. Symptoms of left-sided heart failure develop due to the increased fluid load on the lungs and left side of the heart. If the pressures begin to increase on the right side and within the pulmonary artery, the blood will begin to shift right to left. As a result, right-sided heart failure and cyanosis will occur. In large shunts, deoxygenated blood will be fed to the left arm and lower parts of the body below the ductus, while the upper body continues to receive oxygenated blood without problems. These patients are more prone to endocarditis and may have vegetative valvular growths which may embolize to the lungs. The end result is infarction and death.

Surgical intervention would be required when the patient experiences heart failure or, in children, if the ductus remains open after six months of life. The patent ductus should be closed and on occasion a patch may be required to successfully accomplish this. In severe cases where pulmonary hyptertension and right to left shunting occur, the patient would need a heart–lung transplant. If the patient is unstable and cannot undergo open heart surgery, a transcatheter closure might be performed as an alternative. These procedures may not be successful but pose a lesser risk than a thoracotomy with closure.

Coarctation of the Aorta

This congenital defect typically is described as a narrowing or infolding of the lumen of the aorta. The result is increased resistance to the ejection of blood from the left ventricle proximal to the narrowing, and decreased pressures and diminished blood flow distal to the narrowing. The defect most often occurs just past the branching of the 3rd large vessel from the arch of the aorta, the left subclavian artery.

Similar to other defects, the ventricle enlarges as a result of the increased pressure gradient and can fail due to the increased afterload. Prolonged hypertension can lead to other conditions which result from cardiovascular disease such as strokes, CAD, heart failure, and possibly aortic dissection or rupture. Collateral circulation develops and helps to feed the lower body and extremities with oxygenated blood.

One of the distinct radiological findings of coarctation of the aorta is something called the "3" sign. This triad of findings is a dilated ascending aorta, constriction of the aorta, and a post-stenotic dilation. A cardiac catheterization would be required to identify the degree of coronary artery disease and to assess the depth of the pressure gradients. An aortagram can also be done to assess the narrowing itself.

Surgical correction is required to excise the coarctation, either by an end-to-end anastomosis or an aortoplasty. The approach is via a thoracotomy incision. Complications of this type of surgery are typical for a thoracotomy including hemothorax, chylothorax, paradoxical hypertension, and transient abdominal pain. Spontaneous aortic rupture can occur in an older patient prior to surgical intervention and most often leads to death.

Myxoma Removal

A cardiac myxoma is a benign neoplasm of the heart, most commonly located in the left atrium (75 percent of the cases) along the septum. The myxoma's origin is not known for certain, although it is thought to be a true tumor which originates from an infectious response from an organism such as herpes simplex, human papillary virus, Epstein-Barr virus, or an inherited autosomal trait.

There is a triad of symptoms which are demonstrated in a patient with myxoma, including heart failure (due to obstruction caused by the size of the tumor), evidence of embolism, fever, and weight loss or fatigue. The patient may also experience general malaise or arthralgias.

Surgical resection of the tumor is the only current treatment available for this type of tumor. This is done via a sternotomy incision; the patient must be placed on cardiopulmonary bypass so that the area can be visualized and manipulated to assure adequate resection of the tumor. Often the mitral valve will have to be replaced due to proximity to the tumor and the need to resect a portion of the myocardial wall. Recurrence of the tumor has a low probability even with the predisposition to the tumor due to genetic linkages.

Transmyocardial Laser Revascularization

The transmyocardial laser revascularization procedure is often done in conjunction with other open heart procedures, but may be performed independently in a patient who continues to have unrelieved chest pain. The procedure requires a thoracotomy or sternotomy incision to access the heart tissue, although it can be accomplished via minimally invasive surgery. A specialized instrument which uses a carbon dioxide laser to create small channels in the exposed myocardium is used for this procedure. The external exposed openings close while the internal openings assist in creating channels or bloodlines for the blood to circulate. The expected outcomes of these procedures are to reduce angina chest pain, success in long-term pain control, and improved quality of life.

Thoracic Aneurysm Repair

Thoracic aneurysms are a significant health risk and can cause immediate death if the aneurysm ruptures and there is massive bleeding. Aneurysms do not typically manifest themselves until the patient reaches approximately 60 years of age or older, and they primarily occur in men. Thoracic aneurysms can occur in the ascending, transverse, or descending aorta, or in the iliac, popliteal, or femoral arteries. Patients describe the pain with a dissection or rupture as a sudden ripping pain which radiates the shoulders, neck, and back. There may be evidence of change in the patient's voice such as hoarseness or weakness, and a cough may be produced. As the blood accumulates in the thoracic cavity, there may be pressure placed on the trachea which can cause dysphagia, dyspnea, and physical shifting of the trachea.

The nurse may observe other manifestations of the aneurysm in addition to those listed above. There may be audible bruits over the aorta or other related arteries. The patient may experience hypertension if intrathoracic pressure increases or severe hypotension if bleeding occurs. *Pulse pressures widen* and there may be a significant difference in blood pressures from one arm to the other. Pressure differences of greater than 10 mm Hg indicate the potential for dissection or occlusion of major arteries in the thorax. Shock symptoms may also appear such as cool, pale, diaphoretic skin, absence of central pressures and peripheral pulses, and sluggish capillary refill.

The patient requires immediate surgical intervention for dissection or rupture, as well as fluids and vasopressors to support blood pressure while preparing for surgery. An IABP is *contraindicated* due to the damage to the aorta.

MAZE Procedure for Treatment of Atrial Dysrhythmias/Radiofrequency Ablation for Intractable Supraventricular or Ventricular Dysrhythmias

The MAZE procedure is named for the appearance of an electrical "maze" which occurs as a result of a series of cuts made into the atrial tissues. It is indicated for patients who have *atrial fibrillation* or *atrial flutter* refractory to medical therapy. The goal of the "maze" is to disrupt reentry pathways and direct the impulse of the sinus node to the AV node. The end result is restoration of sinus rhythm and AV synchrony. If there is evidence that the sinus node is non-functional, a pacemaker will be implanted to restore AV rhythm. The MAZE procedure requires open heart surgery and, therefore, has the same risks as a CABG, including bleeding, infection, and cardiac dysrhythmias.

As the MAZE technique developed, another option to the treatment of cardiac dysrhythmia, called *radiofrequency ablation,* was also developed. The origin of the dysrhythmia is localized using specialized pacing electrodes (intraoperative mapping). Once the location is determined, the area of myocardium which is irritable and causing the rhythm disturbance is excised or eliminated by the special ablation catheters and laser or cryosurgery.

CARDIAC TRAUMA

Cardiac trauma occurs as a result of either blunt trauma (motor vehicle injuries, cardiac contusions, falls, or deceleration injuries) to the chest or penetrating trauma (stabbing, gunshot injury, or fractures of the ribs). The injury may be limited to the pericardium, one or more chambers of the heart, the major arteries/veins, or it may be more diffuse such as in cardiac contusions. Obtaining an accurate history of the injury is critical for ascertaining the interventions to be implemented. If the patient is unconscious, attempt to obtain a history from direct observers or the emergency personnel who attended the patient at the site of injury. The nurse should be somewhat of a skeptic when obtaining the history from other sources and maintain a high degree of suspicion for cardiac injury in any of these types of events.

Blunt Trauma

One of the most common causes of blunt non-penetrating injury to the heart is from the steering wheel of a motor vehicle. Patients who are injured in this manner require a 12-lead EKG and continuous cardiac monitoring to observe for myocardial damage. In addition to this type of global injury, blunt trauma can cause shearing or tearing of major vessels, resulting in massive hemorrhage, cardiac tamponade, and potentially cardiogenic shock.

The patient should be hemodynamically monitored for changes in blood pressure, CVP, or PCWP. In addition, continuous cardiac monitoring will allow the nurse to observe for dysrhythmias which may result from muscle damage. Serial cardiac markers (CK, CKMB and Troponin) should be done.

Penetrating Trauma

In penetrating injuries, open wounds can bleed into the pericardial space, or there may be actual damage to the myocardium, heart chambers, or major vessels of the heart. Hypovolemic shock will develop if the bleeding is severe and uncontrolled. Pericardial tamponade occurs in the greatest percentage of stab wounds involving the heart. Additionally, with gunshot wounds there may be extensive myocardial damage, cellular damage to areas adjacent to the myocardium, and emboli which develop when there are remnants such as bullets or metal fragments in the chambers of the heart. Injuries to the coronary arteries can cause pericardial tamponade, acute MI, or death.

The nurse should also be prepared for emergency procedures which may be required in the event of serious complications of cardiac injury. These would include a periocardiocentesis, chest tube insertion, needle thoracotomy, or surgical thoracotomy at the bedside. It is critical to maintain hemodynamic stability with fluid infusion, blood transfusion, and vasopressors, if needed, prior to surgical intervention. The basic ABCs of trauma management should be the first priority with the unstable patient.

CARDIOMYOPATHIES

If the term cardiomyopathy is broken down into word parts and defined, the result is 'disease/condition of the cardiac muscle.' The etiologies of cardiomyopathy vary, but include viral infections, autoimmune disorders, CAD, valvular heart disease, hypertension, and alcohol abuse. Nursing implications for care of the patient with cardiomyopathy incorporate maintaining appropriate fluid balance by monitoring the status of the patient's heart failure, administering medications and monitoring outcomes for improving cardiac function, and individualizing activity for patient's tolerance. For severe cardiomyopathy in the appropriate patient, a heart transplant may be indicated.

Dilated Cardiomyopathy

This type of cardiomyopathy is characterized by dilated ventricles (although it may only be left-sided dilation) without muscle hypertrophy. The result is more global left ventricular dysfunction, a low cardiac output, atrial and ventricular dysrhythmias, and venous pooling that leads to emboli. In severe cases, advanced heart failure and death can occur. Symptoms may also include *narrowing pulse pressures* and *pulsus alternans*.

The goals of therapy in dilated cardiomyopathy are to improve pump function, maintain fluid balance, and control heart failure. Medications which will assist with these goals are diuretics, beta-blockers, anticoagulant and antiplatelet therapy, and antidysrhythmics. In severe cases, where the patient meets criteria, a heart transplant may be indicated.

Hypertrophic Obstructive Cardiomyopathy (HOCM)

In contrast to dilated cardiomyopathy, the ventricles are stiff and noncompliant in hypertrophic cardiomyopathy. In addition, the ventricular septum becomes hypertrophied on a cellular level, resulting in obstruction of the aortic valve outflow tract. This stiffened ventricle also pulls the papillary muscles out of alignment, and causes mitral valve dysfunction.

The symptoms of HOCM vary slightly from dilated cardiomyopathy. The patient experiences dyspnea upon exertion, myocardial ischemia, SVT, VT, syncope, and heart failure. Medication management is used to initially treat these symptoms. These include diuretics, beta-blockers, calcium channel blockers, and antidysrhythmics. Physical activity is limited by the patient's ability to tolerate mobility. In some cases, an implantable cardioverter defibrillator (ICD), surgical myectomy, or a mitral valve replacement may be required.

Restrictive Cardiomyopathy

This is the least common form of cardiomyopathy. Restrictive cardiomyopathy is characterized by ventricular wall rigidity and diastolic dysfunction. It often occurs as a result of myocardial fibrosis. In these cases, ventricular filling is obstructed by the rigid muscular wall. Symptoms are similar to constrictive pericarditis and therefore may be initially treated incorrectly. Right-sided heart failure (backward heart failure), low cardiac output, dyspnea, orthopnea, and liver engorgement are all symptoms of this type of cardiomyopathy. Some of the treatment modalities are similar to the other types of cardiomyopathies and include removal of excess fluid, modification of diet, and improvement of pump function.

It is important for the patient to be engaged and participate in her care, as these conditions have to be managed long-term; they require diligent attendance to symptoms and adherence to medications and dietary restrictions to achieve stabilization. The disease most commonly is not reversed, but the patient may live a reasonable quality of life with appropriate management of signs and symptoms of the disease.

CARDIAC DYSRHYTHMIAS

As a rule, the Advanced Cardiac Life Support (ACLS) guidelines should be used in the critical care unit when dysrhythmias occur. Continuous cardiac monitoring is the standard of care for critically ill patients. In most ICU's the patient is monitored with 5 lead wires, which allows for a variety of lead options for the nurse. The primary lead by which the patient is monitored can be affected by the patient's clinical condition. In most cases the two primary leads used for monitoring are Lead II and MCL_1. For patients with specific heart injury patterns identified on the 12 lead EKG, the primary continuous monitoring lead can be changed accordingly.

For the purposes of this chapter, dysrhythmias will be referred to as either too slow, too fast, regular or irregular, and whether they generate a pulse. Specific pharmacological agents will be discussed in the section on Cardiovascular Pharmacology.

Symptomatic Bradycardia—Too Slow

Symptomatic is defined as a condition where the patient is symptomatic as a result of the dysrhythmia. Symptoms include cool, moist skin, chest pain, hypotension, syncope, fatigue or weakness, decreased level of consciousness, and dyspnea. Bradycardias can be further broken down into dysfunction of the pacemaker for the heart, escape rhythms, drug induced rhythms, or parasympathetic nervous system stimulation.

Conduction defects are the result of dysfunction of the primary or secondary pacemakers of the heart, specifically the SA and AV nodes in the right atrium. Etiologies of these defects can include coronary ischemia, myocardial infarction, degeneration due to age or illness, metabolic disorders, and drug effects. The most common medications which slow heart rate include beta-blockers, calcium channel blockers, and cardiac glycocides (e.g., digoxin). The rhythms which would be observed with these defects are SA exit blocks, sick sinus syndrome, sinus arrest/pause, first degree heart blocks, second degree heart blocks Type I and II, and third degree, i.e., complete heart block.

Treatment of bradycardia is *Atropine 0.5–1 mg IV,* may repeat in 5-minute intervals up to 3 mg and transcutaneous pacemaker. Care should be given not to administer Atropine in doses less than 0.5 mg due to the potential for *paradoxical bradycardia.* Patients with second degree heart block Type II or complete heart block will most likely require a permanent pacemaker.

The critical care nurse must monitor the patient with bradycardia to assure adequate tissue perfusion to vital organs. For severe bradycardia with hemodynamic compromise it is likely that vasosuppressor support will also be required. If the bradycardia is drug related, discussion should be undertaken with the physician regarding dosage and necessity of continued treatment with this medication. Purposeful or accidental overdosages of drugs which cause bradycardia will require reversal agents or, if none are available, hemodynamic support until metabolized and excreted including potentially, dialysis.

Symptomatic Tachycardia—Too Fast

Tachycardia is typically a symptom of another condition and in most cases should be investigated for its etiology prior to intervention. Normally, it is the body's attempt to compensate for a change in cardiac output. However, symptomatic tachycardia with hemodynamic instability will require an immediate conversion either electrically or pharmacologically. It must also be recognized that the loss of atrial kick will result in approximately 15 percent to 20 percent drop in the cardiac output. Tachycardias can be generated by most pacemakers in the heart depending on the etiology.

Atrial fibrillation with rapid ventricular response (referred to by some as "Rapid Atrial Fibrillation") is one of the most common sustained tachycardic rhythms. The immediate goal is to lower the ventricular response rate. Calcium channel blockers such as IV *diltiazem (Cardizem)* or *beta blockers (Esmolol, metorpolol, labetalol* can be administered to treat this dysrhythmia. Cardiac glyosides (such as digoxin) have been used in the past, but are not the standard of care for patients that acutely present with this tachyarrythmia; they may be useful on an outpatient basis. The IV calcium channel blocker works more rapidly at converting the rhythm. *Diltiazem* is administered in an initial bolus of 0.25 mg/kg given over two minutes and can be followed by a second dose if needed. A continuous infusion should then be started at 10 mg/hr. Anticoagulation is required in patients with atrial fibrillation or flutter due to the propensity for clot formation. The INR should be kept between 2 and 3.

In the monitored setting, treatment of the patient with a *narrow complex supraventricular* tachycardia is *adenosine.* The dosage for this drug is a 6 mg rapid bolus, followed by a 12 mg dose, after one to two minutes. When effective, the drug causes a brief asystolic period as the SA or AV node is "reset" from reentry and followed by a return to sinus rhythm. It may also slow conduction briefly so the dysrhythmia can be identified more clearly.

Ventricular or wide tachycardias are treated with an *amiodarone* bolus of 150 mg followed by initiation of a continuous infusion at 1mg/min. The physician may choose to attempt a synchronized cardioversion if the patient remains hemodynamically stable. If the patient deteriorates and becomes unconscious or hemodynamically unstable, immediate defibrillation is required. Torsades de pointes (literally, twisting of the points) is a specific type of ventricular tachycardia which shows a classic polymorphous origination. Treatment for Torsades is IV *Magnesium sulfate* 1–2 grams over 30–60 seconds, which may be repeated in 5 minutes. A continuous infusion can be started at 3–10 mg/min. if required.

Other tachycardias include multifocal atrial tachycardia (MAT), junctional tachycardia, paroxysmal SVT, and Wolfe-Parkinsons-White syndrome (WPW). Vagal maneuvers can be attempted in the stable patient; however, *adenosine and calcium channel blockers* are given for symptomatic rhythms. Care must be used in identification of the rhythm prior to administration of these drugs, as they can cause wide ventricular tachycardias, such as refractory VT, VF and death.

Ventricular Fibrillation/Pulseless Ventricular Tachycardia/Pulseless Electrical Activity/Asytole

All of the above dysrhythmias are considered life threatening and should be treated as a medical emergency with immediate CPR and/or defibrillation. Rhythm should be confirmed and pulses checked. The drug of choice in asystole is either *epinephrine or vasopressin.* Epinepherine is administered 1mg IV every five minutes until spontaneous return of rhythm, while vasopressin 40 units is administered as a one-time dose, in replacement for the first or second dose of epinephrine. Continuous CPR should continue with frequent pulse checks to insure adequate compressions. The patient will most likely require intubation, if not immediately converted to assure adequate oxygenation. Efforts should continue until deemed effective or the physician determines the measures are futile.

Automatic Implantable Cardioverter/Defibrillator (AICD)

The AICD is an implantable device which consists of sensing leads and defibrillator patches attached to the endocardium and to a pulse generator (all implanted internally). The procedure can be done through a thoracotomy incision or transvenous through an incision in the subclavian vein. These devices have the capability of detecting life threatening dysrhythmias such as ventricular tachycardia or ventricular fibrillation and provide defibrillation or they can pace the heart in bradycardic rhythms. The device can be interrogated to ascertain the frequency of delivered shocks, rhythm at the time of shock and battery life.

When educating patients on these devices, the nurse should explain that there is up to a 75 percent likelihood of spontaneous discharges in the first year. They should also be informed that there is no potential harm to their family or medical staff. Patients still will require antiarrhythmic therapy to limit the potential need for the AICD.

Pacemakers

Cardiac pacemakers have become very sophisticated over time and have the ability to pace and sense either or both chambers, and can defibrillate and deliver a shock when appropriate. Pacemakers can be inserted transcutaneously, transvenously, or via permanent placement based on the patient's clinical condition and stability. The primary purpose is to treat bradycardia in patients unable to sustain an adequate cardiac output.

Pacemakers are described by the following parameters: chamber paced, chamber sensed, response to sensing, programmability, and antitachyarrhythmia capability. Sensing and pacing occurs in either one chamber (atria or ventricle) or both chambers. When a pacemaker senses the rhythm it can be either triggered, inhibited, or both. Programmability can be simple, multi-, or rare modulation. Finally, the pacemaker can pace, shock, or do both.

The basic components of a pacemaker are the battery, lead system, and pulse generator. These components are found in both temporary and permanent pacemakers. A transcutaneous pacemaker is placed externally on the skin via external electrodes which adhere to the skin and are connected to the pulse generator, or in most cases, a combination portable defibrillator/monitor/pacing unit. The patient will most likely require analgesia and sedation if the pacemaker is to be required for any length of time, particularly at high mA (milliampheres or output voltage) due to the discomfort the shock causes. Higher mA's will often be required to successfully pace through the thoracic cavity. The rate and mA are set to assure the most effective pacing to produce an adequate cardiac output. The patient's skin must be frequently evaluated for burning.

The transvenous pacemaker leads are inserted via a percutaneous approach through a large vein, typically subclavian or internal jugular, into the right ventricle and/or right atrium for dual chamber pacing. The lead wires are then connected to an external pulse generator. Upon initial insertion the rate is set between 60–80/min. while the mA's are set to the point where capture occurs. Complications of this type of pacing include migration of the lead wires, or perforation of the myocardium. During cardiac surgery the lead wires can be inserted in the epicardium and fed externally via the sternotomy incision for the potential need forpos-operative pacing.

There are three conditions which the critical care nurse must observe while caring for the patient with a pacemaker: failure to pace, failure to capture, and failure to sense. Some of the most common troubleshooting interventions can be accomplished by checking the generator battery, verifying lead placement, checking for inadequate voltage to stimulate conduction, and examining the generator for general failure.

Induced Hypothermia Post Cardiac Arrest

Induced hypothermia was first described in the literature in the late 1950s and was initially used during neurosurgical or cardiovascular surgeries to reduce the incidence of neurological injury during these procedures. However, there was a study done in 1959 where the researcher evaluated hypothermia use in 12 post arrest patients. The survival rate was 50 percent in this group, which was a significant improvement over resuscitation survival during that period. The more current studies were done with some very specific criteria for inclusion, such as VF as initial rhythm, witnessed arrest, adult patient, non-traumatic, and arrest presumed to be of cardiac origin. The majority of these patients suffered out of hospital arrests as well.

Overall initial conclusions indicate that there may be some benefit from induced hypothermia of the post cardiac arrest patient in preserving neurological function and survival. The recommendation from several of these studies is that further study is required to identify the full benefit of this procedure. There are several types of cooling devices which range from a body blanket to intravenous fluid cooling and infusion.

SHOCK

Shock can be defined as a general state where decreased tissue perfusion results in a variety of conditions which impact body functions on the cellular, organ, and system level. It is a complex pathological process that can eventually involve all major organs and systems within the body. The mortality from decompensated shock is extremely high despite aggressive treatment therapies.

Types of Shock

The classifications for shock are based on the type of etiology or pathology. There are three classifications of shock.

Hypovolemic Shock

Hypovolemia is the result of loss of blood or fluid volume primarily in the intravascular space. Etiologies can include hemorrhage, surgery, gastrointestinal bleeding, severe vomiting and diarrhea, massive diuresis, or shifting of fluid volume with the intravascular and extravascular space.

The loss of circulating volume results in a decrease in venous return to the heart (preload). Stoke volume and cardiac output correspondingly decrease. Ultimately tissue perfusion and cellular oxygen supply are diminished, resulting in organ failure. The heart attempts to maintain cardiac output by increasing heart rate in response to sympathetic nervous system stimulation which occurs as a result of the decreased volume. Vasoconstriction occurs to force more volume to the heart and preserve tissue perfusion. The lungs attempt to compensate for decreased oxygen by increasing respiratory rate and respiratory alkalosis develops. Ultimately, the kidneys preserve fluid volume by slowing renal perfusion. Peripheral perfusion decreases and the patient's skin becomes cool, clammy, and pale. Cerebral perfusion will also decrease, causing a change in neurological status. In the refractory stage, the patient's compensatory mechanisms deteriorate and organ failure occurs.

The most appropriate treatment for the patient is to receive rapid fluid volume replacement in the form of red blood cells, crystalloids, or colloids depending on the type of fluid loss. Hemodynamic monitoring of indicators of cardiac output such as HR, blood pressure, CVP, and PAWP are critical to assuring the proper balance is achieved. Accurate documentation of intake and ouput and any further fluid loss is also important. The patient may require vasopressor support; however, agents which increase heart rate and myocardial demand should be avoided. These agents will be discussed in the pharmacological section of this chapter.

Cardiogenic Shock

Cardiogenic shock results from pump failure and the ability to move blood effectively. Right or left ventricular heart failure and inadequate pumping action leads to decreased tissue perfusion. It has a very high mortality rate in patients who have had an acute MI with subsequent heart failure. The etiology of this type of shock is typically cardiac dysfunction such as valvular problems, myocardial infarction, open heart surgery, cardiomyopathies, and dysrhythmias. The pathophysiology of this condition is fairly clear. When the heart is unable to push blood volume forward, there is a decrease in stroke volume and cardiac output. These processes cause a backup of volume into the right side of the heart causing increased pulmonary pressures and pulmonary edema. Oxygenation decreases and in turn oxygen supply to the cellular level also decreases, resulting in impaired tissue perfusion.

Clinically the patient demonstrates hypotension, tachycardia, cool, clammy skin, decreased urine output, chest pain, and evidence of lung congestion. Management of these symptoms requires identification of the cause of the pump failure. Inotropic medications will improve contractility of the heart muscle, while vasodilators will help reduce afterload. Hemodynamic monitoring via pulmonary artery catheter will provide several valuable measurements such as central venous pressure (CVP), right atrial pressure, and pulmonary artery wedge pressure (PAWP) to use for titration of medications and evaluation of the patient's clinical status. An arterial line is beneficial for directly monitoring arterial blood pressure. Ventilator support and potentially IABP and VAD devices might be needed for cardiac support. These are temporary measures which may be undertaken to support the heart and allow healing to occur or to serve as a bridge if heart transplant is an alternative for the patient.

The IABP is a mechanical device which augments diastole and coronary blood flow and reduces afterload. A vascular catheter with a balloon which wraps around the distal end is inserted percutaneously via the femoral artery. The balloon inflates during ventricular diastole concurrent with aortic valve closure. As a result, the blood in the aorta is displaced backward toward the aortic root, thus improving blood flow to the coronary arteries. The blood volume below the balloon is forced peripherally which enhances renal perfusion. When the balloon deflates the blood in the ventricle is ejected against less resistance, unimpeded, and facilitates ventricular emptying. IABP therapy is not without complications and constant observation by the critical care nurse and occasionally in some facilities, a pump technician is required to minimize these as much as possible.

Obstructive Shock

Obstructive shock is defined as impaired tissue perfusion resulting from obstruction of the blood flow. Two of the most common forms of this type of shock are pulmonary emboli and dissecting aortic aneurysm. Most pulmonary emboli are the result of deep vein thrombosis which have broken loose from the original site, typically in the iliofemoral system, and have entered the venous blood flow returning to the heart and subsequently the lungs. The size of the emboli and the force of blood flow determine the impact on the patient's oxygenation. Large emboli can block large pulmonary vessels or smaller emboli can break away from larger emboli and block several small vessels. As a result, pulmonary infarction occurs, and there is altered gas exchange and hemodynamic compromise. Diagnosis is made by patient's clinical condition and spiral CT. Anticoagulation with intravenous heparin is the acute treatment for pulmonary emboli. Dissecting aortic aneurysm has been discussed earlier in the chapter.

Distributive Shock

The definition of distributive shock is decreased tissue perfusion resulting from decreased vascular tone and a pooling of unoxygenated blood in the tissues. Distributive shock may occur as a result of several etiologies that lead to systemic vasodilation: septic, anaphylactic, and neurogenic.

Septic Shock

The frequency of septic shock has increased considerably over the past decade. Despite this and our increased knowledge regarding the disease, the mortality rate remains extremely high at 40 to 60 percent. Septic shock occurs when microorganisms are introduced into the body via a variety of sites (skin, respiratory, blood, gastrointestinal track, etc.). The organisms can be viral, bacterial, and/or fungal. Gram negative bacteria cause over half of all cases of septic shock.

Systemic inflammatory response syndrome (SIRS) is a grouping of symptoms which precede the septic shock state. Early recognition of this response can improve the outcome of septic shock. The patient must demonstrate *at least two of the following criteria* to meet the criteria for SIRS: Temperature > 38 degrees or < 36 degrees, heart rate above 90/min., respiratory rate above 20/min., and a white blood cell count (WBC) greater than 12,000/mm^3 or greater than 10 percent immature (bands) present on differential.

Septic shock is probably one of the most complex processes related to the immune response. It begins with the introduction of the microorganism. The immediate response is release of the plasma enzyme cascade, which includes platelets, neutrophils, and macrophages. The subsequent release of cytokines then initiates a chain of events and interactions within the body, including peripheral vasodilation, increased capillary membrane permeability, microemboli, and selective vasoconstriction. The primary immune response also triggers activation of central nervous and endocrine systems. Stimulation of the sympathetic nervous system (SNS) results in the release of epinephrine, norepinephrine, glucocorticoids, aldosterone, glucagon, and renin. The result is a hyperdynamic state which further causes vasoconstriction and increased cellular metabolic needs. The next effect is the maldistribution of blood flow to the organs and tissues and decreased cellular oxygen level. Ultimately, massive vasodilation results in hypovolemia and decreased tissue perfusion, and end organ failure.

The patient's clinical picture of massive vasodilation is one of a rapid decline in preload and a decline in blood pressure. In contrast to the other shock states, the skin becomes flushed, pink, and warm. The heart rate increases as a compensatory response and the increased metabolic demands. In the lungs there is a mismatch of ventilation and perfusion, resulting in formation of microemboli and pulmonary congestion due to increased capillary membrane permeability. Rapid deterioration in level of consciousness, renal function, and presence of lactic acidosis pursues. The immune response to the invading microorganism is an increase in WBC's and a shift to immature neutrophils as the body tries to mobilize more WBC's to respond to the infection.

The approach in treatment for septic shock has to be comprehensive; it should respond to infection, respond to the pathological cascade of events, provide hemodynamic support, fluid resuscitation, nutritional support, and glucose management. Once the infection source is identified antibiotic, antiviral or antifungal agents should be administered. If the infectious agent is unknown, a broad spectrum antibiotic should be administered. Support of the cardiovascular system with *vasopressors* and *aggressive fluid resuscitation* is critical.

Norepinephrine is used to treat hypotension that does not respond to fluid resuscitation. It can be used in combination with Dopamine to improve renal and visceral blood flow. Mechanical ventilation is often required due to the deterioration in the respiratory status and to assure adequate tissue perfusion. It is felt that early feeding of the patient (preferably via the gut and enteric feedings high in protein) will provide the patient with the needed nutrients to support the high metabolic state, enhance the immune system, and promote wound healing. A newer form of therapy to treat septic shock is being used in acute care facilities. The drug is *drotrecogin alpha,* which is a recombinant form of activated protein C. It has properties that are anti-thrombic, anti-inflammatory, and profibrinolytic. It is a weight-based drug that is infused over a period of 96 hours at 24 mcg/kg/hr.

Anaphylactic Shock

Antigens are protein-based molecules that are introduced into the body via injection, ingestion, through skin, and/or breathing. When these antigens are taken in, there is a chance that they will cause a severe hypersensitive immunological reaction and a life-threatening event. The initial contact of antigens with the body is called a *primary immune response.* Subsequent exposure causes a *secondary immune response* and potentially, anaphylaxis. *Antibodies* in the blood are formed and trigger a cascade of chemical events and reactions with the mast cells and basophils. These chemical reactions cause vasodilation, increased capillary permeability, bronchospasms, excessive mucous secretion, inflammatory response, and constriction of smooth muscle. Subsequently, circulating volume is decreased and oxygenation is not adequate. With the decrease in circulating volume, venous return and stroke volume are also decreased. The ultimate result is decreased tissue perfusion and impaired cellular metabolism.

It is critical that an immediate response is directed toward removal of the antigen, protection of the airway and circulation, administration of medications such as *epinephrine, diphenhydramine, corticosteroids, bronchodilators,* and fluid replacement to prevent further deterioration in the patient's condition and potential death.

Neurogenic Shock

Neurogenic shock is the result of impairment to the SNS and, similar to the other shock states, results in decreased tissue perfusion. It is the least common form of distributive shock. Etiologies of neurogenic shock are trauma, anesthesia, and spinal shock.

The clinical symptoms that the patient manifests as a result of neurogenic shock include alterations in level of consciousness, bradycardia, lack of sweating, apnea, paralysis, hypotension, and decreased urine output. Hemodynamically, the patient evidences decreased CVP, systemic vascular resistance (SVR), CO, CI, and oxygen saturation. The loss of sympathetic tone results in arterial and venous vasodilation and impaired thermoregulation. The cascade continues with decreased venous return, stroke volume, and cardiac output.

Treatment of neurogenic shock is careful fluid resuscitation, and vasopressors may be needed to support blood pressure. Hypothermia is treated with warming measures such as warming blankets and should be done slowly so as to prevent rapid changes in the patient's core temperature. Aggressive pulmonary management is required, particularly in the patient who has evidence of paralysis. Treatment of the underlying condition is also needed and may require stabilization of traumatic injuries and immobilization of spinal injuries.

CARDIOVASCULAR PHARMACOLOGY

Medication administration is a key role of the critical care nurse, and drug titration is often required to stabilize the patient's hemodynamic condition. This section of the chapter will be approached by discussing the classifications of drugs which are used to treat cardiovascular disorders. Some medications have been discussed in previous portions of the chapter and will not be duplicated here.

Preload Reduction Agents

Reduction of preload in the critically ill patient is accomplished that medications which cause *venous dilation,* which will decrease filling pressures in the failing heart. *Diuretics* are the most common form of preload reduction medications. There are several types of diuretics which are categorized by site of the kidneys affected by the drug. **Mannitol** is an osmotic diuretic. Loop diuretics include **furosemide** and **ethacrynic acid and act in the Loop of Henle.** Thiazides such as **hydrochlorothiazide** inhibit sodium reabsorption in the Loop of Henle. Finally, potassium-sparing diuretics promote sodium secretion in the distal tubule and potassium reabsorption. Examples of these include **spironolactone, triamterene,** and **amiloride hydrochloride**.

Nitrates and **morphine** are vasodilators and are discussed in the section on treatment for chest pain associated with MI. Examples of direct smooth muscle relaxants that are direct-acting vasodilators include **nitroglycerin** and **nitroprusside**. Nitroglycerin is used for treatment of heart failure because it reduces cardiac filling pressures and dilates coronary arteries. Initial dosage is 10 mcg/min. and titrated until chest pain relieved and blood pressure remains stable. Nitroprusside is more suitable for reduction of acute hypertension in hypertensive emergencies or afterload reduction in heart failure.

Beta-blockers such as **atenolol, metoprolol, emsolol,** and **labetalol** decrease heart rate and contractility, while increasing diastolic filling pressures. Care should be taken not to withdraw these drugs rapidly to prevent rebound effects such as unstable angina, hypertension, and MI. *Digoxin* is a cardiac glycoside, regulates heart rate, and is classified as a weak inotrope.

Afterload Reduction Agents

ACE (angiotensin-converting enzyme) inhibitors cause vasoconstriction and afterload reduction which results in decreased left ventricular workload. These drugs block the conversion of angiotensin I to angiotensin II. Examples of these medications include **captopril** and **enalapril**. One of the complications of these drugs is hypotension, particularly in volume-depleted patients.

Nitroprusside is discussed briefly above and is classified as a smooth muscle relaxant which can have both arterial and venous vasodilator effects. The dosage is titrated to the desired effect and is typically infused at 0.25–6.0 mcg/kg/min via IV infusion.

Hydralazine is a potent arterial smooth muscle dilator. It is given via slow IV push in dosages of 5–10 mg every four to six hours. The most significant side effect is reflex tachycardia. It can be given intermittently to bridge the period during weaning of IV antihypertensives.

Vasopressor Agents

Dopamine was discussed earlier in the section on heart failure. **Norepinephrine, neo-synepherine** and **vasopressin** are the other vasopressors in the care of the critically ill patient. Vasopressors are primarily sympathomimetic agents which mediate peripheral vasoconstriction. Care must be undertaken when administering these medications in patients with cardiac conditions as they significantly increase afterload by the actions of peripheral vasoconstriction and increased systemic vascular resistance. However, in some shock states, tissue perfusion may be significantly reduced and organ failure is likely to occur without adequate cardiac output and systemic perfusion. The risk must be evaluated against the benefits of the drugs. Vasopressin is useful in patients with gastrointestinal bleeding as it is a vasoconstrictor and decreases blood flow to the visceral bed. It is administered with a loading dose of 20 units over 20 minutes IV and followed by a continuous infusion at 0.2–0.8 units/min.

Inotropic Agents

The function of inotropic agents is to improve cardiac contractility. The end result is improved cardiac output by decreased filling pressures. **Digoxin** is a mild inotrope. Sympathomimetic agents stimulate adrenergic receptors, thus stimulating the sympathetic nervous system. **Dobutamine** has been discussed earlier. **Milrinone** is another example of an inotropic agent. This drug directly relaxes vascular smooth muscle and increases myocardial contractility. It is given in a loading dose of 50 mcg/kg over 10 minutes and followed by an infusion of 0.375 to 0.75 mcg/kg/min. Most inotropes do cause tachycardia.

Lipid Lowering Agents

Some of the most commonly prescribed drugs in the United States are lipid lowering agents. Elevated cholesterol and triglycerides are risk factors for cardiac disease. American Heart Association guidelines recommend these agents when levels for total cholesterol are < 200 mg/dL and for triglycerides < 150 mg/dL. Examples of these agents are

- Atorvastatin (Lipitor®)
- Fluvastatin (Lescol®)
- Lovastatin (Mevacor®, Altoprev™)
- Pravastatin (Pravachol®)
- Rosuvastatin Calcium (Crestor®)
- Simvastatin (Zocor®)

Anti-arrhythmic Agents

Anti-arrhythmics are a diverse category of medications which are used to treat abnormal heart rhythms. These drugs are classified as Class I–IV, and an unclassified grouping. Class I is sodium channel blockers, Class II is beta-adrenergic blockers (beta-blockers), Class III is drugs which slow the rate of phase 3 depolarization, and Class IV is calcium channel blockers. Some examples of specific drugs are listed below.

Class	Drug name
I	Quinidine
I	Procainamide
II	Metoprolol
II	Propranolol
III	Amiodarone
IV	Diltiazem
IV	Verapamil
Unclassified	Adenosine
Unclassified	Magnesium

Anti-anginal

Anti-anginal drugs, as the name implies, are medications that reduce the pain associated with angina pectoris. Angina is typically a reflection of diminished blood or oxygen supply to the myocardium. Examples of these drugs include multiple forms of nitroglycerine, isosorbide dinitrate or mononitrate, nicardipine, amlodipine, and felodipine. Other agents which are in other categories already listed above may also have anti-anginal effects.

Anti-hypertensives

Anti-hypertensives function to reduce blood pressure as a protective mechanism from strokes, renal failure, and coronary artery disease. The general effects of anti-hypertensives are to diminish adrenergic nerve stimulation to the vasculature, vasodilation by relaxing vascular smooth muscle, and reduction of afterload. Examples of anti-hypertensives and the site of primary action include clonidine hydrochloride (central nervous system), reserpine (peripheral nerve endings), labetalol (beta receptor sites), and prazosin hydrochloride (alpha receptor sites).

Calcium Channel Blockers

Calcium channel blockers are considered negative inotropic, negative chronotropic, and dromotropic agents on SA and AV conductive tissue. They are successful in reducing ischemia by increasing the anginal threshold. They also can treat coronary vasospasm. One of the most potent vasodilators in this category of drugs is dihydropyridines, of which nifedipine is an example. Nicardipine and felodipine are examples of second generation dihydropyridines. The other two types of calcium channel blockers are phenylalkylamines (verapamil) and benzothiazepines (diltiazem).

Thrombolytics

Thrombolytics are used to treat acute coronary ischemia as a result of blockage of the coronary arteries and acute myocardial infarction. These can be given peripherally via IV lines or intracoronary via cardiac catheterization and angiography procedures (PTCA). Criteria for treatment with thrombolytics is specific and requires screening of the patient for history for time of onset of symptoms (goal is administration at less than 6 hours after onset of pain and symptoms), any evidence of bleeding, recent surgery or CVA, and evidence of persistent ST elevation despite sublingual nitroglycerine or nifedipine.

There are currently five thrombolytics available for use for treatment of acute coronary ischemia: streptokinase, urokinase, alteplase, reteplase, and anistreplace. The most common drug used at the present time is tPA (alteplase). It is administered 100 mg first hour and 20 mg over the second and third hours.

With any thrombolytic, it is imperative for the critical care RN to monitor the patient for any signs of acute bleeding. Neurological checks should be done minimally every 1 hour for the time of administration and every 2 hours for the next 24 hours. Other observations should be done as for any patient receiving anticoagulant therapy. Should serious bleeding occur, the infusion should be stopped and the patient treated symptomatically for blood loss. Intravenous lines must be placed before the infusion is started and venipunctures should be limited to those as only absolutely necessary. Stress ulcer prophylaxis should be given, especially if the patient complains of epigastric pain.

Evidence of coronary reperfusion can be profound, including reperfusion dysrhythmias, ventricular tachycardia, bradycardias, conduction defects, and occasionally, ventricular fibrillation. ST segments should be normalized during reperfusion, and CK, CKMB, and troponins should also stabilize.

Anticoagulants

Warfarin and enoxaparin have been previously discussed in the section on treatment for atrial fibrillation. INR's should be checked daily while the patient is hospitalized for therapeutic levels and as per primary care physician once patient has been discharged.

Antiplatelets

Two of the most commonly used antiplatelet medications are aspirin (81 mg dose) and clopidrogel (Plavix). Research has demonstrated that these drugs have protective effects and reduce the potential for platelet aggregation at the site of atherosclerotic plaque.

CARDIAC CATHETERIZATION (PERCUTANEOUS TRANSLUMINAL CORONARY ANGIOPLASTY, PTCA)

Cardiac catheterization can be performed on an elective basis to diagnose coronary artery disease and blood flow or can be done emergently in conjunction with PTCA to open a coronary vessel with an obstructive atherosclerotic lesion is causing acute coronary ischemia and infarction. PTCA requires advancement of a balloon-tipped catheter through a percutaneous insertion site such as the femoral artery and vein. The catheter is threaded into the coronary artery system and dye is injected to evaluate the patency of these vessels. If there is an observed obstruction, a guidewire can be inserted through the introducer and the balloon catheter can be threaded to the site of the lesion and inflated to open the vessel. Stents may be placed in the vessel to assure continued patency. The patient does require systemic anticoagulation.

Intracoronary thrombolytics can also be injected through the catheter to the site of the lesion. There is a strong likelihood (30 percent to 40 percent) of restenosis of the vessel within the first 6 months of the procedure. Access to a surgical suite with open heart capability should always be available during this time due to the potential complication for acute coronary occlusion resulting from dissection, acute bleeding at the insertion site, or perforation of a coronary vessel.

There are multiple pressure or closure devices which can be used after the removal of the catheter. Manual pressure at the site of insertion should be held for a minimum of 15 minutes and frequently checked and observed for evidence of hematoma. However, newer closure devices are being used to prevent the need for manual pressure which is not always effective. These include Fem-Stop, C-clamps, and other similar arterial closure devices (Angio-Seal™, Perclose™, StarClose™, and Boomerang™). The affected leg should remain straight and immobile for the next six to eight hours. Continuous cardiac, vital sign monitoring, and CMS checks on the affected extremity should be done as a standard of care.

Complications which may occur post arterial cannulation/cardiac catheterization may include the following: hematoma, AV fistula, pseudoaneurysm, retroperitoneal bleed and acute loss of distal circulation. Typically a hematoma is the result of inadequate or early release of pressure on the insertion site. Care should be taken to assure the artery has closed sufficiently and there is no evidence of subcutaneous bleeding. The patient should be assessed for bruit over the site of sheath insertion at least every eight hours. A positive bruit over the site, in combination with localized pain and a pulsatile mass, is indicative of a pseudoaneurysm—which requires immediate notification to the physician and surgical intervention or ultrasound-guided compression.

The Pulmonary System

5

About 17 percent of questions on the CCRN exam cover pulmonary questions.

ACUTE PULMONARY EMBOLUS

An embolus is an object that occludes a vessel. An embolus can be composed of a detached thrombus or vegetation (mass of bacteria), foreign body, or fat. However, the term *pulmonary embolus* (PE) generally refers to either a detached thrombus or fat.

Pathophysiology

The exact pathophysiology of fat emboli is not completely understood, but it generally occurs approximately *three to four days after the patient experiences a trauma.* Although there are competing theories regarding the pathophysiology, the basic mechanism is that the trauma (generally a long bone fracture, such as a femur) result is the release of fat droplets and/or free fatty acids/chylomicrons in the venous circulation which embolize to the pulmonary vasculature, occluding a pulmonary vein.

Likewise, thromboemboli also generally originate from the extremities from deep vein thrombi (DVT). Essentially, a DVT forms in an extremity, generally the legs, and then a portion of the thrombus detaches and embolizes to the pulmonary vasculature.

Despite the character of the emboli, the effects are similar. There will be an acute increase in the pulmonary vascular resistance and extra strain on the right heart. This may manifest as a *new right bundle branch* on an EKG or *new onset atrial fibrillation.* Other, relatively more minor effects are decreased perfusion to the peripheral lung tissue and mismatch of the ventilation and perfusion of the lung tissue.

Risk Factors

On the history and physical patients will often state that they have "just returned from a long vacation and were in an airplane for a long period of time" or they are truck drivers and their symptoms began after they had been driving for several hours. Hence, one of the biggest risk factors for an acute pulmonary thromboembolism is long-term (generally more than 3–4 hours) immobilization, otherwise referred to as venous stasis. However, other risk factors are *medications* (such as oral contraceptives), *hypercoagulable states* due to antico-agulant deficiencies (such as Protein C and S), the presence of autoantibodies (such as lupus anticoagulant), presence of a *malignancy* (such as breast, lung, colon, etc.) that release proco-agulant hormones, and *damage to the endothelium* of the vasculature (such as inflammation from a vasculitis).

In-patient Prophylaxis

When patients are admitted to the critical care units, they will generally receive gastric ulcer prophylaxis with a proton pump inhibitor or histamine-2 receptor blocker. Likewise, they also receive prophylaxis for DVT since they are likely to be immobile for a prolonged period. This can be done with *"Ted" hose*, i.e., compression stockings, either alone or in combination with *sequential compression devices* (SCD's), which are pneumatic cuffs that wrap around the distal lower extremity and intermittently inflate and decompress to prevent venous stasis. If there is no contraindication to anticoagulation, then patients may also be placed on twice daily subcutaneous injections of heparin, once daily subcutaneous injections *of low molec-ular weight heparin* (LMWH) (e.g., enoxaparin & dalteparin), or *anti-thrombin III binder* (e.g., fondaparinux). If patients are already on anticoagulation with warfarin, then as long as their INR is maintained between 2.0 and 3.0, no other prophylaxis is required.

Symptoms, Diagnosis & Treatment

When patients are present with PE, they will be present with *tachypnea, tachycardia, hypo-tension,* and, sometimes *diaphoresis.*

A detailed description of each test which can be used to diagnose a PE is beyond the scope of this book and the CCRN. However, a critical care RN must understand the reasoning behind certain tests. Hence, here we will briefly list the tests used to diagnose PE's. Gener-ally, the easiest test to order is a *CT of the chest with IV contrast,* sometimes referred to as a "Spiral CT" based on the protocol used by the radiologist. However, if the patient has renal failure or cannot receive IV contrast due to access or allergy, then a *ventilation/perfusion (V/Q) scan* is preferred. In difficult cases where the results of studies are ambivalent, the gold standard is *pulmonary angiography,* which again requires contrast administration. Some physicians may order a *"D-Dimer" blood test.* This test is highly sensitive but has poor specificity, because many inflammatory conditions other than PE result in elevations of the D-Dimer. Hence, this test is useful only in healthy patients with few to no other comorbidities. If this is negative, it is highly unlikely that the patient has a PE.

The treatment of acute pulmonary emboli depends on whether the patient is hemody-namically stable. If hemodynamic stability is not a concern, then either a *heparin drip* (unfractionated heparin) intravenously, subcutaneous injections twice daily of *LMWH* (e.g., enoxaparin, dalteparin, tinazaparin), or *anti-thrombin III binder* (e.g., fondaparinux). *Patients are generally maintained on anticoagulation for three months after their first acute pulmonary thromboembolism once they are discharged from the hospital.* However, recurrent episodes may require more invasive treatment such as an *inferior vena cavae filter* (IVC filter; aka "Greenfield Filter").

ACUTE HYPOXEMIC RESPIRATORY FAILURE

Respiratory failure is generally categorized as defects in either oxygenation or ventilation. If infiltrates are present, the respiratory failure can be further categorized as **cardiogenic** or **non-cardiogenic**.

Cardiogenic Respiratory Failure

Cardiogenic pulmonary edema is the result of *failure of the left side of the heart to maintain forward flow through the left ventricular outflow tract.* This can occur for a number of reasons that are beyond the scope of this section. However, suffice it to say that failure of the left-sided cardiac function results in volume overload in the pulmonary vasculature, which can be measured as *an increase in the pulmonary capillary wedge pressure.* Once the pulmonary capillary wedge pressure is decreased with diuresis, the pulmonary edema resolves.

Non-cardiogenic Respiratory Failure

Non-cardiogenic respiratory failure is due to "leaky" pulmonary capillaries, which result in fluid leaving the vasculature and entering the lung parenchyma/interstitial compartment. This form of pulmonary insult is also known as **acute lung injury** (ALI), when the partial arterial pressure of oxygen (PaO_2) to the inspired oxygen concentration (FiO_2) is ≤ 300. However, if this ratio (PaO_2/FiO_2) is ≤ 200, then it is referred to as **adult respiratory distress syndrome** (ARDS).

Pathophysiology

It is believed that non-cardiogenic respiratory failure results from *damage to the pulmonary endothelium* with or without insult to the epithelium. These insults and damage can come about from *direct toxin exposure, medication side effects,* and/or *inflammation.* Toxic insult can occur from inhalation of aerosolized chemicals, smoking tobacco, etc. Systemic inflammation in sepsis results in widespread release of inflammatory cytokines which cause epithelial damage. Medications such as amiodarone, methotrexate, and carbamazepine (Brand Name: Tegretol) have also been associated with ARDS. Some comorbidities may make patients susceptible to the acquisition of ARDS.

Management & Treatment

The goal in non-cardiogenic respiratory failure is to *maintain oxygenation and provide symptomatic support,* allowing the lungs to recover from the insult. Hence, first remove the insulting agent, e.g., amiodarone. This should occur simultaneously with administration of oxygen and mechanical ventilation, if necessary (almost always). Again, a detailed discussion regarding ventilators is beyond the scope of the CCRN, but a critical care RN should know that the lungs are generally "stiffer" in non-cardiogenic respiratory failure. As a result, the ventilation parameter which will be important is the positive-end expiratory pressure (PEEP). *Increasing the PEEP* will help keep the alveoli open and available for oxygenation.

RESPIRATORY INFECTIONS

"Pulmonary infection" is a broad topic. However, for the CCRN, the scope of this section will be limited to **community acquired pneumonia** (CAP), **aspiration pneumonia**, and **hospital (nosocomial) acquired pneumonia** (HAP).

Symptoms

The presenting symptoms of all respiratory infections are similar: *dyspnea* with or without a *cough.* The cough may or may not be productive. The patient may report *fever, chills,* and/or *night sweats.* The latter should raise suspicion for either septicemia or tuberculosis (TB). Other constitutional symptoms such as body aches and rhinorrhea (runny nose) may be present in viral upper respiratory infections (URI). In the elderly, mental status changes and headache may also be present.

Community-Acquired Pneumonia (CAP)

CAP is defined as pneumonia in a patient who has not recently been hospitalized. A host of organisms can cause CAP. They can be categorized as typical and atypical. Typical bacterial pathogens include Streptococcus pneumoniae, Haemophilus influenza, as well as Moraxella catarrhalis (previously called *Branhamella*). Atypical organisms include Legionella species, Mycoplasma species, and Chlamydia pneumoniae. Organisms that are considered rare, unless the clinical picture is appropriate, are Klebsiella pneumoniae (aspiration in chronic alcoholics), Staphylococcus aureus (post viral pneumoniae), and Pseudomonas aeruginosa (in patients with cystic fibrosis or Bronchiectasis). The antibiotic regiment chosen can vary for CAP. Generally, it will be Ceftriaxone, a quinolone (e.g., levofloxacin; Brand Name: Levaquin), doxycycline, azithromycin, and/or a third- or fourth-generation cephalosporin.

Aspiration Pneumonia

Aspiration pneumonia generally develops in those patients with dysphagia, either due to intrinsic musculoskeletal/nervous system disease or ingestion of medications which cause drowsiness and/or intoxication. Hence, the patient with aspiration pneumonia may be an elderly patient with mild dysphagia or a young patient who is intoxicated and whose state of mental alertness is depressed. In either case, the mechanism and organisms are essentially the same. There will be *multiple oropharyngeal organisms* found in the sputum culture and tracheal aspirate. Further, in aspiration pneumonia, the physicians will often add clindamycin or metronidazole to cover for anaerobes.

Hospital-Acquired (Nosocomial) Pneumonia (HAP)

When patients develop pneumonia during a hospital admission, it can be difficult to determine whether it was a developing pre-existing condition or acquired as a result of the hospital stay. As a result, the definition of hospital or nosocomial pneumonia is a pneumonia that *develops at least 72 hours after being admitted.* Further, since the pathogens within the in-patient setting are much different than those in the community, the antibiotic choices may also vary and include vancomycin, third- and fourth-generation cephalosporins, carbapenems, fluoroquinolones, and aminoglycosides (e.g., gentamycin). Currently, the recommendations are to *treat with a double or triple antibiotic regiment in the setting of hospital-acquired pneumonia.*

Chronic Obstructive Pulmonary Disease (COPD)

Chronic obstructive pulmonary disease (COPD) is a class of lung disease that includes asthma, emphysema, and chronic bronchitis. Within this group, these are the diseases most likely to appear on the CCRN. All of these diseases share common pathophysiology. Namely, they all result in "air-trapping" within the lungs. The etiology behind this "air-trapping" can vary, depending on the disease. In some cases, it is loss of pulmonary elasticity and recoil (e.g., emphysema), narrowing of the airways that may or may not be due to inflammation, thus limiting the amount of expired air (e.g., chronic bronchitis and asthma).

Risk Factors

The risk factors for COPD can be thought of as environmental and genetic. Environmental risk factors include tobacco use, second-hand smoke exposure, occupational exposure (coal, gold, cadmium, isocyanates, silica, and asbestos). Air pollution is also believed to play a role in triggering and, possibly initiating, COPD. Genetic risk factors include, classically, alpha-1-antitrypsin deficiency. This enzyme helps protect the lung from a self-made digestive enzyme (trypsin). The lack of this protein results in unbalanced activity of this digestive enzyme and destruction of lung parenchyma, leading to emphysema (see below). Further, there is evidence that some COPD may be caused by an autoimmune reaction in those with a certain immunological profile. Hence, COPD may also partly be an autoimmune disease.

Symptoms

As one would imagine, the most obvious symptom of COPD is that of dyspnea. *Dyspnea* will gradually worsen over time, to the point that it begins to limit activities of daily living (ADL). A *cough* may or may not be associated with the dyspnea. Likewise, not all patients with COPD have copious *sputum production,* although sputum production increases with time. In the advanced stages, *cyanosis* may be apparent, indicating significant aberration in gas exchange. Finally, in the end stages, cardiovascular circulation in the pulmonary vasculature will be compromised and lead to right-sided heart failure in the absence of left-sided heart failure, otherwise known as **cor pulmonale**. On exam, there may be expiratory *wheezing* (often best heard in the anterior and lateral lung fields), *tachypnea, chest protrusion, use of accessory muscles for breathing* (in exacerbations), breathing with *pursed lips,* and/or the presence of *rales* (crackles) on posterior lung field auscultation.

Chronic Bronchitis

Chronic bronchitis is defined clinically and is characterized by productive *cough on most days for three months of a year and over the course of two consecutive years.* As the name implies, chronic bronchitis results from longstanding inflammation of the airways. As a result, there is hyperplasia and hypertrophy of the mucous-producing cells (goblet cells). Inflammation is histologically dominant. The chronic inflammation also leads to scarring and thickening of the airway, resulting in limited ability to fully expire air. Over time, the chronic obstruction places the patient at increased risk for pulmonary infections, primarily pneumonia.

Emphysema

Emphysema is histologically defined as the *destruction of airspace distal to the terminal bronchioles.* There is also destruction of the walls of the alveoli, in the absence of fibrosis. On imaging, these airspaces are referred to as *bullae.* In emphysema the patient loses elastic recoil of the lung due to the destruction of the parenchyma, and as a result, there is limited ability to expire the inhaled air. Furthermore, there will be gas-exchange abnormalities, since the alveoli are no longer present.

Asthma

Classically, asthma has been defined as *hyper-responsive airways*. There is some overlap with chronic bronchitis. However, there is almost complete reversibility of airway constriction in asthma, where this is not necessarily the case in other forms of COPD. Furthermore, the etiology behind asthma is felt to be environmental, and interestingly, each person with asthma may have a different *environmental trigger*.

COPD and Asthma Exacerbations

Often a "trigger" will cause an exacerbation of pre-existing pulmonary disease. When this occurs, the patient will often be placed in an intensive care setting due to *tachypnea, dyspnea,* and possibly, *hypoxemia.*

In COPD exacerbations, the trigger is a bacterial infection 70–75 percent of the time. Hence, therapy needs to be targeted toward inflammation, airway constriction, oxygenation, and infection. Often, these therapeutic regiments will include *beta agonists* (e.g., albuterol), *anti-cholinergics* (e.g., ipratropium), *intravenous corticosteroids* (e.g., methylprednisolone), and *antibiotics.* The antibiotic/s chosen vary based on each clinical situation and the organism suspected, but include quinolones (e.g., levoflaxacin), doxycycline, Trimethoprim–sulfamethoxazole, macrolides (e.g., azithromycin), cephalosporins (e.g., ceftriaxone), anti-pseudomonas (e.g., piperacillin–tazobactam), and/or aminoglycosides (e.g., tobramycin).

Asthma exacerbations (status asthmaticus) are treated in a similar manner to COPD exacerbations. Understanding that bronchodilation and controlling inflammation is the primary focus of treatment in asthma exacerbations, it comes as no surprise that therapy consists of beta-agonists (inhaled metered dose inhalers or nebulizers) and intravenous corticosteroids (e.g., methylprednisolone). Treatment with antibiotics should take place only in the context of strong clinical suspicion, in contrast to COPD exacerbations, where the trigger is an infection.

"Air-Leaks"

The term "air-leaks" is not a medical or clinical term. Instead it is a term used here to help you remember syndromes where there is *abnormal air collection in the thorax cavity.* For the most part, if you remember that air should be in the airways, lungs, esophagus, and stomach, then if you see air any place else it is abnormal. For example, air between the chest wall and the lung periphery is referred to as a **pneumothorax** ("collapsed lung"); air in the space around the heart is referred to as **pneumopericardium**; air in the space between the two lungs (mediastinum) is known as **pneumomediastinum**; and air in the space around the alveoli is referred to as **perivascular interstitial emphysema** (PIE).

Pneumothorax & Pneumopericardium

The most significant of the "air-leak" syndromes are pneumothorax and pneumopericardium since these can be fatal. Generally, as you remember, there is no air in the pleural space. However, when air enters the pleural space it is referred to as a pneumothorax. As a result, the underlying lung may "collapse." If this occurs, the underlying lung cannot be involved in ventilation and the patient may present with *dyspnea* if the area involved is large. The treatment for a pneumothorax depends on the size, but in cases where the patient will be admitted to the intensive care unit, the rim of air between the lung and chest wall on a cheat radiograph will likely be more than 2 cm. If this is the case, and the patient is short of breath, then a *needle thoracostomy* is performed and a *chest tube* may need to be inserted.

Likewise, a pneumopericardium is air in the pleural space around the heart. The consequences of a pneumopericardium will be the same as a pericardial effusion. Thus, if there is only a small amount of air, then the patient may be asymptomatic. However, if there is a larger amount of air, then there may be compromise of the filling of the heart and, subsequently, the cardiac output, referred to as *cardiac tamponade*. The treatment is similar to that for a large pericardial effusion, needle decompression (pericardiocentesis).

Perivascular Interstitial Emphysema

Normally there is no air between the wall of the alveoli and the surrounding vasculature. However, when air leaks from an alveoli or the alveoli bursts, air can be seen in this perivascular space and is referred to as perivascular interstitial emphysema (PIE). In the majority of cases this is not fatal and patients are asymptomatic. However, the air in this space has the potential to "dissect" through tissues if there is large alveolar pressure. If this air spreads, it has the potential to lead to a pneumothorax and/or pneumopericardium, where the patient may be symptomatic and require immediate intervention as outlined above.

Pneumomediastinum

The space in the thorax demarcated by the medial borders of the lung laterally, the sternum anteriorly, and the spine posteriorly is known as the mediastinum. A pneumomediastinum refers to air in this space. Generally, there is no emergency in a pneumomediastinum, since this space is more than able to accommodate air without compromising pulmonary or cardiac function. However, the patient may feel some discomfort if the pneumomediastinum is large. Further, if there is compromise of the visceral pleura which lines this space, then the patient may develop a pneumothorax and/or a pneumopericardium and require intervention. Hence, pneumomediastinum is not fatal, but should not be taken lightly and needs close follow up. The critical care RN should be aware of tachypnea, tachycardia, hypoxia, and hypotension—signs that may suggest that there is hemodynamic compromise.

Trauma

Trauma to the thorax cavity can be categorized as **non-penetrating (blunt)** or **penetrating**. Further, trauma can also be categorized by site of injury (e.g., airways, cardiac, pulmonary, esophagus, chest wall, diaphragm). The signs and symptoms of trauma to the thorax will generally be the same and may include respiratory distress, subcutaneous emphysema, pneumothorax, hemoptysis, mediastinal emphysema, hypotension, and tachycardia. Hemoptysis will generally occur in penetrating trauma, but if there is compromise of a structure, such as a great vessel or airway in non-penetrating trauma, these patients may also present with hemoptysis.

Non-penetrating trauma to the thorax can occur during motor vehicle accidents, accidents, fights, etc. The force of the trauma, if large enough, will often be transmitted to the internal organs: heart and lungs. This can result in a cardiac or pulmonary contusion. Generally, the patient may be mildly dyspneic and may or may not have oxygenation issues, depending on the severity of the contusion and percentage of the lung involved. The other important structures within the thorax cavity are the great vessels (vena cavae, aorta, pulmonary veins, and pulmonary artery). Depending on the nature and direction of the non-penetrating force, these vessels may experience shearing forces and may rupture. In these cases, it is important that the patient be stabilized immediately and emergent thoracotomy performed. In addition to symptoms of dyspnea, tachypnea, and, possibly tachycardia, the patient may also may experience pulmonary hemorrhage with hemoptysis in extensive pulmonary contusions and/or pulmonary vasculature rupture.

It is important to always look and assess for fractured ribs, as these may compromise the patient's ability to ventilate. Specifically, the most serious condition that can result from multiple fractured ribs is "**flail chest**." The rib fractures need to be in multiple ribs at multiple places. Some sources state that at least two adjacent ribs must be broken in a minimum of two places, while others state three or more ribs must be fractured in two or more places. Either way, there are multiple rib fractures in multiple places. The rib fractures compromise the patient's ability to control the expansion of the thorax cavity, and "flail segment" moves in the opposite direction as the rest of the chest wall, i.e., it moves inward when the chest expands and moves out when the patient exhales. Over 50 percent of patients that present with flail chest will die. Obviously there will most likely be an accompanying pulmonary contusion as well. The pulmonary contusion will compromise the oxygenation, as stated above. The degree to which the oxygenation is compromised will be a determining factor in survival. The treatment of flail chest is positive pressure ventilation, analgesia, supplemental oxygenation, and chest tube placement.

Penetrating trauma is self explanatory. In these instances, the integrity of the thorax cavity has been compromised. An example is a stab wound. In these cases, the risk of bleeding is obviously higher. As a result, the possibility of a hemothorax is likely. A hemothorax is similar to a pneumothorax, but instead of air in the thorax cavity (which may also occur with penetrating trauma) there is blood in the pleural space. The treatment is evacuation and chest tube placement, exactly similar to pneumothorax. If more than 1500 ml of blood is removed from the thorax cavity, it is important to consider injury to a major vessel and pursue thoracotomy. In penetrating trauma, if there is an impailed object present, it is important to remember: DO NOT REMOVE THE IMPAILED OBJECT until the patient is in the operating room and the proper measures have been taken to stabilize the patient as much as possible. This will help deal with the consequences of removing the impailed object (i.e., possibly massive hemorrhage) under controlled circumstances and allow for an immediate thoracotomy.

Finally, you can also have **tracheal perforation** from non-penetrating and penetrating trauma. Tracheal perforation or compromise is more often cervical (above the carina) in penetrating trauma and within 2–3 cm of the lower aspect of the carina in non-penetrating trauma. The symptoms are similar to penetrating trauma in that there is a compromise in the structure of the airway. The treatment of choice is bronchoscopy, if possible, and primary closure with end-end anastomosis.

Mechanical Ventilation

When patients need assistance with ventilation or are unable to ventilate themselves, mechanical ventilation may be utilized. Mechanical ventilation is categorized as non-invasive and invasive. Non-invasive ventilation is also referred to as **noninvasive positive pressure ventilation** (NPPV). The goal of mechanical ventilation is to provide adequate oxygenation (PaO_2) and ventilation ($PaCO_2$).

Noninvasive Ventilation

NPPV is generally used when the patient has a sufficient respiratory drive to breathe on his/her own, but may need assistance in helping keep the airways open. The theory behind NPPV is that positive pressure delivered through a mask can help keep the airways open while a patient is breathing and that this can decrease the work of breathing. There are generally two types of NPPV: **continuous positive airway pressure** (CPAP) and **biphasic positive airway pressure** (BIPAP). In both types of NPPV the patient wears a mask with a seal. In CPAP, the patient receives a constant amount of pressure that is delivered throughout inspiration and expiration. In contrast, in BIPAP, the patient receives a different pressure during inspiration (inspiratory positive airway pressure, **IPAP**) and a different pressure during expiration (expiratory positive airway pressure, **EPAP**).

The types of clinical situations in which NPPV should be considered as a first modality of ventilation are COPD exacerbations, cardiogenic pulmonary edema, acute respiratory failure in immunosuppressed patients, and patients with COPD who are being extubated. The institution of NPPV in the above clinical scenarios has been studied and shown to reduce the need for intubation, decrease mortality, and decrease the length of hospital stay in the intensive care setting. NPPV may also be considered for patients with status asthamaticus, but there are limited numbers of studies looking at the benefit of NPPV with regard to the above endpoints or improvement in pulmonary function (e.g., FEV_1). When instituting NPPV, there are a variety of masks to choose from: full face, oronasal, and nasal.

Invasive Mechanical Ventilation

Invasive mechanical ventilation refers to patients in whom an endotracheal tube (ET) has been placed and a ventilator is being used to ventilate the patient. As with NPPV, there are certain indications to use invasive mechanical ventilation. The obvious cases are where patients are unconscious, cannot protect their airway, or are in acute respiratory distress with or without hemodynamic instability. More specifically, clinical scenarios where invasive mechanical ventilation should be seriously considered are when a patient fails a trial of NPPV, is in acute respiratory distress (as evidence by oxygenation/ventilation and/or the use of accessory muscles for breathing or a respiratory rate of 35 breaths/minute or greater), or in shock.

Ventilators can be confusing and although this section is not designed to transform the reader into an expert, it should provide you with the tools as a critical care RN to understand the basic terminology and modes of ventilation. In short, there are two modes of invasive mechanical ventilation used in the intensive care units: **volume and pressure control**. In *volume control,* the machine simply controls the amount of tidal volume inspired by the patient. Currently, the trend is to use "low-volume ventilation" (also referred to as lung protective ventilation), which is believed to minimize barotrauma to the lung. In volume control, the operator can set the respiratory rate, tidal volume, and the positive end-expiratory pressure (the amount of pressure remaining in the lungs after all the tidal volume has been expired, PEEP). You should note that the PEEP can also be thought of as EPAP. In pressure control, the ventilator allows the patient to determine the tidal volume. However, the ventilator is set to control the IPAP and PEEP or EPAP, as well as the respiratory rate. Whichever mode of ventilation the physician is using, the ventilator will always allow control over the percentage of inspired oxygen that the patient receives (FiO_2). Normally the FiO_2 is 21 percent at room air. Hence, if a patient is requiring the ventilator, it is common for the FiO_2 to be set anywhere from 30–100 percent.

Volutrauma & Barotrauma

When using mechanical ventilation, primarily invasive mechanical ventilation, the patient may experience pulmonary trauma. The simple theory behind the trauma is that the lungs are being over-ventilated, i.e., over-expanded. The two ways in which this occurs are by delivering very *high tidal volumes* (resulting on volutrauma) and by delivering *high airway pressures* (resulting in barotraumas). These forms of trauma damage the parenchyma and may result in pulmonary edema from "leaky" perialveolar capillaries. Hence, using minimal pressures and volume is preferred in invasive mechanical ventilation. Although institutions will vary on which mode (volume or pressure control) they prefer, there seems to be a tendency to use volume control to minimize the risk of barotraumas.

Arterial Blood Gas Analysis

In managing patients in the intensive care setting, it will be important to monitor the arterial blood gas (ABG) and be able to interpret the results. For the purposes of the CCRN, the discussion will be focused on the steps necessary to interpret an ABG. However, a preliminary review of the physiology is important prior to undertaking this discussion.

The body generally has a normal pH in the bloodstream of approximately 7.4 and will attempt to maintain this pH through a number of mechanisms. The key components/organ systems involved in the maintenance of normal blood pH are the bicarbonate (HCO_3^-) buffer system in the blood, the lungs, and the kidneys. The lungs and kidneys can respond to the changing pH of the blood to help correct disturbances in the pH. For example, the lungs can breathe faster and/or increase the tidal volume to make the blood alkaline in response to an acidic change. Conversely the lungs can breathe more slowly and/or decrease the tidal volume to make the blood more acidic in response to an alkaline change in the blood. Likewise the kidneys can reabsorb more or less bicarbonate (HCO_3^-) depending on whether there is an acidic or alkaline change in the blood.

In order to best understand acid-base balance it is important to know the relationship between CO_2 and HCO_3^-, i.e., the chemical equation for the bicarbonate buffer system:

$$H_2O + CO_2 \quad H_2CO_3 \quad H^+ + HCO_3^-$$

Next, in order to interpret blood gases, it is important to first know the components of an ABG and their normal values. The five measurements on an ABG are pH, arterial partial pressure of carbon dioxide ($PaCO_2$), arterial partial pressure of oxygen (PaO_2) , HCO_3^-, and base excess (BE). There are 4 primary acid-base disorders: respiratory acidosis, respiratory alkalosis, metabolic acidosis, and metabolic alkalosis. The normal values for these measurements are listed below.

Normal ABG Values

pH	$PaCO_2$	PaO_2	HCO_3^-	BE
7.35–7.45	35–45 mmHg	80–100 mmHg	22–26 meq/L	–2 to +2 meq/L

Respiratory Acidosis: Low pH and High PaCO$_2$

Respiratory acidosis occurs when the lungs are not sufficiently ventilating. In other words, CO_2 is building up in the bloodstream. Based on the bicarbonate buffer equation above, a build up of CO_2 will lead to an increase in the concentration of H^+, making the blood acidic. Based on this understanding, respiratory acidosis is defined as a pH below 7.35 and a $PaCO_2$ greater than 45 mmHg.

Respiratory Alkalosis: High pH and Low PaCO$_2$

Respiratory alkalosis occurs when the lungs are "over-breathing" and releasing too much CO_2 from the bloodstream. Hence, the CO_2 concentration is decreasing in the bloodstream. Based on the bicarbonate buffer equation above, a decrease in the concentration of CO_2 will lead to an decrease in the concentration of H^+, making the blood alkalotic. Based on this understanding, respiratory alkalosis is defined as a pH above 7.45 and a $PaCO_2$ less than 35 mmHg.

Metabolic Acidosis: Low pH and Low HCO$_3^-$

Metabolic acidosis occurs when the pH of the bloodstream is less than 7.35 and there is a decrease in the HCO_3^- (below 22 meq/L). The decrease in the HCO_3^- can occur as a result of gastrointestinal disorders (e.g. diarrhea), endocrine disorders (e.g., diabetic ketoacidosis), nutritional deficiency, and/or renal disorders (e.g. renal tubular acidosis, acute kidney injury, chronic renal insufficiency, etc.).

Metabolic Alkalosis: High pH and High HCO$_3^-$

Metabolic alkalosis occurs when the pH of the bloodstream is greater than 7.45 and there is an increase in the HCO_3^- (above 26 meq/L). The increase in the HCO_3^- can occur as a result of gastrointestinal disorders (e.g., prolonged emesis), prolonged gastric suctioning with a nasogastric (NG) tube, hypochloremia, administration of diuretics (e.g., furosemide), and/or elevated levels of aldosterone.

Simple Steps to Interpreting ABG

Step 1: Look at the pH and determine whether it is acidic or alkalotic

If the pH is < 7.35 there is an acidosis

If the pH is > 7.45 there is an alkalosis

Step 2: Asses the $PaCO_2$

If the $PaCO_2$ is > 45 mmHg: the primary disorder is respiratory acidosis

If the $PaCO_2$ is < 35 mmHg: the primary disorder is respiratory alkalosis

Step 3: Asses the HCO_3^-

If the HCO_3^- is > 26 meq/L: the primary disorder is metabolic alkalosis

If the HCO_3^- is < 22 meq/L: the primary disorder is metabolic acidosis

	Respiratory Acidosis	Respiratory Alkalosis	Metabolic Acidosis	Metabolic Alkalosis
pH	↓	↑	↓	↑
$PaCO_2$	↑	↓	Normal / ↓	Normal / ↑
HCO_3^-	Normal / ↑	Normal / ↓	↑	↑

PEDIATRICS

Many of the pulmonary disorders of the neonate and pediatric population overlap with that of the adult population. However, the etiology of some pulmonary disorders may vary, e.g., respiratory distress syndrome. In other instances, the neonate and pediatric population experience disorders that are not common to the adult population. This section is designed to briefly cover the above disorders specific to the neonate and pediatric population, as well as those whose etiology are different in these populations.

Respiratory Distress Syndrome (RDS)

Where adult Respiratory Distress Syndrome is caused by pulmonary parenchymal damage and resulting pulmonary edema, RDS of the neonate is caused by lack of surfactant. Almost exclusively, this occurs in premature infants. There also appears to be an increased frequency in male infants and infants born to mothers with diabetes and via caesarean delivery. The lack of surfactant leads to the inability to counter the surface tension on the intraalveolar membrane, resulting in alveolar collapse. The symptoms of RDS are similar to ARDS, with hypoxia, dyspnea, cyanosis, nasal flaring, and tachypnea. Chest radiograph will show bilateral, diffuse reticular granular or ground-glass appearances, air bronchograms, and poor lung expansion. Other tests that are helpful are ABG and continuous pulse oximetry.

There is active treatment of the disease as well as prophylactic measures in the prepartum period. In the prepartum period, when it is clear that there is a risk of premature birth, i.e., before 35–36 weeks, mothers receive antenatal steroids to enhance pulmonary maturity. Resuscitation efforts are aggressively pursued in the peripartum period as well with placental transfusion and immediate use of continuous positive airway pressure (CPAP). In the postpartum period, treatment is directed toward early administration of surfactant and using gentle modes of ventilation to minimize damage to the immature lungs. Sometimes, despite aggressive intervention, RDS may result in bronchopulmonary dysplasia (BPD), patent ductus arteriosus (PDA), apnea, hypertension, failure to thrive (FTT), intracranial hemorrhage, and/or preventricular leukomalacia with neurological deficits.

Acute Respiratory Infections

Neonates and pediatric patients also experience pneumonia, but the pathogens vary based on the age group.

Pathogens more likely to affect **newborns** are group B streptococcus, Listeria monocytogenes, gram-negative rod (GNR). The basis for this group of pathogens is the exposure to the vaginal tract and in utero environment. When the newborn is infected with the above organisms, he/she will generally be febrile and manifest symptoms characteristic of pulmonary disease (e.g., hypoxia, tachypnea, cyanosis, nasal flaring, etc.). However, there are organisms that can infect the newborn and manifest as an afebrile pneumonia. These include *Chlamydia pneumoniae, Ureaplasma urealyticum, Mycoplasma hominis, cytomegalovirus* (CMV), and *Pneumocystis carinii* (PCP). The basis for these pathogen profiles is not only the unique exposure in the birth canal, but neonates are not immunocompetent, making them susceptible to infections with CMV, PCP, and other pathogens that do not affect immunocompetent hosts.

In contrast, where bacterial organisms primarily infect newborns, the majority (90 percent) of acute respiratory infections of **infants and toddlers** are viral. Viral infection in infants and toddlers can clinically be described as bronchiolitis and/or croup. **Bronchiolitis** refers to inflammation in the bronchioles that may result from viral infection, primarily from respiratory syncytial virus (RSV). RSV is the most common viral pathogen and primarily affects infants/toddlers in the winter. Viral infections that are more predominant in the spring include parainfluenza types 1, 2, and 3 and influenza A or B. It is important to note that metapneumovirus has also been identified in this age group and can present similar to the clinical picture of RSV. **Croup** is characterized by a barking cough, inspiratory stridor, and hoarseness due to obstruction in the region of the larynx. In short, the causes of croup are parainfluenzae type 1 and diphtheria, although other types of parainfluenzae can cause similar symptoms. Croup can be prevented by immunization for influenza and diphtheria. An important risk factor in the acquisition of pneumococcal infection is day care attendance. Older toddlers (4–5 years of age) that attend day care are at risk for infection with invasive pneumococcus and can be treated with antibiotics. For reasons that are not completely clear, a history of breast feeding seems to protect against this infection. In cases of croup and bronchiolitis, antibiotics are not useful since the etiology is viral. However, steroids seem to be beneficial, likely due to decreased airway inflammation. Furthermore, a dose of epinephrine, although short-acting, may be indicated in acute hypoxia and respiratory distress due to airway inflammation and edema.

As children become old enough to begin attending school (≥ **5 years of age**), the prevalence of *Mycoplasma pneumoniae* (aka "walking pneumonia") increases with age, accounting for almost 50 percent of reported cases of pneumonia in college-age young adults. Symptoms are gradual and patients may be, in fact, asymptomatic. The term "walking pneumonia" refers to the fact that the chest radiograph appears much worse than the symptoms. If and when school-aged children present with a bacterial pneumonia, it will be clinically very similar to that of adults with tachypnea, fever, possibly chills, and with or without hypoxia. However, mycobacterial infection (tuberculosis) may infect school-aged children and if not treated, will develop into extrapulmonary disease and can have devastating lifelong effects.

Apnea of Prematurity (AOP)

Apnea of prematurity (AOP) is a significant disorder that may present to health care workers in intensive care nurseries. Unfortunately, there is no consensus in the definition, diagnosis, or treatment of AOP. Overall, the discussion behind the etiology of AOP is ongoing and the key point is that premature infants are more prone to apnea than mature infants, and that while many factors contribute to AOP, the common ground seems to be a correlation with *gastroesophageal reflux* (GER). Breathing is regulated centrally; hence, apnea may be central in nature. Central apnea in the newborn is due to decreased respiratory drive to the muscles of respiration. Hypoxia, hyperthermia, and adenosine are believed to initiate apnea in the newborn due to their effect on the respiratory drive of the medulla. This may be part of the reason behind the observation that there is a decreased sensitivity of central chemoreceptors to increased CO_2 concentrations in the blood in premature infants. Finally, upper airway obstruction due to immature development and inability to maintain a patent airway may also contribute to AOP.

Since premature infants will be hospitalized in intensive care settings after birth more frequently, it is important that intensive care health care workers be able to identify AOP. As such, the history will generally be observation of the trained health care worker. It is important to know that infants do experience periodic breathing that may be mistaken with AOP, but should not be confused by the certified health care ICU professional. Further, it is important to look for other changes in vital signs, which is easily done in the ICU since cardiopulmonary monitoring is constant. Hypotension and bradycardia may exist.

Once other possible causes of AOP have been ruled out, the clinical diagnosis of AOP may be made. A proper workup would include EKG, EEG, and possibly intraesophageal pH monitoring (if GER is suspected). The treatment for AOP is supplemental oxygen, tactile stimulation, and possibly CPAP, if the above measures do not result in resolution of the AOP.

Bronchopulmonary Dysplasia

Bronchopulmonary dysplasia (BPD) was formerly known as chronic lung disease of infancy. Clinically, BPD is diagnosed on the basis of dependence on supplemental oxygen beyond 30 days after birth. BPD is most often obvious within the first four weeks of life. BPD is generally associated with RDS. Consequently, it is no surprise that infants who suffer from BPD more frequently have low birth weights, are born prematurely, and have undergone mechanical ventilation. This introduces a certain amount of pulmonary trauma, despite the fact that the benefits outweigh the risks of treatment of RDS. As a result, inflammation and scarring manifest in the lung parenchyma, which are the histological findings characteristic of BPD. Further, the barotraumas from mechanical ventilation can result in necrotizing bronchiolitis with alveolar septal injury. There may also be dilated acini with this alveolar septa without fibrosis. Chest radiographic studies, possibly, with CT and MRI of the chest may be useful studies in determining the severity of the BPD.

Treatment is primarily supportive, including nutritional supplementation, fluid restriction (to limit or prevent edema), diuretics (to treat pulmonary edema), and perhaps inhaled bronchodilators. The treatment of BPD revolves mainly around the treatment of RDS and histologic manifestations of BPD. Hence, surfactant and supplemental oxygen therapy should be initiated with CPAP to maintain patent alveoli and recruit as much of the pulmonary parenchyma as possible for gas exchange. Despite attempts to only use NPPV to avoid baro- and volutrauma, invasive mechanical ventilation modes may be required. There are suggestions that synchronized intermittent mechanical ventilation (SIMV) and high-frequency jet ventilation (HFJV) or high-frequency oscillatory ventilation (HFOV) are useful in minimizing the barotraumas, but there is no consensus behind these recommendations at the moment. Oxygenation is generally monitored by continuous oximetry. However, it is important to refrain from hyperoxygenation of infants and neonates, as this may result in suppression of the respiratory drive. The recommended oxygenation is 88–95 percent—as measured by oximetry. If there is evidence of infection, it is recommended that this be treated.

Transient Tachypnea of the Newborn (TTN, aka Neonatal Wet Lung Syndrome)

Transient tachypnea of the newborn is also known as Neonatal Wet Lung Syndrome. The primary etiology behind TTN is an inability of the neonate to clear excess fluid from the lung parenchyma and is seen in premature infants, term infants delivered by cesarean section, infants with respiratory depression, and term infants born in the presence of meconium-stained amniotic fluid.

Symptoms will be present almost immediately after birth and will include tachypnea, grunting, accessory muscle use with evidence of retractions, and, possibly, cyanosis may develop. Chest radiograph will show hyper-inflated lungs with streaky perihilar markings. Depending on the amount of pulmonary edema, the chest radiograph may show fluid in the fissures between lung lobes.

Since there will likely be an oxygenation deficit, treatment consists of administering supplemental oxygen. However, NPPV, such as CPAP, may be used if neurological deficits or other anatomical deficits are present that hinder the patients respiratory drive. The condition generally resolves after two to four days of treatment. Oxygenation may be adequately monitored by oximetry, but ABG may also be used, if absolutely necessary.

Mechanical Ventilation

For the most part, mechanical ventilation for neonates and pediatrics is similar to adults with some minor notations in details. First, oxygen delivery can be delivered via nasal cannula and facemask (similar to the adult); however, for infants and neonates a hood may also be used to insure oxygen delivery. As stated above, oxygen saturation of 88–95 percent is desirable. Neonates and infants will tolerate a lower saturation, because it will be easier to fully saturate the hemoglobin since fetal hemoglobin will comprise the majority of red blood cells at that time point. Oxygen should also be warmed prior to delivery since neonates and infants cannot self-regulate body temperature; this will also prevent bronchospasms. Where ABGs are obtained primarily from a radial artery puncture in adults, in neonates and infants, an umbilical artery catheter is placed.

NPPV

In pediatrics the premise behind CPAP/BiPAP is the same. However, lower pressures will be needed in neonates, infants, and children.

Invasive Mechanical Ventilation

Again, the premise behind invasive mechanical ventilation is the same, except smaller endo-tracheal tubes and smaller tidal volumes and pressures will be needed than in the adult. For example, adults will generally need an endotracheal tube of about 7.0–8.0 mm whereas infants will need an endotracheal tube of about 2.5–3.5 mm.

Congenital Anomalies

Congenital anomalies are primarily anatomical in nature; some require supportive treat-ment, while others require urgent surgical intervention. For the purpose of the CCRN, it is important to have a general understanding of these anomalies. You do not need to under-stand them in great depth.

At the basic level, you need to understand that the airway is described in relationship to the larynx ("voice-box"). The glottis is the space between the vocal folds, the area above this is referred to as the supraglottis, and below the glottis/larynx the space is referred to as the subglottis. Congenital anomalies may occur in these three areas. Infants/neonates with congenital anomalies may present with cyanosis, tachypnea, weakened cry, feeding abnor-malities (e.g., inability to tolerate feedings due to cyanosis or regurgitation), aspiration, and stridor (inspiratory). These symptoms can be present with anomalies present at all three anatomical locations.

Anomalies of the Supraglottis

The primary anomalies of the supraglottis are laryngomalacia, supraglottic webs, bifid epi-glottis, sacular cysts, laryngocoele, and lymphatic/vascular malformations. Laryngomala-cia is responsible for about 60–70 percent of supraglottic congenital anomalies and refers to underdevelopment of the larynx. This may be associated with an abnormal shape of the epiglottis (omega shape). Laryngomalacia is not fatal, but apnea has been noted due to the weakness of the larynx and its inability to resist collapse when the patient is sleeping. A vari-ety of surgical procedures has been tried in the past, including tracheostomy, but currently supraglottoplasty is performed in symptomatic cases. Supraglottic webs are diaphragmatic growths that vary in size and may occlude the supraglottis. This is a rare disorder (less than 1–2 percent). Treatment consists of surgical excision. Lymphatic and vascular abnormalities such as hemangiomas are similar in their occurrence and treatment. Bifid epliglottis is also a rare disorder and consists of malformation of the epiglottis (as the name implies). These patients need to undergo a complete endocrine evaluation, because this malformation is associated with Pallister-Hall Syndrome (polydactyl, hypothalamic hamaratoma, imperforate anus, kidney anomalies). Saccular cysts are vestigial remnants of fluid filled sacs in the supra-glottic region. They can obstruct the airway and should be surgically excised. Laryngocoeles are air filled, in contrast to the fluid sacular cysts.

Anomalies of the Glottis and Subglottis

These anomalies mimic those of the supraglottis. Laryngeal webs, hemangiomas, and under-development (laryngeal atresia) are the main congenital abnormalities of the glottis. However, since the vocal cords are housed in the glottis, congenital vocal cord paralysis may also occur and accounts for almost 25 percent of glottic anomalies. Treatments are similar to those of the supraglottis. Stenosis can occur at all three levels, but of these three anatomic areas, subglottic stenosis is the most prevalent. Opening with placement of stents may be necessary or surgical correction may be undertaken. Stenosis of the airways can sometimes follow prolonged and/or difficult intubations.

The Endocrine System

The endocrine system is the essential regulator of the body's internal environment. It is important to delineate the difference between endocrine and exocrine glands. Endocrine glands secrete their hormones into the bloodstream, where exocrine glands secrete their hormones/enzymes into ducts. Together with the nervous system, the endocrine system regulates growth, reproduction, sex differentiation, metabolism, fluid and electrolyte balance, and internal homeostasis.

FIGURE 6.1 *The Endocrine System*

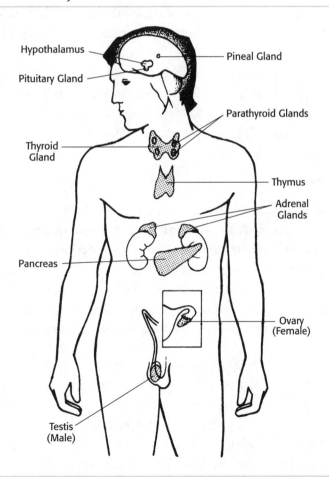

HORMONES

Hormones are chemical messengers that have an effect on target cells distant from the secreting cells. While most hormones travel in the blood, we also know more recently that some hormones never enter the blood and instead act locally in the area where they are released. Hormones that act more locally are described as paracrine (acting on neighboring cells) or autocrine (acting on the cell from which the hormone was secreted) messengers.

Hormones travel to target cells, where they act on specific receptors on the target cell. Some hormone receptors are located on the surface of the cell and act through second messenger mechanisms. Other receptors are located within the cell where they directly influence the synthesis of proteins. After acting on specific receptors on the target cells, hormones are metabolized or inactivated by the target tissues or by the liver. They are excreted by the kidneys to prevent excessive amounts from accumulating in the body over a period of time.

Types

Hormones modulate four broad categories of body function: growth and development, maintenance of homeostasis, energy production during metabolic processes, and reproduction. There are three categories of hormones: peptides, steroids, and amines. Peptides (also called protein hormones) include vasopressin (ADH), thyrotropin-releasing hormone (TRH), insulin, growth hormone (GH), follicle-stimulating hormone (FSH), luteinizing hormone (LH), corticotropin (ACTH), and calcitonin. The steroids include aldosterone, cortisol, estradiol, progesterone, and testosterone. Amines (amino acid derivatives) include norepinephrine, epinephrine, triiodothyronine (T_3), and thyroxine (T_4).

Feedback Mechanisms

Some hormones are needed in very small amounts and act for variable amounts of time, where other hormones have a prolonged period of cellular action; some interact with other hormones producing a very complex and intricate system of control. The levels of many of the hormones are regulated by positive and negative feedback mechanisms, although the majority of hormones are controlled by negative feedback. The levels of many hormones are regulated by feedback mechanisms that involve the hypothalamic pituitary target cell system. The hypothalamus and pituitary provide a more complex control system for some hormones.

The hypothalamus secretes releasing or inhibiting factors such as thyrotropin releasing factor (TRF), which acts on the pituitary gland to secrete thyroid stimulating hormone (TSH). TSH then stimulates the thyroid gland to increase secretion of the thyroid hormones. The release of the thyroid hormones (T_3, T_4) into the circulation results in an increase in metabolism (the biological effect of thyroid hormone). High levels of the thyroid hormones *inhibit* secretion of TSH. This is an example of negative feedback and allows tight control over hormone levels.

ANATOMY AND PHYSIOLOGY

Pituitary Gland

The pituitary gland is located in the sella turcica of the sphenoid bone. It is connected to the hypothalamus by the pituitary stalk and links the nervous and endocrine systems. The two lobes of the pituitary gland are the adenohypophysis (anterior pituitary) and the neurohypophysis (posterior pituitary). Hormones of the anterior lobe (75 percent of gland) are controlled by hypothalamic releasing or inhibiting hormones from the hypothalamus, in response to stimuli received in the central nervous system. These releasing and inhibiting hormones are delivered from the hypothalamus to the anterior pituitary by a portal circulation. Posterior lobe (25 percent of gland) hormones are controlled by nerve fibers beginning in the hypothalamus and ending in the neurohypophysis. The hormones are synthesized in the hypothalamus, stored in the posterior lobe, and then released after activation of the cell bodies in the nerve tract.

The anterior pituitary hormones can be remembered by the pneumonic "FLAT PEG." This acronym stands for **F**SH, **L**H, **A**CTH, **T**SH, **P**rolactin, **E**ndorphins, and **G**rowth Hormone. Posterior pituitary hormones are vasopressin (aka antidiuretic hormone, ADH) and oxytocin (not discussed in this chapter).

FIGURE 6.2 *Hypothalamus and Pituitary Gland*

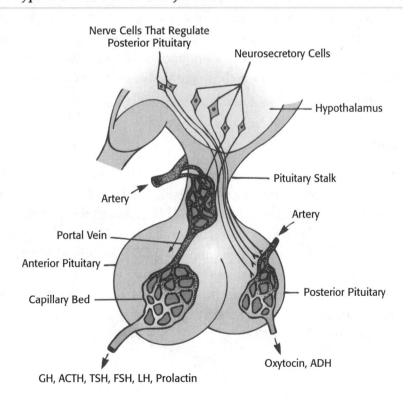

Growth hormone (GH), also called somatotropin, exerts powerful effects on growth and metabolism; it increases protein synthesis, elevates blood glucose levels, increases lipolysis, promotes positive nitrogen balance, and stimulates bone and cartilage growth. Disorders resulting from dysfunction are gigantism or acromegaly with excess and dwarfism with deficiency. Adrenocorticotropic hormone (ACTH) secretion is stimulated by corticotropin-releasing hormone (CRH) in response to physical and/or emotional stress, trauma, hypoglycemia, hypoxia, surgery, and decreased plasma cortisol level. It is inhibited by increased plasma cortisol levels, but stress can override this negative feedback. Disorders resulting from dysfunction are Cushing's disease with excess and adrenal insufficiency or Addisonian crisis with deficiency. TRH stimulates TSH in response to low plasma concentration of thyroid hormones. TRH is inhibited by high plasma concentrations of thyroid hormones. Disorders resulting from dysfunction are hyperthyroidism and thyroid storm from excess thyroid hormones, hypothyroidism, and myxedema coma with deficiency.

Posterior pituitary hormones are ADH and oxytocin (not discussed in this chapter). ADH regulates water balance and plasma osmolality. The site of action of ADH is the collecting ducts and distal convoluted tubules of the nephron. ADH directly increases the reabsorption of water, causes vasoconstriction, and, in the CNS, acts to lower body temperature and facilitate memory. There may be excess ADH secretion or a deficiency of secretion in the body. In instances when ADH is being secreted secondary to causes other than serum osmolality or electrolyte concentration, this is referred to as a Syndrome of Inappropriate ADH secretion (SIADH). The lack of ADH activity is manifested as profuse dilute urination, because water is not being reabsorbed. This is referred to as diabetes insipidus and can be categorized as central (lack of secretion from the posterior pituitary or lack of secretion in the hypothalamus) or peripheral (lack of DH effect in the nephron due to lack of or inactivation of ADH receptors in the kidney).

Thyroid Gland

The thyroid gland is located immediately below the larynx, on either side and anterior to the trachea. There are two lobes connected by an isthmus. Three hormones are produced by the thyroid gland: triiodothyronine (T_3), thyroxine (T_4), and calcitonin. Follicular cells produce T_3 and T_4. Parafollicular cells produce thyrocalcitonin. T_3 and T_4 regulate the body's metabolic rate, influence growth and development, have a positive chronotropic and inotropic effects on the heart, increase erythropoiesis, regulate temperature, and are needed for normal hypoxic and hypercapnic drive in the respiratory center. Disorders resulting from thyroid dysfunction are hyperthyroidism and thyroid storm from excess, and hypothyroidism and myxedema coma with deficiency.

Thyrocalcitonin (calcitonin) affects bone metabolism. It decreases serum calcium by inhibiting calcium mobilization from bone and decreasing calcium resorption in the kidney. Phosphate levels are decreased by inhibiting bone remodeling and increasing phosphate loss in urine.

Parathyroid Glands

Four parathyroid glands are located on the posterior surface of the thyroid gland at the upper and lower ends of each lobe. They receive their blood supply from the thyroid gland and are often damaged by thyroid surgery. Parathyroid hormone (PTH) is released by the chief cells of the parathyroid gland. Stimulation of PTH increases serum calcium levels through direct action in the bone, small intestine, and kidney. Inhibition of PTH decreases serum calcium levels, decreases vitamin D metabolites, and may alter magnesium levels. Disorders resulting from parathyroid dysfunction are hypercalcemia from excess and hypocalcemia from deficiency.

Adrenal Glands

The adrenal glands are located on the upper lobes of each kidney. They are composed of two separate tissues: the adrenal cortex (outer layer) and the adrenal medulla (inner layer). The adrenal cortex (90 percent of the gland) produces three classes of hormones: mineralocorticoids (e.g., aldosterone), glucocorticoids (e.g., cortisol and cortisone), and androgens (e.g., DHEA). Aldosterone helps regulate electrolyte balance by promoting sodium reabsorption and potassium loss. Disorders resulting from dysfunction are primary aldosteronism from excess and Addison's disease or adrenal crisis from deficiency.

FIGURE 6.3 *Adrenal Gland: Cortex and Medulla*

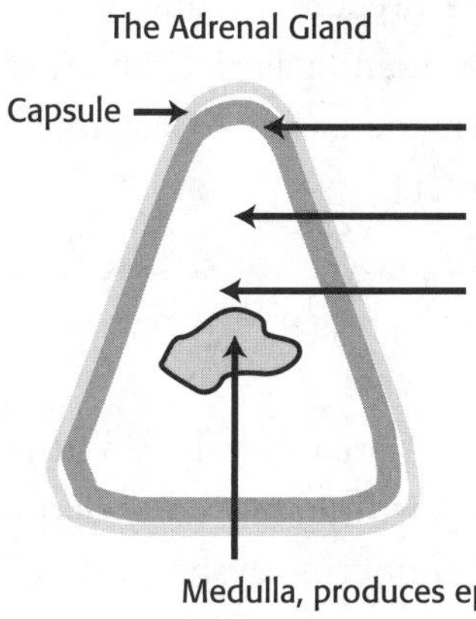

The Adrenal Gland

Capsule

Region	Hormones	Control system
Zona Glomerulosa	Aldosterone	Angiotensin II, $[K^+]_{plasma}$
Zona Fasciculata	Cortisol	ACTH
Zona Reticularis	Androgens	ACTH (LH has no effect here)

Medulla, produces epinephrine, controlled by sympathetic nervous system

Cortisol influences carbohydrate storage, has anti-inflammatory effects, suppresses corticotropin secretion, and increases protein catabolism. Disorders resulting from adrenal cortex dysfunction are Cushing's syndrome from excess and Addison's disease or adrenal crisis from deficiency. Pheochromocytoma is due to excess hormone production by the adrenal medulla.

The adrenal medulla (10 percent of the adrenal gland) produces two catecholamines: epinephrine (e.g., adrenaline) and norepinephrine (e.g., noradrenaline). Epinephrine is a positive inotrope and a major insulin antagonist, and is responsible for the fight or flight (stress) response. Norepinephrine is a potent peripheral vasoconstrictor. Disorder resulting from excess is pheochromocytoma, a tumor that produces epinephrine and/or norepinephrine causing labile hypertension.

Pancreas

The pancreas is located transversely in the left upper abdominal quadrant, behind the peritoneum and stomach. It has both exocrine and endocrine components. The endocrine functions originate from the islets of Langerhans (which constitute two percent of the total pancreatic volume). There are three types of specialized islet cells: alpha, beta, and delta. The beta cells (65 percent of the gland) produce insulin. Insulin decreases blood glucose, promotes synthesis of proteins, carbohydrates, lipids, and nucleic acids, facilitates active transport of glucose across cell membranes, increases glucose uptake by the liver, stimulates glycogen and fatty acid synthesis in the liver, inhibits gluconeogenesis and glycogenolysis by the liver, facilitates the intracellular transport of potassium, and stimulates protein synthesis by muscle cells. Disorders resulting from dysfunction are hypoglycemia from excess and Type I diabetes mellitus (DM-I) from deficiency. Complications of DM-I include diabetic ketoacidosis and hyperosmolar hyperglycemia syndrome. The alpha cells produce glucagon. Glucagon increases blood glucose levels, increases lipolysis, increases amino acid transport to the liver for conversion to glucose precursors, and is a major insulin-antagonistic hormone. Delta cells produce somatostatin and gastrin. Somatostatin inhibits secretion of insulin, glucagon, growth hormone, TSH, and gastrin. Gastrin acts on the stomach and gallbladder and is not discussed in this chapter.

ASSESSMENT

The clinical assessment is primarily carried out by analyzing laboratory values and radiological studies, since most endocrine glands are seated deep within the body. However, the signs and symptoms of an imbalance or malfunctioning endocrine system can also be picked up during the history-taking. Knowledge of the anatomy and physiology discussed in the previous section helps the critical care nurse with interpretation of her assessment findings. Assessment of the endocrine system begins with the history. The health history interview collects subjective data. The second portion is the physical examination of the endocrine system, which collects objective data. Since most of the endocrine glands are deeply encased in the body, direct examination is difficult. The use of indirect measures (laboratory, radiology) allows the critical care nurse to assess the physiology of the gland by monitoring the target tissue.

History of Present Illness

The initial patient presentation determines the urgency and direction of the interview. For patients in acute distress, the history involves questions focusing on the chief complaint and precipitating events. When presenting in a critical care setting, many patients will be in acute distress. This acute distress may or may not be due to a patient's known or unknown endocrine diseases. With this in mind it is important to ask questions, as with all organ systems, during the history-taking process that are directly related to the chief complaint. However, to identify potential endocrine issues, a thorough understanding of the anatomy and physiology is paramount. For example, for those that may present with hypotension and tachycardia, the patient may have atrial fibrillation with rapid ventricular response. In such a case, the patient should be questioned about signs and/or symptoms that may be related to hyperthyroidism (e.g., weight loss, heat intolerance, menstrual cycle abnormalities in women, dry skin, hair loss, vision trouble, etc.). Questions in the history taking process regarding prenatal history, such as exposure to drugs, alcohol, infections, radiation, and pregnancy complications may be useful, but should be reserved only for situations where the patient is not in acute distress and has been stabilized. The neonatal history should include gestational age, delivery method, Apgar scores, complications of labor and delivery, congenital anomalies, and any postnatal complications. History for a child includes factors such as, height and weight, diet, developmental milestones, and growth patterns. These later types of questions play a small role in the treatment of acutely ill adult patients. However, for those working in pediatric critical care, this information may be more useful and is often readily available from parents or guardians and the medical record.

The patient's chief complaint is why he is seeking help and how long the problem has existed. Have the patient describe when the problem started, what symptoms were experienced, any treatments tried, and the effect of the treatments. This helps to focus the interview and physical examination. A review of the patient's past medical and surgical history helps to identify any preexisting or traumatic endocrine dysfunction. Next, a review of any medications taken regularly or as needed, including prescription, over-the-counter, and herbal remedies may identify occult problems. Indicators of altered health patterns include:

- Cognitive changes (vision, personality, depression, memory)

- Nutrition/metabolism (weight change, GI upset, edema, heat/cold intolerance)

- Elimination (diarrhea, constipation, polyuria, nocturia, excessive sweating)

- Activity/exercise (fatigue, weakness, impaired activities of daily living)

- Sleep/rest (restlessness, insomnia, excessive sleeping)

- Sexual (decreased libido, impotence, menstrual irregularities, infertility)

- Coping/stress (past or present psychiatric history, coping mechanisms)

Then, determine the patient's perception and what behaviors he uses to manage his health. Next, review any family history of endocrine disorders and social history, including the use of tobacco products, alcohol, or illicit drug use.

The focus and extent of the examination is dependent on the patient's symptoms and the probable or actual diagnosis. Assessment begins with observation of the patient's level of consciousness. The nurse takes note of the patient's speech pattern, mental status, intellectual functioning, reasoning ability, and movement or lack of movement of all extremities while obtaining a health history. If the patient is alert, able to state his name, where he is, and what day it is, proceed with the health history. When the patient is comatose or too lethargic to cooperate, the nurse must access secondary sources such as family or significant others.

Physical Examination

Inspection and palpation start with a general inspection of the patient including stature and posture; fat distribution; any gross deformities or asymmetry; hair distribution and texture; and any visible scars, goiter, or edema. Vital signs including blood pressure (lying, sitting, standing); heart rate and rhythm; respirations (rate, depth, rhythm); temperature; and height and weight should be obtained. Examination of the head and neck involves checking eyes for exophthalmos, strabismus, facial or periorbital edema, visual acuity, facial bone structure, and thyroid gland (enlargement, palpable mass, nodules, tenderness, and palpable thrill). Skin, hair, and nail examination includes color, texture, turgor, temperature, evidence of bruising, striae, thinning, edema, acne, spider angiomas, alopecia, brittle nails, and tongue enlargement or protrusion. In addition, cardiac point of maximal impulse; heaves; breath odor; mental status; pupil size, shape, and reactivity; and any visible tremors should be assessed. Deep tendon reflexes are assessed next. Ascultation includes:

- Neck: bruits over thyroid gland

- Heart: distant heart sounds; third heart sound

- Lungs: crackles or stridor

- GI: hyperactive or hypoactive bowel sounds

Diagnostic Studies

Laboratory studies of blood and urine includes the following: chemistry (electrolytes, renal panel, ketones, glycosylated hemoglobin), hormone levels (TSH, T_3, T_4, ACTH, random cortisol, ADH, activated PTH, FSH, LH, testosterone), CBC, arterial blood gases (ABGs), nutritional labs (vitamin D, B1, B6, B12, folate), plasma and urine osmolality/osmolarity, and urinalysis. Radiology studies include x-ray (skull, chest, abdomen); scans (thyroid, pancreas); CT; MRI; angiography; and a bone mineral densitometry (DEXA scan). In addition, an ECG and visual field testing should be done.

PATHOLOGIES

Diabetes Insipidus (DI)

Diabetes insipidus is defined as either a deficiency of or insensitivity to ADH. This leads to an inability to concentrate urine with the resultant volume depletion. The presenting signs and symptoms are the result of dehydration and hypernatremia. DI can complicate the course of the critically ill patient and result in acute, life-threatening fluid and electrolyte disturbances.

Three types of diabetes insipidus have been identified: **neurogenic, nephrogenic and dipsogenic**. *Neurogenic* (hypothalmic or central) DI is due to damage of the posterior pituitary gland by tumors or trauma, causing insufficient amounts of ADH to be synthesized, transported, or released. *Nephrogenic* DI (peripheral) is an inadequate response by the kidneys to ADH, usually related to kidney disorders or drug toxicity and is fairly uncommon. *Dipsogenic* DI (primary polydipsia) results from the oral intake of large amounts of water, which suppresses the release of ADH, causing polyuria. Impaired ADH activity causes rapid excretion of large amounts of dilute urine, increasing plasma osmolality and decreasing urine osmolality.

Causes of Diabetes Insipidus

Neurogenic (central) Congenital	Nephrogenic Pyelonephritis	Dipsogenic Idiopathic
Idiopathic	Amyloidosis	Psychoses (compulsive water drinking)
Trauma	Sarcoidosis	Impaired thirst mechanism
Surgery	Polycystic kidney disease	
Primary/Metastatic malignancies	Multiple myeloma	
Autoimmune diseases	Sickle cell disease	
Infections	Nephrotoxic drugs	

When DI is seen following brain surgery or head trauma, it usually occurs in the first one to three days after the inciting event. Trauma (including brain surgery) may lead to edema of the hypothalamus and/or the neurohypophysis, causing a decreased secretion of ADH. The reason this takes time to manifest is that the posterior pituitary often has reserve amounts of ADH stored and it takes some time to deplete these stores. If there is damage to the supraoptic nuclei in the hypothalamus and/or proximal end of the pituitary stalk, then permanent DI will ensue; however, in most cases it is transient and resolves with resolution of the edema. *Primary polydipsia* is the inappropriate drinking of water, despite normal hydration or even over-hydration. It can occur due to hypokalemia, hypercalcemia, or increased angiotension II levels. It is usually **psychogenic** in origin and found, most often, in patients with a history of psychosis, hysteria, or depression. They often have irrational faith that more water will rid them of a real or imagined disease (hiccups, worms, poisons, or cancer). Dipsogenic patients have a plasma osmolality lower than normal.

Clinical manifestations include *polyuria, polydipsia, hypernatremia, hyperosmolality, hypotension,* and *mental status changes.* Initially urine output may exceed 300 ml per hour (2 to 20 liters per day), regardless of intake. Alert patients have excessive thirst and may consume as much as 5 to 20 liters of fluids per day. When the patient is unable to replace the fluid lost by responding to thirst, signs of hypovolemia will develop: hypotension, decreased skin turgor, hypernatremia, dry mucous membranes, tachycardia, low central venous (CVP), low venous oxygen saturation (SVO_2), and pulmonary artery occlusion pressures (PAOP, otherwise also known as wedge pressure). Hypernatremia results from hypovolemia due to concentration of the serum sodium from polyuria. Hyperosmolality is the increased concentration of solutes in the serum. This will correspond with a decreased urine osmolality, since the urine should be correspondingly dilute. Mental status changes such as confusion, irritability, and seizures are related to the increased serum osmolality and hypernatremia, causing neural cells to shrink. Hypotension is secondary to volume depletion (polyuria).

Diagnostic Procedures

- Negative running fluid balance

- UA: Colorless, odorless, specific gravity < 1.005, sodium < 20 mEq/L, and osmolality < 300 msom/L.

- Serum osmolality > 295 mosm/L, sodium > 145 MEq/L increased BUN and creatinine.

- Water Restriction test can help discriminate between neurogenic and nephrogenic DI. Baseline values for serum ADH, serum and urine osmolalities, and serum sodium concentrations are obtained. Then measure the urine volume, urine osmolality every hour and the serums' sodium and osmolality every two hours. If the urine

TABLE 6.1 *Interpreting the Results of Water Restriction Tests and Exogenous ADH*

Primary Polydipsia	• Urine osmolality > Plasma osmolality • Urine osmolality increases minimally (<10%) after exogenous ADH
Central Diabetes Insipidus	• Urine osmolality remains less than plasma osmolality after water restriction • After ADH is given, urine osms increase 50–100% in complete CDI
Nephrogenic Diabetes Insipidus	• Urine osmolality remains less than plasma osmolality • After ADH, urine osms increase by less than 50%

osmolaity reaches 600 mOsm/kg, then the ADH secretion and response are both intact and there is no DI. However, the test should be stopped earlier to prevent harm to the patient. The criteria to stop the test are if a normal response is obtained as stated above, the urine osmolality remains the same on two to three consecutive hourly assessments despite rising serum osmolality, and the serum osmolality exceeds 295–300 mOsm/kg. In a normal patient, the urine osmolality can be concentrated upwards of 1000–1200 mOsm/kg when deprived of water.

- Vasopressin test differentiates between neurogenic and nephrogenic DI. First give no fluids. Measure output hourly to get a baseline. Then give Pitressin (ADH) five units SQ, IM, or IV or desmopressin (DDAVP) 10 mcg nasal spray or 1 mcg SQ. Urine is measured at 30-60-90-120 minute intervals. If the urine volume decreases *and* the urine osmolality increases more than 50 percent, the test is positive for neurogenic DI. The patient with nephrogenic DI will either not respond or will respond with less than 50 percent increase in the urine osmolality.

- Serum osmolality can be estimated by the following formula:

$$\text{Serum osmolality} = 2(\text{serum Na}) + \text{BUN}/2.8 + \text{Glucose}/18 = (275–295 \text{ mOsm})$$

Treatment

The goals of treatment are to identify and correct the underlying cause and restore normal fluid volume, osmolality, and electrolyte balance. If the patient is alert and able to respond to thirst, she will generally drink enough fluids to avoid symptomatic hypovolemia. Patients in the critical care unit and the elderly with cognitive impairments are unable to respond appropriately to thirst and fluid replacement is necessary. Volume replacement, especially if the patient is hypotensive, is rapid infusion of *hypotonic* (e.g., D5W) intravenous solutions and careful monitoring without a rapid reduction of serum sodium. Since the volume that is lost is simply extra water, we refer to this clinically as "free water," which means water without any solutes. The serum sodium (Na) is the marker that we use to measure the "free water deficit" in such patients. The amount of free water deficit can be estimated based on normal fluid stores and usual body weight, using the formula:

$$\text{Body water deficit in liters} = (0.6) \times (\text{weight in kg}) \times [(\text{serum sodium}/140) - 1]$$

The formula assumes that 60 percent of an individual's weight is fluid. The amount of estimated fluid deficit can be used as a guide for replacement fluids.

Medications used to successfully treat DI include desmopressin (DDAVP) and vasopressin (Pitressin) given as replacement for the decreased ADH. Pitressin is synthetic, but is identical in structure to naturally occurring ADH. Desmopressin is a structural analogue of ADH. Vasopressin has powerful vasoconstrictor actions and can cause adverse cardiovascular effects. By constricting arteries of the heart, it can cause angina pectoris or myocardial infarction. In addition, it may cause gangrene by decreasing the blood flow to the periphery. Desmopressin has very few vasoconstrictive (i.e., "pressor") effects and is the agent of choice because it has a long duration of action, is easy to administer, and lacks significant side effects. Potential adverse effects include: abdominal pain, transient headache, nasal congestion, rhinitis, nausea, and water intoxication especially young children and older adults. Caution patients to drink only enough to quench their thirst.

Nursing Responsibilities

Establish a baseline (weight, blood pressure, serum/urine osmolality, serum electrolytes, and strict intake/output) from which to monitor the effects of the drug, and coordinate testing throughout therapy. Monitor for possible cardiac adverse effects and possible nasal septum ulceration. Remove/stop offending chemical(s), if patient has nephrogenic DI. Maintain accurate input and output records and perform the testing as ordered by the physician at the proper times, as the osmolality will change with time and timing is essential in interpreting the results of the water restriction and DDAVP administration.

Syndrome of Inappropriate Antidiuretic Hormone Secretion (SIADH)

Syndrome of inappropriate antidiuretic hormone secretion is the excessive release of ADH without regard to plasma osmolality or fluid volume status. The normal inhibition of ADH by the posterior pituitary is absent, resulting in excessive reabsorption of water by the renal tubules and collecting ducts of the kidney. The presenting signs and symptoms are the result of hypervolemia and hyponatremia. SIADH can complicate the course of the critically ill patient and result in acute, life-threatening fluid and electrolyte disturbances.

Etiology

There are multiple causes of SIADH including ectopic ADH production, central nervous system disorders, and medications that increase or potentiate ADH secretion. Excess ADH production or utilization is seen in patients with malignant cancers (lung, pancreas, prostate, thymus, duodenum, Hodgkin's, and leukemia), nonmalignant pulmonary conditions (tuberculosis, pneumonia), CNS disorders (brain trauma, tetanus, meningitis, vascular lesions, Guillian-Barré syndrome), and medications (nicotine, TCAs, chemotherapeutic drugs, ADH therapy, lismapril, metoclopramide, narcotics, SSRIs, anesthetics).

Clinical signs and symptoms of SIADH are related to the hypovolemia and hyponatremia and may present as mild to severe. Symptoms of mild hyponatremia (serum sodium level less than 135 mEq/L) include low urine output, dark concentrated urine, thirst, dulled sensorium, dyspnea on exertion, hypertension, weight gain without edema, headache, and nausea. Central nervous system symptoms are due to cellular swelling, as a result of a reduction in the serum osmolality and hyponatremia. The severity and the rate of onset of the hyponatremia determine the extent of the mental status changes. As the water and sodium imbalance continue (sodium levels below 120 MEq/L), progressive neurological deterioration includes irritability, confusion, lack of concentration, apprehension, seizures, loss of consciousness, coma, and death.

Diagnostic Procedures

Laboratory values provide the diagnostic hallmarks of SIADH:

- UA: Dark, concentrated, specific gravity >1.025, sodium >20 mEq/L, and osmolality >300 msom/L

- Serum osmolality <275 mosm/L, sodium <135MEq/L, low BUN, creatinine, and albumin

- Water-loading test with elimination of less than 50 percent of the fluid challenge

Treatment

The goals of treatment are to identify and correct the underlying cause, eliminate excess water, and increase serum osmolality. In many instances, treatment of the underlying cause returns the patient's condition to normal. In mild to moderate SIADH (sodium 125 to 135 mEq/L), fluid restriction is calculated on the basis of individual needs and losses, a general criterion is 500 ml less than average daily output. Patients with severe hyponatremia (less than 115 mEq/L) or those experiencing seizure may be given hypertonic saline (3 percent or 5 percent). Hypertonic saline administration should be no faster than 1 to 2 ml/kg per hour to raise the serum sodium no more than 0.5 to 2 mEq/L per hour. Administration of a loop diuretic such as furosemide (Brand name: Lasix) prevents urine concentration when given with hypertonic saline, increasing the removal of the excess fluid.

Nursing Responsibilities

Establish a baseline (weight, blood pressure, serum/urine osmolality, serum electrolytes, and strict intake/output) from which to monitor the effects of treatment and coordinate testing throughout therapy. Monitor for possible cardiac adverse effects, including, distended neck veins. Remove/stop offending chemical(s). Correct electrolytes, slowly.

Thyrotoxic Crisis (Thyroid Storm)

Thyrotoxic crisis is a severe form of hyperthyroid disease often leading to systemic decompensation and can result in death within 48 hours without treatment. It occurs most often in patients with Grave's disease that is either undiagnosed or undertreated and is precipitated by another illness, injury, or surgery. Theories regarding the occurrence of thyrotoxic crisis include a change in the binding of thyroid hormone to albumin, a change in the thyroid hormone receptors of the target tissues, or an exaggerated response to sympathetic activity. Hyperthyroidism can produce a hyperdynamic, hypermetabolic state that disrupts major body functions.

The most frequent clinical symptoms of thyrotoxic crisis are high fever, tachycardia, palpitations, arrhythmias, altered respirations, fatigue, tremors, delirium, stupor, coma. Temperature regulation is lost and the patient's temperature may be as high as 106° F (41.1° C). The increased heat production and accumulated metabolic end products causes dilation of the blood vessels of the skin, the reason for warm moist skin. The increased metabolism and stimulation of catecholamines causes a hyperdynamic heart and may be severe enough to produce heart failure and cardiovascular collapse. Neurological disturbances are secondary to hypermetabolism, causing hyperactivity of the nervous system. The respiratory system responds to the hypermetabolism by increasing respirations to increase the oxygen supply. However, the increased protein catabolism reduces the muscle mass of the diaphragm and intercostal muscles, which can prevent the patient from meeting the increased oxygen demand causing hypoventilation, carbon dioxide retention and respiratory failure. The patient's ability to survive thyrotoxic crisis is determined by the severity of the hyperthyroid state and his general health.

Diagnostic Procedures

There are no specific laboratory tests to differentiate thyrotoxic crisis from uncomplicated hyperthyroidism. TSH, T_3, T_4, and resin T_3 uptake should be measured. Resin T_3 uptake is an indirect measure of free T_4 levels (free T_4 is the portion that is biologically active) and is elevated in hyperthyroid states.

Treatment

Patients with suspected or diagnosed thyrotoxic crisis should be managed in the ICU. Goals of treatment are to inhibit thyroid hormone biosynthesis, block thyroid hormone release, antagonize of the peripheral effects of thyroid hormone, supportive care, and treat the precipitating cause. Inhibition of thyroid hormone biosynthesis is accomplished with antithyroid medications. Propylthiouracil (PTU) is the preferred agent because it prevents the peripheral conversion of T_4 to T_3. A loading dose of 600 mg is given and followed by 200 mg every four hours until production of thyroid hormone is blocked. PTU must be given orally, via a nasogastric tube, or rectally, since there no parenteral preparation available in the United States. Patients not able to take PTU are given methimazole (Brand name: Tapazole), 20 mg orally every four hours until inhibition is achieved. Since PTU and Tapazole lack immediate effect, iodine agents are administered to block the release of the thyroid hormones from the gland. Sodium iodine is given by slow IV drip or Lugol's solution (saturated solution of potassium iodine) may be given orally. Serum T_4 levels fall by 30–50 percent and stabilize in three to six days. Radiographic contrast media such as ipodate (Brand name: Oragrafin) or iopanoic acid (Brand name: Telepaque) may also be used. For patients with iodine allergy, lithium carbonate may be used, but it has worse side effects and must be monitored regularly to maintain therapeutic levels. It is given orally or via a nasogastric tube every six hours.

Hormone synthesis inhibition and blockade may take days or weeks, therefore antagonism of the peripheral effects is required to minimize injury to the major organ systems and decrease the signs and symptoms of beta-adrenergic stimulation. The mortality rate of thyrotoxic crisis (20 percent) has been significantly reduced with the use of beta-blockers. The most frequently used is propranolol (Brand name: Inderal), but esmolol (Brand name: Brevibloc) or Atenolol (Brand name: Tenormin) may also be used. Results including reduction of tachycardia, restlessness, sweating, tremors, and agitation may be seen within 1 hour when given IV. Supportive care includes stress doses of hydrocortisone; Tylenol®, cooling blankets, or ice packs for fever; fluid replacement to prevent dehydration; and anticoagulation if necessary. Treatment of the precipitating cause will prevent the reoccurance of thyrotoxic crisis.

Nursing Responsibilities

Nursing responsibilities include monitoring the effects of treatment, cardiovascular status, monitor and treat hyperthermia; administering fluids, oxygen, and medications; and providing adequate nutrition and injury prevention.

Myxedema Coma

Myxedema coma is a life-threatening emergency, seen in *hypothyroid* patients, resulting from the addition of a stressor such as infection, trauma, exposure to cold, intake of tranquilizers, barbiturates, or narcotics. These stressors increase the patient's metabolism and deplete any stored thyroid hormone from the body, causing a crisis. Myxedema coma occurs more often during the winter, is seen in women and the elderly, and has a mortality rate estimated to be 20 percent to 50 percent.

Presenting signs and symptoms include hypothermia, hypoventilation, hypotension, bradycardia, hyporeflexia, hyponatremia, and generalized interstitial edema. The patient's hypothermia is due to the decreased metabolic rate and low thermal energy production. 80 percent of patients presenting with hypothermia have temperatures between 80° F (26.7° C) and 88.6° F (32° C) and have a grave prognosis. Depressed cardiac function causes bradycardia, decreased contractility, low stroke volume and cardiac output, and hypotension. Respirations are depressed causing hypoventilation and CO_2 retention, leading to decreased mentation. Slowed neuron conduction depresses the deep tendon reflexes. The hyponatremia is due to water retention. Fluid collects in the tissues of the face, joints, muscles, and can cause pericardial effusion.

Diagnostic Procedures

Laboratory testing should include thyroid function tests, complete blood count (CBC), biochemical profile (electrolytes, hepatic functions tests, renal indices), random cortisol, creatine kinase (CK), blood cultures, arterial blood gases (ABGs), and urinalysis (UA). Chest X-ray, electro-cardiogram (ECG), abdominal ultrasound, and CT of the head may also be required. Serum T_3, T_4 and T_3 resin intake levels will be low. TSH will be elevated if the patient has primary hypothyroidism, and normal or low if the problem is in the hypothalamus or pituitary gland (secondary hypothyroidism). Serum glucose and sodium levels will be low. Cortisol levels may be low. If cortisol levels are low, then a cosyntropin stimulation test will be ordered to rule out the possibility of adrenal insufficiency. In a cosyntropin stimulation test, cosyntropin is injected parenterally and the cortisol level is drawn before administration and 30–60 minutes after administration. If there is a rise in the cortisol levels following administration of the cosyntropin, then the patient does not have adrenal insufficiency; however, if there is not an adequate rise in the cortisol level, then the patient is diagnosed with adrenal insufficiency and needs exogenous steroid administration.

Treatment

Patients with suspected or diagnosed myxedema coma should be managed in the ICU. The goals of treatment include hormone replacement, correct fluid and electrolyte balance, provide supportive care, and identification and treatment of the precipitating cause. Thyroid hormone replacement should be started early using both T_4 and T_3. The loading dose of T_4 [levothyroxine (Brand name: Synthroid)] is 2 mcg/kg body weight, given IV over 5 minutes and then 100 mcg every 24 hours. This is followed by a loading dose of T_3 [liothyronine (Brand name: Thyrolar)] of 10 to 25 mcg IV, every 12 hours until the patient responds with an elevation of body temperature, pulse, blood pressure, and improved mental status and

ABGs. While the thyroid hormones are being loaded, the patient may require intubation and mechanical ventilation due to airway obstruction. Patients with cardiac dysrhythmias may require continuous cardiac monitoring. Symptomatic bradycardia may require temporary pacing using transvenous or transcutaneous methods. Hyponatremia (serum sodium less than 120 meq/L) may be treated with hypertonic saline and limited water using a central venous catheter. Hypothermia is best monitored with core temperature. Glucose may be added to the IV solution and stress doses of steroids will help to increase both blood pressure and serum glucose. Hydrocortisone (Brand name: Solu-Cortef) 100 mg IV is given every 8 hours for 48 hours.

Nursing Responsibilities

Nursing responsibilities include monitoring the effects of treatment and cardiovascular status; monitoring and treating hypothermia; administering fluids, oxygen, and medications; and providing adequate nutrition and injury prevention.

Acute Adrenal Insufficiency (Addisonian Crisis)

Addisonian crisis is the acute form of chronic adrenal dysfunction resulting in inadequate adrenal secretion of glucocorticoids (cortisol) and mineralocorticoids (aldosterone). Dysfunction of the adrenal glands may result from primary, secondary, or tertiary causes. Primary insufficiency may be due to idiopathic autoimmune disease, granulomatous disease (tuberculosis, sarcoidosis, histoplasmosis), metastatic cancer, trauma, sepsis, acquired immunodeficiency syndrome (AIDS), drugs (ketoconazole, trimethoprim, phenytoin, barbiturates, rifampin), or a developmental abnormality. At least 90 percent of the adrenal cortex must be destroyed before clinical signs and symptoms become evident. Secondary causes interfere with hormone secretion, including pituitary tumors, hemorrhage, radiation, Sheehan's syndrome (postpartum hemorrhage), trauma, surgery, and hypothalamic disorders. Tertiary adrenal insufficiency is iatrogenic, secondary to long-term use of steroids, causing failure of the adrenal glands to resume hormone production of cortisol when exogenous administration stops.

The lack of cortisol results in decreased glucose production, decreased metabolism of protein and fat, decreased appetite, decreased intestinal motility and digestion, decreased vascular tone, and diminished catecholamine effectiveness. When patients with deficient cortisol are stressed, profound cardiovascular collapse can result. Low levels of aldosterone cause decreased retention of sodium and water, decreased circulating blood volume, and increased potassium and hydrogen ion reabsorption.

Presenting signs and symptoms are often nonspecific and can be attributed to other medical disorders. Since acute adrenal insufficiency is a medical emergency, it must be considered in any patient with fever, vomiting, hypotension, shock, decreased sodium, increased potassium, or hypoglycemia unresponsive to standard therapy. The most common presentation in the ICU is hypotension refractory to fluids and requiring vasopressors. Other symptoms may include decreased cardiac output, dysrhythmias, cold/pale skin, headache, confusion, lethargy, anorexia, nausea, vomiting, vague abdominal pain, and decreased urine output.

Diagnostic Procedures

Laboratory testing should include complete blood count (CBC), biochemical profile (electrolytes, hepatic, renal), ABGs, cortisol, and aldosterone levels. Common laboratory results with acute adrenal insufficiency are hypoglycemia, hyponatremia, hyperkalemia, eosinophilia, elevated BUN, hypercalcemia, and hyperuricemia. A decreased serum cortisol level is suspicious for adrenal insufficiency. In acute adrenal crisis, there is no time to wait for the laboratory results to confirm the diagnosis before beginning treatment. If cortisol levels are low, a cosyntropin stimulation test will be requested by the physician to rule out the possibility of adrenal insufficiency. Failure of the cortisol level to adequately rise 30–60 minutes after parenteral administration of 250 mcg of cosyntropin is diagnostic of adrenal insufficiency.

Treatment

The treatment goals for acute adrenal crisis include hormone replacement, correct fluid and electrolyte balance, supportive care, and identification and treatment of the precipitating cause. Fluid deficit should be replaced with 5% glucose with 0.9% normal saline (D5.9NS) providing both volume replacement and enough glucose to minimize hypoglycemia. The patient may require as much as 5 liters of fluid in the first 12 to 24 hours. Glucocorticoid replacement is the most important hormone to be given first. Hydrocortisone (Brand name: Solu-Cortef) is given as a bolus of 100–300 mg IV and followed by 100 mg every eight hours. Mineralocorticoid replacement may also be required with fludrocortisone (Brand name: Florinef) 0.1 to 0.2 mg daily.

Nursing Responsibilities

Nursing responsibilities include monitoring the effects of treatment and cardiovascular status; administer ing fluids and medications.

Hypercorticism (Cushing's Syndrome)

Hypercorticism is an increased production of mineralocorticoids, glucocorticoids, and androgen steroids. Causes include adrenal cortex tumor, pituitary tumor, ectopic ACTH-producing pulmonary neoplams, or long-term use of steroids. Adrenal cortex tumors (usually adenomas) produce excess cortisol. A pituitary tumor stimulates increased release of ACTH causing hyperplasia of the adrenal cortex and increased hormone production. Ectopic ACTH-producing tumors (usually oat cell carcinomas) stimulate excess cortisol production. Long-term exogenous steroid administration for other medical diseases, such as chronic obstructive pulmonary disease or inflammatory bowel disease, may cause Cushing's syndrome.

Presenting signs and symptoms include truncal weight gain with a pendulous abdomen; facial, supraclavicular, and dorsocervical deposition of fat (hump); purple striae on the abdomen and breast; acne; hirsutism and male pattern hair loss in women; extreme muscle wasting; hypertension; abnormal glucose intolerance; poor wound healing; sodium and water retention, altered libido, and poor wound healing.

Diagnostic Procedures

A 24-hour urine free cortisol level is the gold-standard screening test. Serum cortisol and ACTH levels (drawn between 8 AM and 10 AM) help to differentiate between pituitary and adrenal sources. MRI of the head, chest and abdomen may identify a tumor source.

Treatment

Treatment of pituitary adenoma may include transsphenoidal resection of the pituitary adenoma or radiation therapy if surgery is not possible. Adrenal adenomas and ectopic ACTH-producing tumors are usually surgically removed.

Nursing Responsibilities

These patients may be cared for in the ICU after surgery and require stress doses of corticosteroids. Their immune systems will be depressed due to the high levels of steroids prior to surgery, and they will require close monitoring for signs of infection.

Pheochromocytoma

Pheochromocytoma is a rare cause of hypertension (0.3 to 1 percent), but it is malignant in 3 to 36 percent of the patients found to have this tumor. Fifty percent of the patients with malignant pheochromocytoma die within five years. The disease can be life threatening due to the possibility of cerebrovascular accidents (CVA) and heart failure. It is an encapsulated vascular tumor of neuroendocrine chromaffin cells of the adrenal medulla and it secretes norepinephrine and/or epinephrine.

Presenting signs and symptoms include sustained or paroxysmal (intermittent) hypertension (90 percent), postural hypotension, chest pain, headache, sweating, palpitations, tremor, and hyperglycemia. The symptoms may last for just a few seconds to hours, and the episodes occur with irregular frequency. Triggers for the attacks may include diagnostic procedures, anesthesia, medications, or foods (chocolate).

Diagnostic Procedures

Measurement of serum and urine free metanephrines (catecholamine metabolites) is the first priority for diagnosis. The urine sample should be collected after a symptomatic episode. A second test, if the first is nonspecific, involves clonidine suppression (0.3 mg/kg), then measurement of norepinephrine levels in three hours. Failure to suppress the level of norepinephrine would suggest pheochromocytoma. Once the diagnosis is made, tumor localization is done using either CT or MRI imaging. The newest method uses the positron emission tomography (PET) for identifying both primary and metastatic lesions.

Treatment

Surgical excision of the tumor(s) is the best treatment method for pheochromocytoma. Two weeks prior to surgery, catecholamine blockade is started using alpha-adrenergic blockers [phenoxybenzamine (Brand name: Dibenzyline)] and beta-adrenergic blockers [atenolol (Brand name: Tenormin)]. Preoperative volume expansion is used to prevent hypotension from the alpha and beta blockade. When diagnosed and treated early, 90 percent of the cases are cured. Left untreated, pheochromocytoma is usually fatal from arrhythmias, myocardial infarction or cerebrovascular accidents.

Nursing Responsibilities

These patients may be cared for in the ICU after surgery. Monitor closely for shock, hypotension, hemorrhage, and hypoglycemia.

Diabetic Ketoacidosis (DKA)

Diabetic ketoacidosis (DKA) is defined as acute hyperglycemia with acidosis. Incidence ranges from 4.6 to 8 episodes per 1,000 hospital admissions and appears in four to nine percent of all hospital discharge summaries. Mortality rates range five to nine percent. The most common causes of DKA are failure to take sufficient insulin, stressful events, trauma, surgery, infections, pregnancy, alcohol intoxication, and undiagnosed DM. DKA is almost always the first presentation of Type I diabetics and although it is possible for Type II insulin dependent diabetics to present with DKA, DKa is almost exclusively limited to Type I diabetes (also known as juvenile onset diabetes).

DKA has four hallmark pathologies: hyperglycemia, hypovolemia, ketonemia, and anion gap metabolic acidosis. Hyperglycemia is caused by a lack of insulin, preventing cellular glucose utilization. Thus, although blood glucose rises, the negative feedback to the cells producing glucagons cannot be activated; hence, glucagon is released and breaks down glycogen and stimulates gluconeogenesis, releasing more glucose and further increasing the blood glucose. The high glucose level in the blood exceeds the renal threshold, spilling glucose into the urine. Ketonemia results from the accumulation of ketones (from fat metabolism, beta-oxidation) in the bloodstream contributing to metabolic acidosis. To compensate, the lungs attempt to eliminate the excess carbonic acid by hyperventilation (Kussmaul respirations). Excess serum glucose produces osmotic diuresis extracting water from the vascular space and causing rapid dehydration. The body attempts to buffer the excess hydrogen ions, causing a decrease in bicarbonate levels. Excess cellular hydrogen ions cause the potassium ions to leave the cells, increasing the serum potassium levels. Altered consciousness is related to acidosis and dehydration.

Clinical signs and symptoms include acetone breath, altered sensorium, hypothermia, Kussmaul breathing, tachycardia, abdominal pain, nausea, vomiting, polyuria, polydipsia, weakness, weight loss, and fever. The patient with DKA may be lethargic, stuporous, or unconscious depending on the extent of dehydration and electrolyte imbalance. Physical examination reveals flushed, dry skin, dry mucous membranes, skin 'tenting' greater than 3 seconds, hypotension, tachycardia, Kussmaul respirations, 'fruity'-smelling breath, abdominal tenderness on palpation, and temperature alterations.

Diagnostic Procedures

Laboratory tests should include serum biochemical panel (lytes, renal, liver function), CBC, ABGs, serum ketones, serum osmolality, urine for glucose and ketones, and serum ketones (beta-hydroxybutyrate) and lactic acid. An ECG may show tachycardia. Blood sugar will be greater than >300 mg/dl. Elevated sodium, potassium, and magnesium levels will be due to dehydration and acidosis. Serum ketones of greater than 3 mOsm/kg. BUN will be increased with a BUN/creatinine ratio greater than 20:1, which is strongly indicative of dehydration. Metabolic acidosis with pH less than 7.30, bicarbonate less than 15 mEq/L, $PaCO_2$ less than 35 mm Hg, and anion gap greater than 12–16 mEq/L. Ketones will be elevated in both urine and blood. Hematocrit and white blood cell count will be elevated. Serum osmolality will be 295–330 mOsm/kg.

Treatment

Treatment of the patient with DKA requires an aggressive approach. Management goals include correction/restoration of hypovolemia, hyperglycemia, acidemia, electrolytes, and the insulin-glucagon ratio. Volume replacement is accomplished with rapid infusion of 0.9% normal saline (Normal Saline, NS): 1 liter in the first hour, then 300–500 ml per hour, until the serum osmolality returns to normal. When the serum glucose is 250 mg/dl, the IV solution is changed to 5% dextrose with 0.45% NS (D5/ ½ NS) to avoid hypoglycemia, hypokalemia, and cerebral edema caused by the glucose diuresis. Correction of hyperglycemia requires the administration of insulin. Regular insulin is administered at 10 to 20 units IV bolus and followed by a continuous infusion of 0.1 unit/kg/hr. Hourly blood glucose monitoring and insulin infusion rate adjustments should be done. When the blood glucose levels are between 100 and 200 mg/dL, begin subcutaneous insulin for one to two hours before stopping the insulin infusion. Replace potassium, phosphorus, and magnesium as needed.

Complications Associated with Treatment of DKA

- Hypoglycemia is reported in 10 to 20 percent of the patients during insulin therapy. Most common causes are failure to reduce the insulin infusion rate and failure to use dextrose-containing solutions when glucose levels reach 250 mg/dL.

- Hypokalemia occurs when insulin therapy and correction of acidosis decreases the serum potassium levels. Reduce the risk by using low-dose insulin protocols and aggressive potassium replacement.

- Relapse can occur with a sudden interruption of IV insulin, when patient is not given concomitant subcutaneous insulin, or with a lack of frequent monitoring.

- Etiology, pathology, and ideal method of treatment of cerebral edema are unknown.

- Treatment of acidosis includes frequent assessment of respiratory compensation and level of consciousness. It is usually corrected by fluids and insulin. Give bicarbonate if the pH is less than 7.1.

Nursing Responsibilities

These patients may be cared for in the ICU for cardiac, respiratory, and hemodynamic monitoring. Assessment of intake and output, skin turgor, mucous membranes, and neurologic status should be done hourly. Continuous cardiac monitoring may reveal U waves with hypokalemia, "peaked" or "tented" T-waves with hyperkalemia, and tachycardia that converts to bradycardia with increasing hyperkalemia. Maintaining a patients' airway, suctioning to prevent aspiration, and evaluating the ABGs will identify and prevent hypoxia. Frequent blood pressure, CVP, and SVO_2 monitoring will identify the effectiveness of fluid administration. Urine should be checked every one to two hours for glucose and ketones. Use of a diabetic flow sheet helps to quickly identify changes, trends, and potential complications.

Hyperosmolar Hyperglycemic State (HHS)

Incidence rate is lower than DKA and accounts for approximately one percent of adult hospital admissions. Where DKA is generally an illness of Type I diabetics, HHS is an acute illness, primarily, of Type II diabetics. HHS is very rare in children; however, the recent increase of Type II diabetes in children and adolescents may increase the incidence rate. Mortality rates range 10 to 15 percent from HHS. It is often seen in geriatric patients with decreased compensatory mechanisms. The most common causes of HHS are stressful events, infections, medications, trauma, surgery, and undiagnosed or inadequately treated Type II diabetes.

HHS has three hallmark pathologies: hyperglycemia, hypovolemia, and hyperosmolality. Hyperglycemia is caused by insufficient insulin production and decreased cellular glucose utilization. As blood glucose rises, glucagon is released and breaks down glycogen and stimulates gluconeogenesis, releasing more glucose and further increasing the blood glucose. The high glucose level in the blood increases the extracellular osmolality and exceeds the renal threshold, spilling glucose into the urine. Excess serum glucose produces osmotic diuresis extracting water from the vascular space and causing profound dehydration. HHS develops more slowly than DKA, sometimes over weeks or months. Alterations in neurologic status are due to the cellular dehydration. The average total body deficit in HHS is 9 to 10 liters.

Clinical signs and symptoms include *altered sensorium* (paresthesia, paresis, plegia, aphasia, decreased deep tendon reflexes, seizure), *hypothermia, tachycardia, tachypnea, abdominal pain, nausea, vomiting, polyuria, polydipsia, weakness, weight loss,* and *fever.* The patient with HHS may be lethargic, stuporous, or unconscious depending on the extent of dehydration and electrolyte imbalance. Physical examination reveals warm, dry skin, dry mucous membranes, skin 'tenting' greater than three seconds, hypotension, tachycardia, abdominal tenderness on palpation, and temperature alterations.

Diagnostic Procedures

Laboratory tests should include serum biochemical panel (lytes, renal, liver function), CBC, ABGs, serum osmolality, and urine for glucose and ketones. An ECG may show changes and tachycardia. Blood sugar *600–2000 mg/dl* with average of 1100 mg/dl. Serum sodium is normal to slightly elevated. Decreased potassium, calcium, phosphorous, and magnesium levels are due to dehydration. Serum ketones are normal or slightly elevated. BUN increased with a BUN/creatinine ratio greater than 20:1. ABGs have a normal or mildly acidotic pH. If acidosis is present it is lactic acidosis related to hypoperfusion not ketoacidosis. Ketones in urine are negative or trace. Hematocrit and white blood cell count elevated. Serum osmolality is often greater than 330 mOsm/kg and may be as high as 450 mOsm/kg.

Treatment

Treatment of HHS requires an aggressive approach. Management goals include correct hypovolemia, correct hyperglycemia, replenish electrolytes, and restore the insulin-glucagon ratio. Volume replacement is accomplished with rapid infusion of 0.9% normal saline: one liter the first hour, then 300–500 ml per hour, until the serum osmolality returns to normal. When the serum glucose is 250 mg/dl, the IV solution is changed to 5% glucose with 0.45% NS (D5/ ½ NS) to avoid hypoglycemia, hypokalemia, and cerebral edema caused by the glucose diuresis. Correction of hyperglycemia requires the administration of insulin. Regular insulin is administered at 10 to 20 units IV bolus and followed by a continuous infusion of 0.1 unit/kg/hr. Hourly blood glucose monitoring and insulin infusion rate adjustments should be done. When the blood glucose levels are between 100 and 200 mg/dL, begin subcutaneous insulin for one to two hours before stopping the insulin infusion. Replace potassium, calcium, phosphorus, and magnesium as needed.

Complications Associated with Treatment of HHS

- Hypoglycemia is reported in 10 to 20 percent of the patients during insulin therapy. Most common causes are failure to reduce the insulin infusion rate and failure to use dextrose-containing solutions when glucose levels reach 250 mg/dL.

- Hypokalemia occurs when insulin therapy and correction of acidosis decrease the serum potassium levels. Reduce the risk by using low-dose insulin protocols and aggressive potassium replacement.

- Relapse can occur with a sudden interruption of IV insulin, if patient is not given concomitant subcutaneous insulin, or with a lack of frequent monitoring.

Nursing Responsibilities

These patients may be cared for in the ICU for cardiac, respiratory, and hemodynamic monitoring. Assessment of intake and output, skin turgor, mucous membranes, and neurologic status should be done hourly. Continuous cardiac monitoring may reveal U waves with hypokalemia, peaked or tented T waves with hyperkalemia, and tachycardia that converts to bradycardia with increasing hyperkalemia. Maintaining a patent airway—suctioning to prevent aspiration—and evaluation of ABGs will identify and prevent hypoxia. Frequent blood pressure and CVP monitoring will identify effectiveness of fluid administration. Urine should be checked hourly for both glucose and ketones. Use of a diabetic flow sheet helps to quickly identify changes, trends, and potential complications.

Acute Hypoglycemia

Acute hypoglycemia can be a life-threatening event if left untreated. Hypoglycemia is a blood glucose level less than 60 mg/dL and is a common endocrine emergency. It is an imbalance between glucose production and glucose utilization. Glucose is the metabolic fuel of the brain and since it is not synthesized or stored in the brain, the brain is dependent on blood glucose concentration. When the serum glucose concentration drops below normal levels, the physiologic effect on the brain can be profound, leading to coma or death.

The etiology of hypoglycemia includes endogenous, exogenous, and functional causes. Endogenous hypoglycemia is caused by tumors (pancreatic, insulinoma) or inborn metabolic errors. Exogenous low blood glucose is caused by insulin excess, insulin secretagogues, oral antidiabetic agents (sulfonylureas, meglitnides), alcohol use, and other drugs (salicylates, pentamidine). Functional hypoglycemia causes include dumping syndrome, spontaneous reactive hypoglycemia, other endocrine deficient states, and prolonged muscle use (exercise, seizures).

Neonatal hypoglycemia can be transient. Causes include decreased exogenous supply, defective gluconeogenesis, immature fasting adaptation, or hyperinsulinemia. Approximately 10 percent of normal newborns will experience hypoglycemia, when the first feeding is delayed more than six hours after birth or if there is inadequate breastfeeding. Pediatric hypoglycemia has multiple causes: inborn errors of metabolism, decreased growth hormone, decreased cortisol, stress, liver dysfunction, excess insulin or lack of oral intake, infections, drugs, or severe malnutrition.

Clinical signs and symptoms are related to the activation of the sympathetic nervous system (epinephrine release) and neuroglycopenic indicators. Most commonly seen are palpitations, tachycardia, diaphoresis, anxiety, nausea, pallor, weakness, hunger, restlessness, difficulty thinking or speaking, visual disturbances, tremors, piloerection, slurred speech, staggering gait, seizures, and coma.

Diagnostic Procedures

Laboratory studies include electrolytes, renal panel, liver function studies, and serum drug screen. ECG is used to screen for cardiac causes. Blood glucose level less than 60 mg/dl (varies with individual patients) is diagnostic for hypoglycemia. Serum glucose of 20 to 40 mg/dL is associated with seizures. Less than 20 mg/dL is usually seen in comatose patients.

Treatment

Treat adult hypoglycemia with 15 g carbohydrate orally, if the patient is alert and able to swallow, or IV D50 (25 grams of dextrose in 50 ml water), if the patient is unconscious. Assess response. Recheck blood glucose in 20 to 30 minutes. Repeat treatment is necessary. Provide longer acting carbohydrate source (cheese, crackers) or a meal to prevent recurrence. Identification and treatment of the cause of the hypoglycemia is done after the patient stabilizes. Monitor for complications such as myocardial ischemia or infarction, seizures, coma, or irreversible neurologic injury. Newborns may require early feedings or supplemental nutritional support.

Emergency Foods for Hypoglycemia

- 4 oz apple or orange juice
- 4 oz carbonated cola
- 8 oz skim or 1% milk
- 4 cubes or 2 packets of sugar
- 2 oz corn syrup, honey, grape jelly
- 6 life savers or jelly beans
- 10 gumdrops
- 2 tablespoons of raisins
- ½ cup regular gelatin
- 2 to 3 graham cracker squares
- 3 glucose tablets (5 grams each)

These amounts have 10 to 15 grams of carbohydrates.

NEONATAL & PEDIATRIC ENDOCRINE PATHOLOGIES

Inborn Errors of Metabolism

Inborn errors of metabolism comprise a large class of genetic metabolic diseases. The majority are due to defects of single genes that code for enzymes which facilitate conversion of various substances into other products. Problems occur because of accumulation of substances which are toxic or interfere with normal function, or due to the reduced ability to synthesize essential compounds. Major classes of congenital metabolic diseases are listed in table 6.2.

The following are examples of potential manifestations affecting each of the major organ systems:

- Growth failure, failure to thrive, weight loss
- Ambiguous genitalia, delayed puberty, precocious puberty
- Developmental delay, seizures, dementia, encephalopathy, stroke
- Deafness, blindness
- Skin rash, abnormal pigmentation, lack of pigmentation, hirsutism, lumps and bumps
- Dental abnormalities
- Immunodeficiency, thrombocytopenia, anemia, splenomegalia, lymphadenopathy
- Many forms of cancer
- Recurrent vomiting, diarrhea, abdominal pain
- Excessive urination, renal failure, dehydration, edema
- Hypotension, heart failure, cardiomyopathy, hypertension, myocardial infarction
- Hepatomegaly, jaundice, liver failure
- Unusual facial features, congenital malformations
- Excessive breathing (hyperventilation), respiratory failure
- Abnormal behavior, depression, psychosis
- Joint pain, muscle weakness, cramps
- Hypothyroidism, adrenal insufficiency, hypogonadism, diabetes mellitus

Specific diagnostic tests include blood, urine, tissue biopsy or specific DNA testing. Laboratory abnormalities can be transient. Therefore, values within the reference range do not rule out an IEM and may require multiple testing points. Treatment that involves a single or several strategies such as enzyme replacement, gene transfer, and organ transplantation

TABLE 6.2 *Congenital Metabolic Disease Classification*

Substrate	Dysfunction
Carbohydrate	Glycogen storage disease
Amino acids	Phenylketonuria
	Maple syrup urine disease
	Glutaric acidemia type 1
Organic acids	Organic acidurias
	Alcaptonuria
Kreb's Cycle	Glutaric acidemia type 2
Porphyrins	Acute intermittent porphyria
Purines	Lesch-Nyhan syndrome
Steroids	Congenital adrenal hyperplasia
Mitochondria	Kearns-Sayre syndrome
Peroxisoma	Zellweger syndrome
Lysosomal storage	Gaucher's disease

have become available and beneficial for many previously untreatable disorders. Some of the more common or promising therapies are reduction of dietary protein, dietary supplementation or replacement, dialysis, enzyme replacement, gene transfer, and bone marrow or organ transplantation.

Infant of Diabetic Mother

Diabetes has long been associated with maternal and perinatal morbidity and mortality. Fetal and neonatal mortality rates were as high as 65 percent before the development of specialized maternal, fetal, and neonatal care. Since then, infants of diabetic mothers (IDMs) have experienced a nearly 30-fold decrease in morbidity and mortality rates. Between 3 percent and 10 percent of pregnancies are affected by abnormal glucose regulation and control. Of these, 80 percent are related to abnormal glucose control of pregnancy or gestational diabetes mellitus. Infants born to mothers with glucose intolerance are at an increased risk of morbidity and mortality secondary to respiratory distress, growth abnormalities, polycythemia, hypoglycemia, congenital malformations, and electrolyte disturbances.

Pathophysiology

Increased levels of estrogen and progesterone affect glucose homeostasis as counter-regulatory hormones in early pregnancy. As a result, beta-cell hyperplasia occurs in the pancreas, stimulating an increased release of insulin. Increased insulin levels stimulate glycogen deposition and decrease hepatic glucose production. The release of increasing amounts of contra-insulin factors as placental growth continues, causing up to a 30 percent increase in maternal insulin needs as pregnancy progresses. Mothers with previous borderline glucose control, obesity, or frank diabetes may require initiation of or an increase in their insulin requirements to maintain glucose homeostasis.

The fetus is subjected to high levels of glucose during times of maternal hyperglycemia. Before 20 weeks' gestation, fetal islet cells are incapable of responding, subjecting the fetus to unchecked hyperglycemia and decreased fetal growth. Poor growth is especially noted in mothers with diabetic vascular disease. After 20 weeks' gestation, the fetus responds to hyperglycemia with pancreatic beta-cell hyperplasia and increased insulin levels. Fetal growth acceleration can be noted on ultrasound by 24 weeks' gestation, especially with fluctuating maternal glucose levels. The combination of hyperglycemia and insulin increases fat and glycogen stores, resulting in weight increases marked by hepatosplenomegaly and cardiomegaly without an increase in head circumference.

Chronic fetal hyperglycemia and hyperinsulinemia increase the fetal basal metabolic rate and oxygen consumption, causing hypoxia. The fetus responds by increasing oxygen-carrying capacity by increasing erythropoietin production, leading to polycythemia. The fetus redistributes iron from developing organs, including the heart and brain, to support this expanded blood mass, leaving these organs iron deficient and with possible long-term functional consequences.

Prior to birth, elevated insulin levels may inhibit the maturational effect of cortisol on the lung, putting the fetus at risk for developing respiratory distress syndrome after birth. The first one to three hours after birth are the most critical for the development of hypoglycemia.

The Hematologic & Immunological Systems

7

The hematology and immunology portion of the CCRN exam is approximately three percent of the total number of questions.

Critical care nurses need to be able to *identify alterations in the hematology and immunology systems* to appropriately manage patient conditions related to these systems and reduce unexpected outcomes. This requires a general knowledge of the processes related to the anatomy and physiology of those systems, including formation of cells, hemostasis, coagulation, oxygenation, immune responses, and antibody formation. In addition, the nurse must be able to plan for the care of the critically ill adult with abnormal conditions in these systems, including appropriate goals, interventions, and evaluation of those interventions.

This chapter will provide an overview of the basic hematologic components and anatomical structures, primary organs of the immunological system, pathophysiology, management of patients with hematologic and immunologic disorders, and care of patients receiving transfusions or undergoing organ transplantation. Generally, the hematological and immunological systems provide support for the other major systems in the body (oxygenation and acid-base balance); however, when there is a malfunction of the normal processes in these systems such as abnormal bleeding due to a coagulopathy or an anaphylactic response, significant complications can occur and these patients are often treated in the critical care setting.

BASIC HEMATOLOGICAL COMPONENTS/ANATOMICAL STRUCTURES

Human blood is comprised of several types of cells which are responsible for a range of functions within the body. The primary precursor to the cells outlined below is the *pluripotent stem cell*. In the adult, this cell is produced in the bone marrow of the membranous bones within the body (vertebrae, sternum, ribs and ilia) and moves through various stages of cell division to form the different cells in the circulating blood volume.

RBC/Erythrocytes

The first of these are the *red blood cells* (RBCs) or erythrocytes. Typically RBCs remain alive and active for approximately *120 days*. Upon death of the cell, the spleen or liver filters out these products of the primary circulation. Iron is retained from the RBC, put back into circulation with transferrin as the transporter, and returned to the bone marrow for reuse. Normal RBC count in the blood for the male is $4.5–5.0 \times 10^6$/L and $4.0–5.0 \times 10^6$/L in the female. The pluripotent stem cell differentiates into three phases of colony forming units: the colony forming unit—spleen (CFU-S), the colony forming unit—blast (CFU-B), and the colony forming unit—erythrocyte (CFU-E) which transitions into the erythrocyte. The regulation of this process is guided by the glycoprotein; *erythropoietin.* This protein is produced primarily in the kidneys. In the event there are decreased oxygen levels in the blood, the kidneys will stimulate the release of erythropoietin, which acts upon the bone marrow to produce more RBCs.

Blood and Rh typing is determined by antigens located on the RBC membrane. The two main antigens are named A and B. From these, the four major blood groups are created: A, B, AB, and O, which are based on the presence or absence of these antigens. For example, the "A" antigen is present in people with Type A blood. Conversely, since the B antigen is NOT present in Type A blood, a person with Type A blood will have antibodies AGAINST the "B" antigen. The Rh antibody develops if the Rh negative person is exposed to Rh positive blood such as in pregnancy or in transfusion.

	Antigen	Antibodies	Donate To	Receive From
Type A	A	Anti-B	A, AB	A, O
Type B	B	Anti-A	B, AB	B, O
Type AB	AB	None (no antibodies are present)	AB only	All Blood Types (UNIVERSAL RECEIVER)
Type O	None (no antigens are present)	Anti-A & Anti-B	All Blood Types (UNIVERSAL DONOR)	O only

WBC/Leukocytes

Another primary type of cell is the *white blood cell* (WBC) or leukocyte. Unlike RBCs there are several subtypes of WBC's which are based on the developmental stage and function of the WBC. The precursor of the WBC is also the pluripotent stem cell and the CFU-S or colony forming unit—spleen which forms the *granulocytes (neutrophils, eosinophils, and basophils), monocytes, megakaryocytes, and platelets and the lymphoid stem cell (LSC)* which forms the T-lymphocytes and the B-lymphocytes. The average life span of a WBC is four to eight hours and another four to five days in the tissues. WBCs are formed partially in the bone marrow and partially in the lymph tissue. Leukocytes are considered mobile units as they are transported in the blood to various sites where they are needed, the most important function of which is to provide defense against inflammation and infection. There are also complementary substances which assist in the function of these cells and include the factors of the complement system (composed of serum proteins C1–C9), cytokines, and eicosanoids. These will be discussed later in this chapter.

When measuring WBCs in the complete blood count (CBC), two measurements are done: the total number of WBC's (4,500–10,000/µl) and the differential which includes the percentage of the following types of WBC's: bands, neutrophils, esosinophils, basophils, lymphocytes, and monocytes. These percentages total 100 percent. Leukocytosis is defined as an overall WBC count greater than 10,000. White counts greater than 30,000 typically indicate a massive infection unless there is an overproduction of immature cells, which can demonstrate conditions such as leukemia. In contrast, when a patient has a WBC less than 4,000, she is referred to as leukopenic. When analyzing the blood, the CBC will also be accompanied by a microscopic differential, where the approximate number of each of type cell will be estimated. If the neutrophils component of the WBC is less than 500, then the patient is referred to as leukopenia and also neutropenic. Since patients with leukopenia and/or neutropenia are susceptible to infections, they present with a fever. A febrile neutropenic patient is a clinical emergency and warrant immediate hospitalization. Unless she has hemodynamic compromise, such as signs of septic shock, she can generally be managed in reverse isolation on a general floor, but should receive immediate broad spectrum antiobiotics such as Cefepime. Prior to antibiotic administration, patients should have a chest radiograph, blood cultures × 2 from the periphery, blood cultures from each chronic IV or central line, urinalysis, and urine culture.

There are several types of granulocytes as mentioned above. The first of these are the **neutrophils.** Neutophils are those cells which are the most proliferate of the types of WBC's and move to sites of infective invasions to destroy microorganisms. They are often destroyed in the process as well. When one sees pus at the site of an infection, this is evidence of cellular debris that is formed at the destruction site. **Monocytes and macrophages** mature once they leave the bone marrow and also function as phagocytes. The difference in these cells is that there are some which are specific to localized tissue, e.g., Kupffler cells are macrophages located in the liver, while Langerhaus cells are located in the skin. There are also macrophages specific to the lungs, kidneys, and central nervous system (CNS). Another difference with these types of cells is that they often survive the initial destruction of microorganisms and will survive many months and sometimes years. Another type of granulocyte is the **basophil**; these are nonphagocytic cells located just outside the capillaries and serve to release substances such as *heparin, histamine, bradykinin,* and *serotonin.* Their role is primarily to attract immunoglobulin E (IgE) and antibodies to their cell membranes which serve an important role to stimulate the allergic reaction and inflammatory response.

Monocytes are produced in the bone marrow; however, the maturation process occurs in the circulation. When they are transported and enter the tissue they become macrophages. Macrophages can appear in various forms depending on the site in which they act, including histiocytes in the subcutaneous tissue, alveolar macrophages in the lungs, or microglia in the brain. When triggered by infection and inflammation, they first enlarge and then break loose from their attachments and go to the site of the infection. They are typically the first preliminary line of defense against infection, yet it is a weak response which is not considered life-saving. The process for ingesting these organisms is phagocytosis. Since, monocytes/macrophages engulf foreign bodies and organisms, they are also referred to as "phagocytes." Phagocytes must be selective of the organisms they destroy; otherwise, normal healthy cells and structures within the body will be ingested. There are three selective procedures which occur to prevent this from happening. The first two of these is that most natural substances in the body have a smooth and protective coating which discourages and repels the phagocytes. On the other hand, most foreign invading organisms have rough surfaces and no protective coating which enhance phagocytosis. The final procedure is that antibodies are formed when infectious agents such as bacteria enter the body and adhere to the membranes of the invading agent, making it more susceptible to phagocytosis. In order to accomplish this, the antibody molecule combines with C3, which is a product of the complement cascade. The combined molecule attaches onto the phagocyte membrane and initiates phagocytosis. This "tagging" of foreign particles and invading organisms for phagocytosis is referred to as *opsonization*.

Eosinophils are a small portion (only about two percent) of the total blood leukocytes. The number of eosinophils increases in patients with parasitic conditions. Although the eosinophil is not large enough to phagocytize the parasite, it attaches itself to the parasite and releases a substance that kills the parasite. Parasites found in Third World countries such as schistosomiasis, trichinosis, and trichinella are affected by these cells. The eosinophil also has the ability to collect in tissues where allergic conditions occur and detoxify some of the inflammation-producing substances. In turn, they phagocytize and destroy allergen-antibody complexes, preventing the spread of inflammation.

Mast cells also work similarly to basophils, in that they attract IgE antibodies to their cell membranes. An inflammatory response is stimulated when the mast cells release histamine as the IgE binds antigens. There is one significant difference between mast cells and basophils: the mast cells are located in the tissue and survive weeks, sometimes months, while the basophil circulates in the blood and survives only a few days.

Other forms of leukocytes are the lymphocytes or the lymphoid series of leukocytes. The most common of these are the **B lymphocytes** (B cells) and the **T lymphocytes** (T cells). *B cells* are responsible for the manufacture and release of antigen-binding proteins called immunoglobulins or antibodies. When antibodies bind with a specific antigen, it is stimulated to divide into plasma cells and memory B cells. The plasma cells continue to synthesize antibodies which bind to the antigen, while the memory B cells sit and wait dormant until more plasma cells are needed. These antibodies provide "humoral immunity." Four types of immunoglobulins can be secreted: IgM (Immunoglobulin M), IgG (Immunoglobulin G), IgA (Immunoglobulin G), and IgE (Immunoglobulin E). Each of these immunoglobulins has a role in the immune response.

T cells migrate to and are reprocessed in the **thymus** where they mature. They are responsible for formation of the activated cell lymphocytes that provide "cell mediated" immunity. These cells develop specificity to the antigen in association with cell membrane proteins. The proteins are known as *major histocompatibility complexes* (MHC). There are two types of MHC proteins which work with the T cells that function within the bodies immune to provide protection against intracellular microorganisms, viruses, and cancers. They may also provide delayed hypersensitivity reactions and rejection of transplanted tissue.

Precursors

As discussed previously in the chapter, during the genesis of cells, there are precursors to various cell forms. The primary precursor is the pluripotential hematopoietic stem cell from which most all circulating blood cells are formed. This cell is formed in the bone marrow. The pluripotential hematopoietic stem cells differentiate into intermediate stage cells and become committed stem cells based on which colonies of specific blood cell types they will form into. These are the myelo-erythroid, myeloid, and granuloctye-monocyte progenitor cells which give rise to the white and red blood cells, and the lymphoid progenitor which forms B and T lymphocytes and plasma cells.

There are processes which help in the transport of the newly formed cell or its precursor from the bone marrow to other areas of the body such as tissue and organs. Diapedesis is one means by which the cells pass from the bone marrow to the circulation. This process is literally squeezing through the pores of the capillary membrane.

Hemoglobin/Hematocrit

Hemoglobin is a protein which is formed within the red blood cell. The heme molecule is a portion of the hemoglobin which is comprised of *iron* and *protoporphyin IX* (this is formed from pyrrole molecules generated during the Krebs cycle). The globulin portion of the molecule is a polypeptide synthesized by the ribosomes. The heme and the globulin form a chain and in turn, *four chains* bind to form the hemoglobin. One of the most significant functions of the hemoglobin is oxygen transport. When the hemoglobin is concentrated in the cell fluid it can be measured. The normal concentration of hemoglobin is 15 grams per 100 ml of cells for men and 14 grams per 100 mL.

Hematocrit is a calculation of the percentage of hemoglobin in the blood. It is based on the hemoglobin and the volume of blood. This concentration varies with the age and sex of the individual, with the highest concentrations appearing in neonates and stabilizing as the person matures. In adult men, the hematocrit is 42–52 percent, while in adult women it is 36–48 percent. The primary reason why women have a lower hematocrit is related to menstruation.

Plasma/Platelets

Plasma is the substance in which blood cells are suspended, and serves as a transporting media. It is comprised primarily of water, but also contains other particles such as dissolved proteins, glucose, mineral ions, hormones, carbon dioxide, as well as the blood cells. Plasma also contains coagulation factors and proteins such as fibrinogen, which are critical to hemostasis in the body. Plasma which is taken via phlebotomy from a single donor may be frozen for future use. It is especially helpful to patients with coagulopathies related to blood loss or bleeding diathesis.

Platelets are fragments of megakaryocytes which are formed in the bone marrow. These thrombocytes are very small discs approximately 1–4 micrometers in diameter. Platelets have no nuclei and cannot reproduce. Their life span is fairly short at approximately 10 days. A unique characteristic of platelets is that their cell membrane has a coat of glycoproteins which reduces their adherence to normal endothelial cells but actually increases their ability to adhere to injured cells or vessel walls. Platelets are transported to the site of blood vessel or tissue injury and form a "plug" which adheres to the site of injury. At that site, the platelets release cytokines which help to stimulate the recruitment of additional platelets and additional clotting factors. Upon death of platelets, macrophages in the spleen remove them from the circulation.

Clotting Factors

Research has discovered more than 50 substances which may cause or affect coagulation either in the blood or tissue. Those which promote coagulation are called *procoagulants,* and those which prohibit coagulation are called *anticoagulants*. Not all of these substances will be discussed. Table 7.1 describes the most common of these factors.

Anatomical Organs of the Hematologic System

Bone Marrow

The majority of the blood cells originate in the bone marrow of the vertebrae, ribs, skull, pelvis, and proximal epiphyses of the long bones in the leg and arm, femur and humerus. Bone marrow is the spongy interior of the bone. An infant's bones contain only red marrow

TABLE 7.1 *Clotting Factors and Components*

Factor	Description/Function
Thrombin	A compound split from prothrombin
Prothrombin	Plasma protein, formed in liver, assists in blood clotting
Fibrinogen	High molecular weight protein, formed in the liver, essential factor in the coagulation process
Tissue factor (Factor III)	Composed of phospholipids plus a lipoprotein complex, functions as proteolytic enzyme
Calcium	Required for promotion/acceleration of all blood-clotting reactions
Factor V	Combines with Factor X to form a complex called prothrombin activator
Factor VII	Prothrombin conversion accelerator
Factor VIII	Participates in the intrinsic pathway for clotting
Factor IX	Component of plasma thromboplastin
Factor X	Activation of this factor results in formation of prothrombin activator
Factor XI	Second step in the intrinsic pathway for blood clotting
Factor XII	Converts to protelytic enzyme when exposed to collagen
Factor XIII	Fibrin stabilizing factor
Platelets	Assists in forming "plug" at the site of bleeding; abnormally low platelet count is called thrombocytopenia

where the blood cells are formed. As individuals age, fatty yellow marrow forms and replaces the red marrow. Amazingly the bone marrow releases approximately 10–15 million erythrocytes *every second* and the same amount are destroyed by the spleen as they become inactivated. Blood vessel membranes serve as a barrier to prevent immature blood cells from leaving the marrow.

Liver

The liver is the largest solid organ in the body and is located in the right upper quadrant of the abdomen. The liver receives approximately one third of the cardiac output. This organ serves to synthesize plasma proteins such as globulins and albumin which are important to the function of maintaining osmotic balance of the blood. Additionally, many of the coagulation factors including fibrinogen, prothrombin, and factors (II, V, VII, IX, and X) are synthesized in the liver. The production of these factors is significantly dependent on the presence of vitamin K. Kupffer's cells in the liver assist in the removal of worn red blood cells, while hepatocytes conjugate bilirubin, a by-product of this cell destruction, so that it can be excreted.

FUNCTIONS OF THE HEMATOLOGIC SYSTEM

Formation of RBCs and Hemoglobin

One of the most important functions of the hematological system is the formation of blood cells. During fetal development red blood cells are produced in the yolk sac and toward the third trimester of gestation, the liver becomes the main organ for production of RBCs. Finally, in the few weeks before birth, RBCs are produced primarily in the bone marrow which continues until the time we die. As age increases, the production of RBCs decreases. Earlier in this chapter, the process for development of erythrocytes, leukocytes, and lymphocytes from precursor and intermediate cells was discussed. All blood cells originate from the pluripotential hematopoietic stem cell.

The regulation of red cell production is done within very tight limits with the goal of providing sufficient oxygen via transport by the hemoglobin and to assure that the actual volume of RBCs does not impede blood flow. The principle stimulator of RBC production is erythropoietin. This hormone responds to decreased oxygen levels in the blood by increasing production of RBCs. About 90 percent of the erythropoietin is formed in the kidneys. In a patient who has either one or no functional kidneys, the residual 10 percent of the formation of erythropoietin is sufficient only to stimulate the production of 30–50 percent of the needed RBCs. Epopoietin alpha is an amino acid glycoprotein manufactured by recombinant DNA technology and has the same biological effects as endogenous erythropoietin. This drug is administered to dialysis patients who suffer from anemia to stimulate the production of RBCs, and also to other patients with anemia partially or all completely due to deficiency in the circulating level of erythropoietin.

Synthesis of hemoglobin begins in the proerythroblasts (a precursor to erythrocytes) and continues through the reticulocyte stage. The process is a chemical process. During the Kreb's cycle of metabolism, succinyl-CoA binds with glycine to a pyrrole molecule. The heme molecule is formed from four pyrroles (protoporphyrin) and iron. The final stage of synthesis occurs when the heme molecule combines with a long polypeptide chain (globin, formed from ribosomes). Four of these chains become the hemoglobin molecule.

Hemostasis

Hemostasis is the ability of the body to stop bleeding. Typically the first stage of this process is vasoconstriction of the smooth muscle of the vascular wall to reduce blood flow to the area of injury and preserve blood volume. The endothelium releases biochemical mediators which promote vasoconstriction upon injury. The two primary agents are endothelin and thromboxane A2. Platelets are then mobilized to the site of injury, where they adhere to the damaged vascular surface. Platelets are activated by many conditions or substances, such as shear stress, collagen, serotonin, thrombin, epinephrine, or ADP (adenosine diphosphate). The platelets morph, swell and become sticky, which continue to make the platelets adhere to each other and allow for attachment of many factors, thus forming a platelet plug. Platelets degranulate, release serotonin, von Willebrand factor, adenosine diphosphate (ADP), fibrinogen, and thromboxane from cell vesicles. These substances serve to recruit more platelets and clotting factors to the site of injury. If the site of injury is small, this will usually be successful in blocking further blood loss. A stronger plug is generated when fibrin threads attach to the platelets. The coagulation cascade is initiated based on phospholipids in the platelet membrane.

Oxygenation

Each hemoglobin molecule can transport four molecules of oxygen which bind with the iron on the molecule chain. The types of hemoglobin chains in the molecule determine how readily the molecule binds oxygen. Oxygen which is combined with hemoglobin in the lungs is released in the peripheral capillary tissues where the oxygen tension is lower. Approximately 97 percent of the oxygen is transported in this manner; the other three percent is dissolved in plasma. PaO_2 measures the oxygen carried in the arterial plasma.

The propensity for the release of oxygen is determined by the oxyhemoglobin dissociation curve which is described in the pulmonary chapter. The dissociation is based on several factors, but primarily hemoglobin saturation and PaO_2. Other factors influencing or causing shifts on the curve are pH, temperature, levels of 2, 3 DPG, PCO_2, and carbon monoxide poisoning.

Coagulation

Another critical function of the hematology system is *hemostasis*. Hemostasis is the ability to control bleeding. The coagulation cascade is the process which is initiated when there is insult or injury causing bleeding. There are two pathways within the coagulation cascade: the extrinsic and intrinsic pathways. Many of the factors described in the table above function in some capacity in the cascade. In the **extrinsic pathway** (Common Pathway), the insult as a result of trauma or damaged tissues initiates the release of Factor III. Factor VII then combines with Factor X and converts Factor III to Factor Xa. With assistance of Factor V, prothrombin (Factor II) is converted to thrombin (Factor IIa). Thrombin then converts fibrinogen (Factor I) to fibrin (Factor Ia) which is what helps bind with the initial platelet plug to strengthen the bond at the site of the injury to form a stable fibrin clot.

The **intrinsic pathway** (Alternative Pathway) starts slightly differently, but the end result is the production of fibrin. The intrinsic pathway starts with endothelial damage or venous stasis. One of the differences in this pathway is that it is a *slower pathway*. The intrinsic pathway begins with the endothelial damage and collagen exposure to Factor XII. This exposure converts Factor XII to XIIa. At each stage in the cascade, the inactive proenzyme is converted to the active enzyme by a process whereby the bond between amino acids in the protein is broken down by substances called peptidases, proteases or proteolytic cleavage enzymes. Additional substances such as calcium, coenzymes, or phospolipids may be required to participate in the process. The cascade continues with Factor XIIa combining with Factor XI to convert it to Factor XIa. Factor XIa converts to Factor IX. At this point, with the assistance of factor VIII and platelets, the intrinsic pathway continues in the same manner as the extrinsic pathway by converting Factor XIa to Factor X. Vitamin K is required for this conversion.

Eventually the fibrin clot is removed by plasmin which is a proteolytic enzyme. The body is constantly forming and dissolving clots. Activated protein C and anti-thrombin II are endogenous anticoagulants which play a big role in clotting. Thrombin is broken down by various factors into plasminogen, plasmin, and stable fibrin. One of the tests which can determine if the clot is beginning to break down is a blood test called serum fibrin split products, which is the final product in this process.

Iron Metabolism

Iron is a critical element in the body which is required for synthesis of hemoglobin and for other substances within the body such as myoglobin or cytochromes. Approximately 65 percent of the total amount of iron in the body is in the hemoglobin and 4 percent is in myoglobin. A person obtains iron through dietary intake which is then absorbed through the intestine. There it combines with the plasma and binds loosely with apotransferrin to become *transferrin*. The transferrin is transported by the plasma to cell cytoplasm where it also combines with apoferritin to form *ferritin*. This iron is stored for future use. When iron is needed within the body at any point, it is converted back to transferrin to be transported. This includes being transported to the cell membrane of erythroblasts. A syndrome which can develop due to the inability of the body to transport transferrin to the erythroblast cell membrane is called hypochromic anemia.

Reticuloendothelial System

Earlier in this chapter, it was discussed that macrophages function as a mobile unit that serve as a phagocyte. However, there is another more long-term function of the macrophages which aids the body in phagocytosis of bacteria, viruses, necrotic tissue and other foreign particles by becoming attached more long term to the tissues. The body has this capability in nearly all tissues within the body. These cells can become detached at any time and function in their original role as macrophages.

The reticuloendothelial system is the combination of the following: monocytes, mobile macrophages, fixed tissue macrophages (as described above), and specialized endothelial cells in the bone marrow, spleen, and lymph nodes. The Kuppfer cells in the liver and the Langerhaus cells in the skin are examples of these specialized cells.

TRANSFUSION OF BLOOD AND BLOOD COMPONENTS

In this section, the indications for *the primary types of blood and blood product transfusion* will be discussed. Additionally, a brief discussion will be done regarding *transfusion reactions* and potential *complications of blood transfusion*. Commonly in the critical care unit many of these products are administered in emergent situations. Patients who are susceptible to transfusion reactions or who have known antibodies may be premedicated with diphenhydramine and acetaminophen to prevent febrile reactions.

Probably one of the most common components administered in the critical care unit is **packed red blood cells** (PRBCs). The first indication for PRBCs is anemia, particularly anemia associated with symptoms of hypoxia such as shortness of breath, tachycardia, hypotension, chest pain, hypovolemia, etc. Another indication for administration of PRBCs is a decreased ability to oxygenate a patient due to diminished oxygen carrying capacity. In the latter, care must be taken to assure that the patient does not show evidence of fluid overload in the event multiple units are required. In most institutions, the Hgb must be significantly decreased, < 8.0 g/dL, to indicate the need for transfusion due to the risks. Considerations must be taken during the transfusion of PRBCs to prevent complications if multiple units are given. If multiple units are required in a short period of time, fresh frozen plasma should be administered to prevent dilutional coagulopathies. Another consideration is that PRBCs are preserved in citrate; therefore, multiple transfusions of PRBCs may cause a reduction in serum calcium due to the binding of the patient's calcium with the citrate.

Fresh frozen plasma (FFP) is another common component administered. Fresh frozen plasma contains the clotting factors needed to maintain hemostasis. Patients with clotting factor deficiencies such as hemophilia or those who have elevated bleeding times due to warfarin will benefit from transfusion of this component. Patients may also have coagulopathy from liver disease (e.g., cirrhosis) since the majority of the clotting factors are synthesized in the liver. In these patients, as well as those on warfarin (Brand Name: Coumadin), the administration of vitamin K will help synthesize clotting factors. This is not an immediate reversal of the anticoagulation, but can be followed with the PT/INR over days. In contrast, administration of FFP will immediately reverse the anticoagulation, which may be necessary for invasive prodedures. Another blood component which may be administered to the hemophiliac is cryoprecipitate. There are two clotting factors in this preparation that are not present in FFP in appreciable quantities: Factor I (fibrinogen) and Factor VIII.

Thrombocytopenia is the condition of decreased platelet count and is the primary indication for transfusion of platelets. Typically the platelet count is less than 50,000 to require transfusion. Platelets may be administered rapidly and often can be pooled in a multipack for more efficient transfusion.

Albumin is a plasma protein which is synthesized in the liver. When levels of albumin drop, the most common causes are a failure to produce adequate levels of plasma proteins (liver diseae, such as cirrhosis) or conditions which cause leakage of protein from plasma (renal disease, such as nephrotic syndrome). Edema may be present in these patients due to this leakage of fluid into the extracellular spaces. Administration of albumin may increase osmotic pressure and assist in shifting the fluids from the extracellular spaces to the intracellular spaces. Albumin is also indicated for patients in shock, those who have serious burns, or those with cerebral edema. Unfortunately, the half-life of albumin in the bloodstream is short due the body's enzymatic digestion of exogenously administered albumin. Further, if a person is suffering from nephrotic syndrome, the exogenously administered albumin will be subject to capillary loss as was the original albumin. The end result is that the administration of albumin is a transient solution that is quickly revered within a few days.

Finally, the last product to be discussed is **intravenous immunoglobulin (IVIG)**. There are a few differences with this component with regard to set up and administration. IVIG does not have to be typed with the patient's blood. Additionally, it is administered with D_5W rather than normal saline like all other blood products. IVIG is indicated in patients with idiopathic thrombocytopenic purpura (ITP), acquired immunodeficiency syndrome (AIDS), bone marrow transplant, severe combined immunodeficiency disease (SCID), as well as a host of autoimmune disorders which are beyond the scope of this book and the CCRN.

During initiation of all blood components, the infusion should be started slowly for the first 15–30 minutes while the patient's vital signs are monitored for transfusion reaction. If there are incompatibilities with the component administered and the patient's own blood, there is a chance that the patient will develop one of **four types of transfusion reaction**: *hemolytic, anaphylactic, febrile,* and *circulatory (volume) overload*. It is rare that a person would develop an agglutination of the recipient's red blood cells due to the patient's own plasma diluting the donor blood or the patient still being able to agglutinate mismatched donor cells due to the actual percentage of blood volume in the donor blood versus the total volume of blood.

Hemolytic reactions develop shortly after the initiation of the blood, and are caused by the antigen-complement reaction which occurs with ABO-incompatible blood. The patient will evidence symptoms of *fever, shortness of breath, chest or back pain, and hypotension*. The nurse must *immediately stop the transfusion* and notify the physician. Supportive care should be provided to maintain hemodynamic stability.

Hypersensitivity reactions or **anaphylactic reactions** occur when there is an *allergic reaction* to the plasma proteins. Common symptoms of this type of reaction include *hives, wheezing, shortness of breath, or hypotension*. These reactions may be slightly delayed, up to 30 minutes, but immediate actions must be taken if they develop: stop the transfusion, call the physician, and prepare to administer emergency drugs such as epinephrine or steroids to prevent continuation of the reaction.

Febrile reactions can sometimes be prevented with pre-medication, but occasionally the patient's antibodies react with the donor's leukocytes causing fevers and chills. This reaction doesn't often start until 60–90 minutes into the transfusion. As above, the component needs to be stopped and the physician notified of the reaction.

Circulatory (volume) overload can occur if the transfusion is administered too quickly or the patient cannot tolerate the additional fluid overload. This is a challenge in patients with decreased oxygen carrying capacity due to anemia with a decreased ejection fraction. A very fine balance must be maintained. This condition may occur during or even post transfusion. Commonly a dose of furosemide is administered between units to prevent the fluid overload. Oxygen should be administered in patients with these conditions. This should be suspected and caution taken in the administration of blood products in patients with systolic cardiac dysfunction. The patient may develop hypoxia, edema, and/or fevers. A chest radiograph may be useful if hypoxia is present. If the patient has developed circulatory overload, diuresis is the main stay of therapy.

HEMATOLOGICAL CONDITIONS OF THE CRITICALLY ILL PATIENT

Anemia

Anemia is simply a decreased RBC level, quantity of hemoglobin, or volume of RBCs. The causes of anemia are varied, but the manifestation of anemia is most always hypoxia which can subsequently cause end tissue damage if severe. The body compensates for anemia by increasing heart rate, which in turn increases cardiac output, and respiratory rate to increase oxygenation. Additionally, blood supply to other key organs such as gastrointestinal, skin, and kidneys will decrease. This can produce symptoms such as cold, clammy skin, ileus, or decreased urine output.

Anemia can be acute or chronic. **Acute anemia** typically occurs with trauma, gastrointestinal hemorrhage, or hemolysis. Immediate, extensive blood loss can significantly alter the hemodynamic status of an individual and requires emergent intervention to decrease the potential for adverse outcomes. Rapid administration of PRBCs and FFP is required to maintain hemostasis. Stabilization of the bleeding should be undertaken as well; typically this is done surgically or endoscopically. **Chronic anemia** results from conditions such as acute renal failure, dietary deficiencies, menorrhagia, or sickle cell anemia. The treatment for these conditions is based on the etiology of the disease, but may include transfusion, injection of erythropoietin, or surgical interventions.

During history taking it is important to question the patient regarding subjective symptoms of hypoxia. The physical examination should include observation for signs and symptoms of anemia including *pallor, shortness of breath, tachycardia,* and *hypotension. Orthostatic blood pressures* should be taken. Examination of laboratory testing results is done to ascertain the degree of anemia and to determine the potential cause of the bleeding and/or hemolysis.

Thrombocytopenia

Thrombocytopenia is a decreased level of platelets in the blood. As a result the patient is at an increased risk of bleeding when the platelet count drops below 50,000. Conditions which cause thrombocytopenia are categorized into two categories: conditions that result in *decreased production of platelets* and conditions that result in the *increased destruction of platelets.*

Malignancies such as leukemia and lymphoma are examples of the decreased production, where the increase in cancerous cells limits the production of healthy platelets in the blood. Two of the most common conditions that result in destruction of platelets are *disseminated intravascular coagulation (DIC)* and *immune thrombocytopenic purpura (ITP).* Both of these will be discussed in more detail in this section. Many medications can also cause thrombobcytopenia.

Administration of platelets is the treatment for thrombocytopenia. The patient most likely receive transfusion of platelets is one who has a platelet count less than 50,000 *and* evidence of bleeding. Other manifestations of thrombocytopenia include a skin rash called petichiae, conjunctival bleeding, and oozing from peripheral IV sticks.

Hypercoagulable Disorders

In this condition, there is evidence of a disruption of the normal coagulation processes, and the patient clots more readily. On occasion as a result of a hypercoagulable disorder, the patient may also develop a secondary bleeding disorder when platelets and clotting factors are exhausted, referred to as consumptive coagulopathy.

In acute conditions such as ischemia, infarction, or venous stasis, where there is decreased blood flow to specific locations, the coagulation cascade will be initiated and a hypercoagulable state may occur. Additionally, any condition which increases the activity of platelets such as atherosclerosis, hypertension, diabetes, or smoking may cause hypercoagulopathy. Venous thromboses may occur as a result of this state. In the event the thrombus breaks loose, arterial emboli occur and pulmonary embolus or CVA may result. Other conditions which can initiate a hypercoagulable disorder include vessel wall injury and thrombotic thrombocytopenic purpura (TTP). TTP results when there is a vessel wall injury with a resultant exaggerated immunologic response. The symptoms vary slightly in this type of response and include *fever, thrombocytopenia, acute kidney injury, altered mental status, and/ or hemolytic anemia.* Additionally, the treatment is different and primarily consists of plasmapheresis and infusion of FFP.

The treatment for hypercoagulable disorders is anticoagulation which in and of itself has a certain degree of risk in these patients. Careful monitoring of prothrombin times (PTT) while on heparin, and INRs while on warfarin, is important to assure a patient does not hemorrhage from supratherapeutic anticoagulation. The treatment that one would anticipate with TTP, i.e., administration of platelets, is contraindicated because of its potential to worsen the hypercoagulable and thrombotic state.

Sickle Cell Disease

Fortunately, the incidence of sickle cell anemia is very small; however, there is a small group who shows a more prevalent incidence: West Africans and African Americans. Individuals with sickle cell anemia have an abnormal type of hemoglobin called *hemoglobin S.* From earlier discussion of the formation of hemoglobin, a polypeptide chain is formed from alpha and beta chains. The hemoglobin S molecule has defective beta chains. When exposed to hypoxia, these molecules form crystals in the red blood cell. The RBC, as a result, becomes disfigured into the shape of a sickle versus the normal concave disc. The membrane of the cell also becomes damaged and hemolysis is often present, which leads to anemia.

The patient with sickle cell disease presents with *generalized pain,* most often in the joints, abdomen, chest, and back which is often sudden in onset. He *may show evidence of infection* including *tachycardia and tachypnea.* The patient may also experience *congestive heart failure,* which is a result of chronic anemia and hypoxia.

The patient with sickle cell anemia can suffer crises, which essentially is a continuous circle of the above processes causing low oxygen tension and anemia and more conversion of healthy red blood cells into sickled cells. The situation can become so severe that the patient's life is in jeopardy. The treatment for this condition is *blood transfusion and supportive care,* including oxygen, fluids, and analgesics.

Hemophilia

Approximately 85 percent of all cases of hemophilia are in males, because these are X-linked recessive disorders. There are three types of hemophilia: **hemophilia A** (classic hemophilia), **hemophilia B**, and **hemophilia C** (factor XI deficiency—Ashkenazic Jews). Hemophilia A is an abnormality or deficiency in factor VIII, while hemophilia B patients have a deficiency in factor IX. Even though the male is the individual who suffers from hemophilia in the majority of cases, it is actually the mother who carries the chromosome which has the deficiency. When the mother is a carrier and the father is normal, then the male children will have a 50 percent chance of manifesting the disease and the female children will have a 50 percent chance of becoming a carrier.

Hemophilia causes the individual to have a propensity to bleed. There are various levels of this disease and symptoms. Most often the child is taught how to prevent trauma which may cause bleeding. The treatment for excessive bleeding is administration of Factor VIII. Factor VIII is limited in supply and is used primarily when severe bleeding occurs.

Iron Deficiency Anemia

Iron deficiency anemia is the most common form of anemia and is most often caused by *chronic blood loss* such as menorrhagia, renal failure, or gastrointestinal bleeding from chronic use of NSAIDs. One of the most interesting symptoms of iron deficiency anemia is a craving for unusual foods/substances. These include ice, dirt, chalk, or plaster.

The treatment for iron deficiency anemia is supplemental iron in an oral form. Patients who are known to have chronic blood loss conditions can be given supplemental iron to prevent anemic states.

Disseminated Intravascular Coagulopathy (DIC)

DIC occurs frequently in critically ill patients and is extremely hard to manage due to the combination of both hypercoagulable states and hemorrhage. DIC does not occur in isolation but rather as the result of other serious precipitating factors: sepsis/septic shock, major trauma/crash injuries, shock states, obstetrical emergencies; abruptio placentae or fetal death, and malignancies including acute tumor lysis syndrome.

The precipitating factor causes *stimulation or initiation of the coagulation cascade* as discussed earlier in the chapter. This often results from large amounts of traumatized or damaged/dying tissues. The clotting factor which is initially released to initiate the cascade is the tissue factor/tissue thromboplastin/factor III. Small clots begin to form and begin to clog the smaller peripheral blood vessels. One example, which is common in the critical care unit, is the septic patient with circulating endotoxin from the infecting bacterial organism when overwhelming infections occur. The release of endotoxins initiates the clotting cascade. Subsequently, as the peripheral vessels become obstructed with clots, the oxygen carrying capacity of the vessels diminishes and nourishment to the cells is limited. This causes shock and circulatory collapse.

In addition to the clotting cascade initiation, the patient also demonstrates evidence of bleeding. It is felt that the precipitating factor for the bleeding is the widespread consumption of the clotting factors. Hence, the supply (synthesis) of the clotting factors does not match the rate of consumption.

The patient must be provided with supportive care to assure that hemodynamic stability is maintained. Treatment of the cause of the coagulopathy should be a primary focus. Heparin therapy may be required to inhibit the clotting cascade by limiting the conversion of prothrombin to thrombin. Support with platelet transfusion may also be required if the platelet count is below 50,000 **and** there is evidence of bleeding. In the situation where the cause of bleeding is not known, FFP should also be given. In patients with low fibrinogen levels, cryoprecipitate should be given. Oxygenation must be maintained including intubation if required to assure an adequate airway and exchange of blood gases.

Leukemia

Leukemia is a complex malignant disease of the white blood cells. There are several kinds of leukemia based on the speed of the progression of the cloning of the white blood cell into the malignant white blood cell. The two most common types of leukemia are **acute myelogenous leukemia** (AML) and **acute lymphocytic leukemia** (ALL). There are chronic forms of the disease; however, most often these are not managed in the critical care unit. Additionally, most acute leukemias can be managed on the oncology unit; however, when serious complications arise such as sepsis and acute tumor lysis syndrome, admission to the critical care unit is required. The cloned white cells are not functional, healthy cells, but rather, multiple in quantity and overtake the space that normal healthy white blood cells occupy.

The cloned white blood cells in leukemia do not have the ability to function as normal white blood cells; therefore, patients have an increased likelihood of infection. They have no ability to initiate an immunologic response even to simple bacterial exposures that otherwise healthy individuals could ward off fairly easily. Patients with leukemia, WBC counts less than 4,000, and an absolute neutrophil count of less than 500 are placed in neutropenic precautions to limit exposure to infectious agents. Further, as mentioned earlier, neutropenic fever is a clinical emergency and the patient should be hospitalized, an infectious workup undertaken, and started empirically on broad spectrum antibiotics.

Tumor lysis syndrome occurs when a patient with malignancies is administered chemotherapy. In the case of both leukemia and lymphoma, the malignant cells are being produced quickly and they develop a large tumor burden even before the diseases are diagnosed. Chemotherapy is typically effective on these cells and causes significant lysis. Upon lysis the cell contents are released into the bloodstream and the byproducts (uric acid, potassium, phosphorous, and calcium) can cause renal failure if they obstruct the distal tubules or collecting ducts in the kidneys.

Lymphoma

Lymphoma is another malignancy condition of tissues of the lymphatic system. The two primary types of lymphoma are **Hodgkin's disease** and **non-Hodgkin's lymphoma**. In lymphoma the T and B lymphocytes are abnormal. The production of these abnormal cells increases dramatically because they are carried by the lymphatic system and are distributed throughout the body. Recalling from earlier discussion, the T and B lymphocytes protect the body against infection from viruses, fungi, and some bacteria. Therefore, without healthy cells of this type the patient is less likely to develop an immune response to these organisms.

The patient is often treated with chemotherapy to eradicate the abnormal cells. Most patients admitted to the critical care unit with lymphoma have a complication such as an overwhelming infection or sepsis.

Other Conditions of the Hematologic System

Deep Vein Thrombosis

The precipitating factors that cause deep vein thrombosis (DVT) are called Virchow's triad, named after the German professor Rudolf Virchow. The three factors are 1) alterations in blood flow, specifically stasis, 2) injuries to the vascular endothelium and 3) alterations in the coagulopathy of blood. One of the most common sites of DVT is the iliofemoral vascular system, although DVT can occur in any vessel. Immobility due to post-operative recovery on bedrest, long air flights, obesity, and advanced age are some of the most common causes of DVT.

At the site of the DVT, the extremity may become swollen, painful, and hot to touch. Diagnostic testing includes Doppler studies, d-dimer, CBC, and coagulation studies. Treatment is low molecular weight heparin or unfractionated heparin for renal patients. The risk for patients with DVT is that the thrombus will break loose and travel to the lungs, causing pulmonary embolus.

Pulmonary Embolus

Pulmonary embolus is an obstruction of the pulmonary vasculature caused by emboli, most often from a DVT in the iliofemoral system. The potential impact of this obstruction is based on the size and location of the embolus, as well as the patient's current cardiopulmonary health.

If the embolus completely occludes a pulmonary vessel, most likely infarction of the pulmonary tissue occurs. Partially occluding embolus can cause hemorrhage and atelectasis, though the tissue remains viable. The effects of pulmonary embolus include *alterations in gas exchange* and *hypoxia, hemodynamic compromise* based on the extent of the blockage, *pulmonary hypertension, pulmonary edema,* and *right ventricular dysfunction.* Diagnosis is made with ventilation perfusion scans, spiral CT scan, and evaluation of clinical symptoms including *chest pain, shortness of breath, and feeling of impending doom in severe cases.* The treatment for pulmonary embolus is *low molecular weight heparin or unfractionated heparin* depending on the extent of the obstruction, symptoms, and support of hemodynamic stability including oxygenation.

Immune (Idiopathic) Thrombocytopenic Purpura (ITP)

Initially this condition was named idiopathic thrombocytopenia, as the specific cause of the disease was not known. As more research has been done, the potential causes of the disease are becoming known. It is thought that the body develops an immune response and creates antibodies which destroy platelets. Specific drugs may elicit this response and can cause ITP. These include sulfanamides, thiazide diuretics, chloropropamide, quinidine and gold.

There are two treatments depending on the severity of the disease. The first is transfusion of whole blood which improves the anemia and the thrombocytopenia, as whole blood contains both red blood cells and platelets. The more invasive treatment is a splenectomy. The spleen removes platelets from the circulation on a normal basis; hence, removing the organ will prevent this from occurring.

Sepsis

Sepsis is a complex disease which is multisystem in nature. A massive systemic inflammatory response develops as a result of exposure to infectious agents, which in turn, initiates the immune response and massive phagocytosis occurs. On occasion the coagulation cascade is initiated as well, due to the widespread cell endothelium and tissue damage from hypoxemia, perfusion abnormalities (vasodilation), lactic acidosis and renal failure. This can lead to microcirculatory coagulation and continued hypoxia. Endotoxins also stimulate a cytokine and mediator release which produces a multitude of cellular responses, including increased cellular permeability, further vasodilation, activation of B and T lymphocytes, and many other systemic effects.

Treatment of sepsis includes antibiotic therapy (or therapy dependent upon type of organism), support of hemodynamic stability with vasopressors, fluids, and ventilation, medication to treat bleeding disorders, monitoring and treatment of blood glucoses, and transfusion of appropriate blood components based on applicable laboratory data. Sepsis is discussed in more detail in the chapter on multisystem disorders.

Heparin Induced Thrombocytopenia (HIT)

Heparin induced thrombocytopenia is platelet deficiency which develops after the initiation of heparin therapy. There are two types of HIT: *Type I* where mild thrombocytopenia develops within a few days after initiation of heparin therapy, and *Type II* where an immune syndrome develops and IgG attaches to the platelet causing clumping and subsequently thrombosis. The second type develops approximately 5–14 days post exposure to heparin.

In **Type I HIT**, the heparin may continue and the patient should be observed for symptoms for bleeding due to low platelets. In **Type II HIT**, the heparin must be stopped and symptomatic treatment begun. Type II HIT occurs in only about 3–5 percent of the patients on unfractionated heparin and 0.5 percent of patients on low molecular weight heparin.

The critical care nurse must be aware of this syndrome and of the potential for formation of thrombus. Venous or arterial clots may form, although venous clots are more likely. The patient should be treated with *direct thrombin inhibitors* (e.g., argatroban and lepirudin).

SPECIAL SITUATIONS

Organ Transplantation

As the medical science of organ transplantation develops, the tissue rejection challenges of the early years have diminished considerably. However, when donor cells or tissue are implanted into a recipient, it is a natural and important process which produces an immune response to the invasion of foreign cells. Significant attempts are made during matching to get the closest ABO match as is possible between the donor and the recipient.

Prevention of rejection of donor tissue is done primarily through suppression of the immune system prior to transplantation and administration of anti-rejection medications throughout the patient's life post transplantation. The primary cells which initiate rejection of transplanted tissue are the *B and T lymphocytes* as these are the cells responsible for production of antigen-binding proteins called immunoglobulins. These cells essentially kill grafted cells and therefore suppression of these cells is important to prevent rejection. The challenge becomes that the patient is then unprotected against infectious organisms. Additionally, patients who are immunosuppressed have a greater likelihood of developing cancerous cells due to the normal function of the immune system to destroy early cancer cells.

Drugs typically used in transplant patients include glucocorticoid hormones, azathioprine, cyclosporine, and other agents (Cyclophosphamide) which have a toxic effect on the lymphoid system.

Bone Marrow and Stem Cell Transplantation

Patients with malignancies who have received chemotherapy and radiation in doses high enough to destroy their bone marrow will often benefit from bone marrow and peripheral stem cell transplantation. These processes reconstitute the patient's hematological and immunological systems with healthy cells which can reproduce. The donor marrow or stem cells are harvested and infused intravenously into the recipient and travel via a natural homing mechanism to the patient's bone marrow.

There are *three types of transplantation* in this category. The first is what is referred to as an **allogenic** bone marrow transplant. A donor is identified via HLA-matching (human leukocyte antigen) to assure compatibility with recipient. A relative is the most likely donor in this type of transplantation. A sibling has a 25 percent chance of a match. There is only a small chance that an unrelated donor will match. The second type of bone marrow transplant is the **autologous** donation. Prior to treatment with chemotherapy or radiation, the patient's own marrow is harvested then later infused back into the patient. With this type of transplantation the risk of rejection is eliminated; however, there is always the potential that the transplanted marrow contains the malignant cells the patient was being treated for. Therefore, this option is more successful in patients with solid tumors and unaffected bone marrow. The final type of transplantation is done by **stimulation of the patient's own marrow to produce colony-stimulating factors**. The stem cells produced from this process are then harvested through pheresis. After the chemotherapy or radiation, the stem cells are reinfused to the patient. Similarly to the autologous donation, the risk of rejection is absent. There is a slight benefit with this type of transplant in that the ability for the stem cells to re-engraft is quicker than marrow, thus lessening the time the patient is unable to illicit an immune response.

One of the most significant complications of transplantation of bone marrow or stem cells is potential for infection due to the absence of a cellular immune function while the patient is being prepared for the transplantation. This compromise can last up to a year. A complication of chemotherapy and radiation is thrombocytopenia which can place the patient at risk for bleeding. There is also a risk of renal insufficiency from many of the medications required to either address infection or rejection. Damage can also occur to the venous system of the liver from high dose chemotherapy or radiation. Graft vs. host disease (GVHD) can occur as long as 100 days post-transplantation due to grafted T lymphocytes attacking the recipient. This can occur in up to 40–50 percent of the recipients.

PRIMARY ORGANS OF THE IMMUNOLOGICAL SYSTEM

Bone Marrow

Bone marrow has been discussed in the earlier section on organs of the hematological system.

Thymus

The thymus is a gland that is located in the upper chest under the sternum. Early in an individual's life, the lymphocytes are produced in the bone marrow and released, travel to the thymus where they mature into T cells prior to being released into the blood circulation. The thymus gland actually changes size over the life of a human. In fetal development and infancy it grows very quickly as the T cell maturation process is active, and the gland slowly degenerates as the person matures into adulthood.

Spleen

The spleen is also considered a lymphoid organ which functions to filter RBCs from the circulation, but it also filters antigens to be evaluated by the lymphocytes. The spleen is a very vascular organ. It provides lymphocytes and a source of plasma cells and therefore antibodies for cellular and humoral specific immune responses.

Lymph Vessels/Lymph System

The lymph system is a series of vessels and nodes which serve to collect plasma and leukocytes from the tissues that are not returned to the circulatory system. The combined substances are called lymph and play a role to balance fluid levels in the tissues and prevent edema from retained fluids in the tissues. Propulsion of the lymph is done by skeletal muscles. Because lymph does not contain any of the clotting factors, it coagulates slowly. The lymph fluid returns to the circulation via the right subclavian vein and thoracic duct and eventually to the left subclavian vein. On occasion the lymph nodes swell either due to WBC's or leukocytes responding to an infectious process or malignant cells which have migrated away from the primary site.

Tonsils and Adenoids

There is a mixed debate about the effectiveness of the role of the tonsils and adenoids in immunity. It is felt that in the first year of life these glands do provide some protection against infection by trapping bacteria and viruses. Years ago it was fairly common to have the tonsils and adenoids removed; however, today surgical removal is done only with repeated, frequent infections.

Skin

The skin is one of the largest organs in the body, and serves as the first line of defense to protect the body against infections. The outermost layer of epidermis serves as a tough protective barrier against environmental hazards. Additionally, the dermis contains mast cells which are in the connective tissue and function to perform the functions of secretion, phagocytosis, and production of fibroblasts.

FUNCTIONS OF THE IMMUNOLOGICAL SYSTEM

The immunological system is a very sophisticated set of organs and processes that protect the human body against nearly all types of invasive organisms. The capability to resist infection with these organisms is called *immunity*. In this section, we will discuss the two types of immunity: *acquired/adaptive immunity* and *innate immunity*. As stated above, the first line of defense to protect the body against the invasion of infectious microorganisms is the skin. It is a *mechanical barrier*. The second line of defense is *inflammatory*. Inflammatory responses are considered more rapid responses in comparison to the immune response.

Innate Immunity

Initial Primary Barriers

Innate immunity is considered to be a set of processes which are directed to respond as a first line of defense and are non-specific with regard to the organism being targeted. These include the anatomic and physiological barriers to infectious agents. As mentioned above, the skin is the first line of defense against microorganisms and is part of the innate immune response. Another simple barrier is the pH of the skin and stomach which is slightly negative. Some body functions serve as a means of a mechanical defense through flushing or mechanical removal of the organism. Examples of these include the emptying of the bladder, coughing and sneezing to remove respiratory pathogens, or gastrointestinal motility. All of these are examples of the innate immune response. Immune cells that react non-specifically to foreign particles and organisms such as macrophages, neutrophils, eosinophils, baspohils, and natural killer cells are also part of the innate immune system.

Inflammation

When inflammation occurs, the innate immune response brings about a hallmark set of events. This begins with vasodilation of the capillary bed of the site of inflammation. The capillary membrane becomes more permeable allowing fluid and immune cells to move into the area. Mediators of inflammation called eicosanoids, specifically thromboxane and leukotriene, help to increase the movement of additional inflammatory cells to the area. The physical symptoms include *erythema* (redness at the site), *edema, warmth at the site of inflammation,* and *pain.*

Phagocytosis

The next stage of the response is phagocytosis. Neutrophils and macrophages are phagocytes, described earlier and function to ingest and digest antigens such as microorganisms, dead cells, and cellular debris. During this process, the cell is able to recycle useable products and allow evaluation of the protein pieces by T cells.

Along with the above processes, a complement system is initiated which is a group of proteins that when activated or triggered by an immune response, transform specific proteins into cytokines. These products stimulate further transformations which ultimately result in massive cell destruction of the invading organisms.

Acquired (Adaptive) Immune Response

The human body also has the ability to develop a more specific response to individual antigens which include bacteria, viruses, toxins, and foreign tissue. Acquired immunity is more focused on extracellular organisms or hypersensitive reactions to allergens. Immunizations are a type of acquired immunity and provide a level of protection which is significantly stronger (as much as 100,000 times). There are two types of acquired immunity: humoral immunity and cell-mediated immunity. Both of these types of immunity are initiated by antigens. An antigen is described as a substance which, when introduced into the body, stimulates the production of an antibody.

Development of Antibodies

Antibodies are essentially proteins that sit on the surface of a B lymphocyte which is secreted into the blood at the time of exposure to an antigen. Immunoglobulins on the B cell bind the antigen on the cell surface. Antibodies are normally not present at birth but are transferred passively from the mother to the baby via the placenta or colostrum in breast milk. Antibodies are also introduced into the body by immunizations or following natural infections.

Humoral Immunity

Humoral immunity is named after the term "humours" or body fluids where the immune response is stimulated by substances known as antigens. In response to the antigen, the body stimulates the B cells to produce antibodies which bind with the antigen on the surface of the cell. Prior to stimulation, the clones of the B lymphocytes stay dormant in the lymphatic tissue. Upon presentation of the antigen, macrophages phagocytize the antigen and "present" it to the B lymphocyte and the T lymphocyte. The T cell assists as a helper cell, while the B cells specific for the antigen enlarge and transform eventually into gamma globulin antibodies (immunoglobulins). These immunoglobulins then perform specific functions to protect the body, including agglutination, precipitation, neutralization, and lysis.

Formation of the T Lymphocyte

Refer to the earlier section on formation of leukocytes, including T lymphocytes.

Cell-Mediated Immunity

Cell-mediated immunity is focused primarily on the intracellular microorganisms, viruses, and cancer cells, and is responsible for delayed hypersensitivity or allergic reactions, and tissue rejection. This type of immunity does not involve antibodies or the complement pathway, but rather involves cytotoxic T lymphocytes. With repeated exposure to allergens, activated helper and cytotoxic T cells are formed. Within a day of a subsequent exposure, the activated T cells diffuse from the circulating blood into the skin (or other areas such as the lungs) to respond to the toxins from the allergen. This produces a local response where tissue damage can occur.

Cytokines

Cytokines are secreted by cells and are considered vasoactive and biologically active mediators. There are many types of cytokines which have various activities including proliferation of B and T cells and antiviral and thrombopoietic actions. Some of the most commonly known cytokines include Interleukin-1, Interleukin-2, Tumor necrosis factor alpha (TNF-α), Interleukin-6, Interluekin 8, and Interleukin 10. Interferons are another category of cytokines that play a larger role in viral infections. Most cytokines play a role in the initial inflammatory response and are triggered by the innate immune system. The presence of these cytokines then play a differential role in the orchestration of other lymphocytes.

Eicosanoids

Eicosanoids are fatty acids which regulate processes within the body. Examples of these substances are prostaglandins, thromboxanes, and leukotrienes. These are short-lived compounds which signal cells in specific areas. For example, thromboxanes have both cardiovascular and hematological effects. The hematological effect of this eicosanoid is platelet aggregation. Medications can inhibit eicosanoid production, and can in fact, affect other physiological processes. NSAIDs (non-steroidal anti-inflammatory drugs) block the enzyme cycolooxygenase, which converts arachidonic acid to prostaglandins and thromboxanes.

CONDITIONS OF THE IMMUNOLOGICAL SYSTEM

Allergic/Hypersensitive Reactions

An allergy is sensitivity to a substance most commonly known as an allergen. There are various levels of allergic reaction to these allergen, ranging from a simple mild sensitivity to a severe anaphylactic life-threatening reaction.

In hypersensitive reactions, it is the frequency and degree of exposure which can cause subsequent more severe reactions over time. At the time of the first exposure to an allergen, abnormally large amounts of IgE antibodies are formed. When the individual has a repeated exposure, IgE triggers the release of histamine, heparin, and other cytokines which can cause more systemic symptoms such as bronchiole constriction, peripheral vasoconstriction, airway obstruction, pulmonary edema, hypovolemia, shock and circulatory collapse.

The treatment of these types of reactions includes medications such as epinephrine, diphenhydramine, bronchodilators, and steroids. Hemodynamic support may be required if the reaction causes serious hypotension or compromising arrhythmias such as supraventricular tachycardias.

Anaphylactic Shock

Anaphylactic shock is a type of distributive shock which is the result of a severe hypersensitivity reaction. This is a life-threatening event which requires immediate intervention to prevent complications and poor outcome. The ultimate effect of anaphylactic shock can be altered tissue perfusion and hypoxia, and subsequent initiation of the general shock state.

Allergens which are ingested, inhaled, or absorbed through the skin cause an antibody-antigen response which precipitates the immune response. The first time the individual is exposed to the antigen, the antigen-specific IgE (immunoglobulin) is stored as an attachment to the mast cells and basophils. The more frequently the individual is exposed to the allergen, the secondary immune response is initiated which triggers the release of chemical mediators. On occasion the individual who is not sensitized can have an anaphylactic response to the allergen.

During these severe reactions, eosinophils phagocytize the antibody-antigen complex and other debris. These antigens release enzymes which inhibit vasoactive mediators, in term secondary mediators which can increase capillary permeability and favors vasodilation. This initiates the cascade whereby peripheral vasodilation results in decreased venous return, loss of intravascular volume and hypovolemia. Altered tissue perfusion occurs as a result of the loss of cardiac output, and if left untreated or treated ineffectively, can result in airway obstruction or cardiovascular collapse.

The treatment for anaphylactic shock is to treat the patient symptomatically and immediately respond with hemodynamic support: securing the airway, mechanical ventilation, vasopressors, fluids, and removal of the allergen.

Human Immunodeficiency Virus (HIV) & Autoimmune Deficiency Syndrome (AIDS)

The treatment for HIV and AIDS has dramatically changed over the years due to extensive research in an attempt to find a cure for these diseases. Individuals who may have succumbed to these diseases in the past are living many years beyond initial expectations. The first known diagnosed case of AIDS occurred in 1981. AIDS is the disease which is caused by HIV, which progressively destroys the immune system, exposing the individual to infections.

Exposure to HIV occurs through unprotected sexual contact or intravenous needles which are shared by individuals who have HIV. It is considered a blood borne pathogen disease. The scientific name for the virus is human T lymphocyte virus-3 (HTLV-3). Once HIV has attached to the cell membrane of a CD4 T-lymphocyte, its RNA from the virus enters the cell, undergoes enzymatic transformation to DNA and this DNA is inserted into the genome of the CD4 T-lymphocyte. The CD4 T-lymphocyte then produces virion when it is activated to respond to another infection or inflammatory response. The above description is a gross oversimplification of the replication cycle of HIV, but a more detailed discussion would be futile for the purposes of the CCRN. Once the immune system has been compromised significantly (monitored by the CD4 count), the patient is susceptible to a number of opportunistic infections, such as fungal, parasitic, and viral infections.

Typically, treatment is at first a combination of drugs targeted toward HIV, as well as empiric antibiotics. The HIV medications typically include those which inhibit the replication of the RNA protein as inhibitors, and new drugs which prevent the virus from entering the cell. If patients also have evidence of infection, they are treated appropriately with antibiotics, anti-fungals, or antivirals as appropriate. At this time there is still no cure for the disease, though patients may have a much longer lifespan than they would have years ago.

Immunosuppression

Immunosuppression is simply a deficit in the immunological system which prevents an individual from launching a defense against infection. There are physiological conditions which cause immunosuppression, as well as medications which stimulate immunosuppression. Patients are often admitted to the critical care unit due to a condition which has caused immunosuppression as an adverse effect.

During organ transplantation, patients are purposefully immunosuppressed to prevent the likelihood of rejection. Anti-rejection medications work primarily on B cells and T cells in attempt to suppress not only the donor allograft but also the individual's own immune system. The challenge with this process is that the patient is then exposed to the potential for opportunistic infections, and therefore must be protected such as with neutropenic precautions.

NURSING CONSIDERATIONS IN PATIENTS WITH HEMATOLOGICAL OR IMMUNOLOGICAL CONDITIONS

The critical care nurse plays an important part in the care and management of the patient with these two types of conditions. As mentioned earlier, hematological and immunological conditions are not often the primary reason why a patient presents to the critical care unit; however, they do become conditions which dramatically impact the care of the patient throughout his stay.

History and Physical

During the course of taking the patient's history, it is imperative that the critical care nurse focus her questions to determine if the patient has evidence or symptoms of hematological or immunological conditions. The following are areas in the history which may be indicative of these conditions:

1. Current, past, or recurrent infections, including HIV

2. Malignancies

3. Liver abnormalities

4. Renal abnormalities

5. Any problems with prolonged bleeding or clotting disorders, including splenectomy

6. Past history of blood or blood component transfusion

7. Replacement of heart valves

8. Recent surgeries including dental surgery

A review of systems should also be done with the patient, or if the patient is unable to respond to the questions including signs and symptoms, the family.

1. Any evidence of fever, chills, weakness, malaise, night sweats, pain, altered mental status

2. Conditions of the skin including petechiae, changes in color, rashes, bruising

3. HEENT: headaches, vision changes, bleeding from nose or gums, problems or pain with swallowing

4. Cough, hemoptysis, dypnea, orthopnea

5. Feelings of palpitations, dizziness when standing, chest pain

6. Nausea, vomiting, passing blood in stool, weight changes, anorexia, or bloating

7. Hematuria, menorrhagia, enlarged nodes at any location (groin, axillary, neck)

8. Changes in musculoskeletal system, pain, swelling

Along with these observations and questions, family history, social history, and list of current and recent past medications should be taken. A complete head to toe physical assessment should be done, including observations which relate to evidence of bleeding or clotting disorders, infectious processes such as skin breakdown, abnormal lung sounds, etc., and any evidence of hemodynamic instability.

Diagnostic Testing

A chart of normal laboratory data relating to these systems is shown in table 7.2. Recognizing that this is not a complete listing of all laboratory tests is important. Additionally, each laboratory has a custom set of normal values (based on the calibration of instrumets used) and therefore, and these should be verified by the critical care nurse.

Cultures will be done if there is suspicion of an infection so that the site can be determined and treated appropriately. If transfusion of blood products is required, the patient will need to be typed and cross matched. If the patient has unusual antibodies, more extensive testing will be required to get a safe blood match.

Radiological testing should include chest films if a respiratory infection is suspected. Ultrasound testing is helpful if there needs to be an assessment of the spleen or liver, particularly if there is suspicion of malignancy.

TABLE 7.2 *Normal Lab Values*

Test	Expected Normal Value
WBC	4000–10000/µl
Neutrophils	50–65%
Bands	3–6%
Monocytes	3–7%
Basophils	0–1%
Eosinophils	0–3%
Lymphocytes	25–40%
RBC	Men $4.5–5.5 \times 10^6$/L
	Women $4.0–5.0 \times 10^6$/L
Hgb	Men 14–17.4 g/dL
	Women 12–16 g/dL
Hct	Men 42–52%
	Women 36–48%
Platelets	140,000–440,000/mm^3
Bleeding time	3–10 min.
INR	0.9–1.2
PT	11–13 sec
PTT	30–45 sec
FSP	Negative at 1:4 dilution
Iron	Men 75–175 µg/dl
	Women 65–165 µg/dl
TIBC	240–450 µg/dl
Fibrinogen	200–400 mg/dl

Another common test for patients with suspected leukemia or lymphoma will be the bone marrow aspiration and biopsy. Surgical biopsy of lymph nodes may also be required.

Skin tests will be helpful to determine if the patient has sensitivity to allergens or antigens. Some infections such as tuberculosis and coccidiomycosis can also be helpful for diagnosing.

Appropriate Nursing Diagnoses

Critical care nurses have the ability to identify the highest priority in patient care needs and devise a plan of care which will address the goals and interventions for those priorities. It is helpful also to have a multidisciplinary team who evaluates these priorities on a daily basis and engages in the recovery of the patient.

Key nursing diagnoses for patients with hematological and immunological conditions include:

1. Risk for infection related to disease or treatment, e.g., neutropenia

2. Risk for hemorrhage related to disease or treatment, e.g., thrombocytopenia

3. Altered gas exchange related to anemia, abnormal loss of RBCs

4. Alterations in hemodynamic stability relating to shock states, e.g., septic shock, anaphylactic shock, hemorrhagic shock

5. Coping difficulties related to new diagnosis of malignancy or abnormality in blood components

With the information the critical care nurse has gained with the physical assessment and the above nursing diagnoses, specific interventions can be determined and put into place. Many times due to the nature of the conditions these are emergent interventions which should be implemented immediately to prevent complications. Most often with conscientious and meticulous care these patients can recover with good outcomes.

The Neurologic System

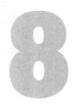

The nervous system is a complex network of cells, tissues, and specialized organs. It is the center of thinking, judgment, memory, cognition, communication, behavior, emotion, sensation, and movement. There is both direct and indirect control of the body systems. For example, a traumatic brain injury affecting the motor strip of the temporal lobe may result in seizures and/or loss of limb movement.

ANATOMY REVIEW

The entire nervous system is made up of two types of cells: **neurons**, which transmit or conduct nerve impulses, and **neuroglial cells**, which support the neurons. Each neuron consists of a **cell body**, an **axon**, and **dendrites**. Myelinated axons are called **white matter**. Nonmyelinated axons are called **gray matter**. The myelin sheath is interrupted at intervals by the **nodes of Ranvier**. The nodes of Ranvier allow movement of ions across the cellular membrane.

FIGURE 8.1 *Neuron*

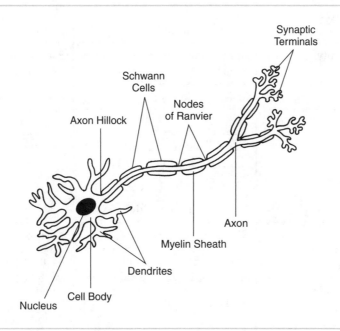

Neurotransmitters

In the central nervous system, **neurotransmitters** are chemical substances that inhibit, excite, or modify the responses of another cell. In general, each neuron releases the same transmitter at all of its terminals.

TABLE 8.1 *Neurotransmitters: Site and Action*

Amines		
Classes	**Site**	**Action**
Acetylcholine	Brain, brainstem, basal ganglia, and autonomic nervous system	Usually excitatory; some inhibitory effects of parasympathetic nervous system (e.g., heart by vagus)
Serotonin	Medial brainstem, hypothalamus, dorsal horn of spinal cord	Inhibits spinal pain pathway; helps control mood and sleep

Catecholamines		
Classes	**Site**	**Action**
Dopamine	Substantia nigra to basal ganglia	Usually inhibitory
Norepinephrine	Brain stem, hypothalamus	Usually excitatory, sometimes inhibitory
Amino acids	Sympathetic nervous system	Some excitatory; some inhibitory
Aspartate	Brain, spinal cord	Excitatory
Gamma-amino-butyric acid (GABA)	Brain, basal ganglia, cerebellum, spinal cord	Some excitatory; some inhibitory
Glutamic acid	Sensory pathways	Excitatory
Glycine	Spinal cord	Inhibitory
Substance P	Pain fibers of dorsal horns of spinal cord, hypothalamus	Excitatory

Polypeptides		
Classes	**Site**	**Action**
Endorphins	Pituitary gland, thalamus, spinal cord, hypothalamus	Excitatory to systems that inhibit pain
Enkephalins	Spinal cord, brain stem	Excitatory to systems that inhibit pain

Neuroglial Cells

The second types of cells in the nervous system are **neuroglia (glia)**. They support the neurons by providing protection, structural support, and nutrition. In the central nervous system, there are four types of neuroglia: **astrocytes**, **ependymal cells**, **oligodendroglia**, and **microglia**. The neuroglia are very important for their support of the neurons but also for their capability of division and replication throughout adulthood. This ability makes glial cells susceptible to abnormal cell division (cancer).

The central nervous system (CNS) has two major divisions: the **brain** and **spinal cord**. The brain is composed of the cerebrum, the brainstem, and the cerebellum. The spinal cord is the conduit for the ascending sensory and descending motor neurons. This is the pathway for two-way communication between the brain and the periphery.

Bones

The bones of the skull and the vertebral column prevent injury to the brain and the spinal cord. The skull is the bony, rigid framework of the head. It is composed of the 14 bones of the face and the eight bones of the cranium. In the newborn, fontanelles (areas between the bones) remain open for approximately 18 to 24 months. They fill with fibrous tissue that is gradually replaced with bone to form suture lines. The four major suture lines are **sagittal**, **coronal**, **lambdoidal**, and **basilar**.

Meninges

The brain and spinal cord are covered with a series of membranes called the **meninges**. These include the **dura mater**, the **arachnoid**, and the **pia mater**.

Brain

The **cerebrum** is the largest part of the brain. Each hemisphere has an outer layer of neurons called the white matter and an inner layer of gray matter. These two hemispheres are connected by a thick band of white fibers called the **corpus callosum**. The corpus callosum allows the two hemispheres to communicate. Each hemisphere receives sensory and motor impulses from the opposite side of the body. The majority of people are left brain dominant. The left side controls language, while the right side controls perception.

Ventricles

There are **four ventricles** (or chambers) within the brain. The chambers are filled with cerebrospinal fluid and are linked by ducts (also called foramen), that permit circulation. **Cerebrospinal fluid** (CSF) is a clear, colorless fluid produced by the **choroid plexus**, located in the ventricles. Reabsorption occurs via the **arachnoid villi**.

FIGURE 8.2 *Cross-Section of Spinal Cord and Components of a Spinal Nerve*

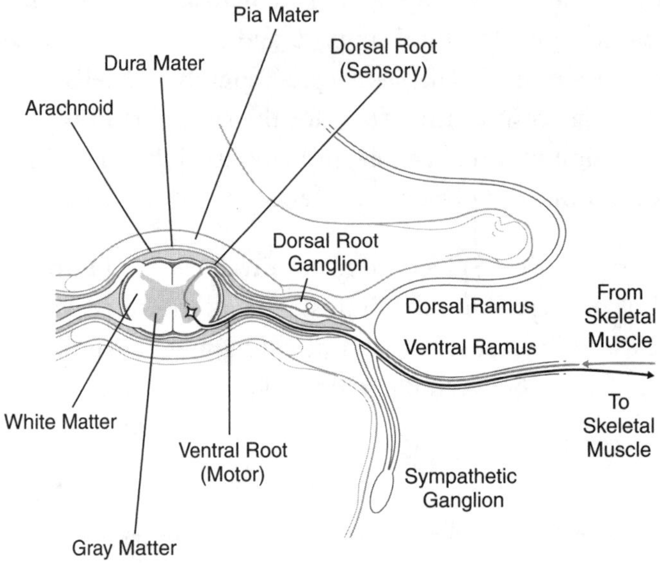

Pia Mater

Dura Mater

Dorsal Root
(Sensory)

Arachnoid

Dorsal Root
Ganglion

Dorsal Ramus

Ventral Ramus

From
Skeletal
Muscle

To
Skeletal
Muscle

White Matter

Ventral Root
(Motor)

Sympathetic
Ganglion

Gray Matter

FIGURE 8.3 *Brain*

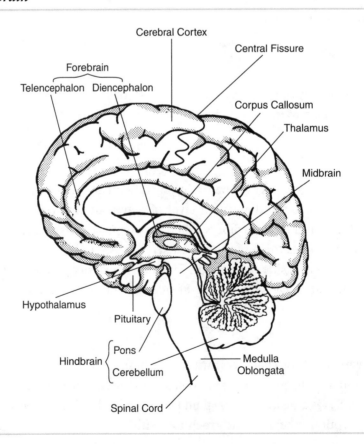

Cerebral Cortex

Central Fissure

Forebrain

Telencephalon   Diencephalon

Corpus Callosum

Thalamus

Midbrain

Hypothalamus

Pituitary

Pons

Hindbrain

Cerebellum

Medulla
Oblongata

Spinal Cord

FIGURE 8.4 *CSF Circulation*

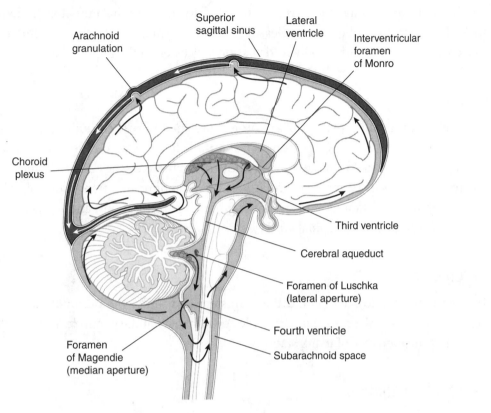

Basal Ganglia

The **basal ganglia** are found deep within the cerebral hemispheres. They consist of several collections of nuclei: the **lenticular nucleus**, the **caudate nucleus**, the **amygdaloid body**, and the **claustrum**. The basal ganglia coordinate communication between the cerebral cortex and the cerebellum that controls motor activity. Lesions of the basal ganglia produce abnormal movements including chorea, althetosis, hemiballismus, and dystonic posturing.

Lobes

The lobes of the cerebral hemispheres are **frontal**, **parietal**, **temporal**, and **occipital**.

Diencephalon

The diencephalon is composed of the **thalamus**, **epithalamus**, and **hypothalamus**. The thalamus is the initial processing area for sensory input. The epithalamus forms the roof of the third ventricle and the pineal gland. The hypothalamus regulates temperature, appetite, water metabolism, emotional expression, thirst, and a portion of the sleep-wake cycle.

Hypophysis

The **hypophysis** (pituitary gland) is connected to the hypothalamus by the hypophyseal stalk. There are two lobes, each releasing specific hormones into the systemic circulation (see chapter 6). It is controlled by information processed in the hypothalamus.

Brainstem

The brainstem includes the **midbrain**, **pons**, and **medulla**. The midbrain is the center for auditory and visual reflexes. The pons is responsible for arousal and sleep, assistance in controlling autonomic functions, and relays information between the cerebrum and cerebellum. The medulla plays is the main control center for autonomic functions (control of heart rate, blood pressure, respirations, and swallowing.), such as respirations, and relays neural signals between the brain and the spinal cord.

Cerebellum

The **cerebellum** is located behind the brainstem and under the occipital lobe of the cerebrum. Functions of the cerebellum include coordinate voluntary muscle movement, equilibrium, and maintenance of trunk stability.

Cerebral Circulation

The source of blood to the brain occurs via the **internal carotid arteries** (anterior circulation) and the **vertebral and basilar arteries** (posterior circulation). These arteries join at the base of the brain to form the **Circle of Willis** (cerebral arterial circle). The two anterior cerebral arteries (ACA) supply the medial portion on the frontal lobes. Two middle cerebral arteries (MCA) supply the outer portions of the frontal, parietal, and superior temporal lobes. The two posterior inferior cerebral arteries (PICA) supply the medial portions of the occipital and inferior temporal lobes.

Venous blood drains from the brain via the dural sinuses that drain into the two jugular veins. Knowledge of the major arteries of the brain and the areas supplied is necessary for understanding and evaluating the signs and symptoms of brain tumors, cerebral vascular disease, and trauma.

Blood-brain Barrier

The **blood-brain barrier** maintains a functionally stable environment for the central nervous system. It does this by selectively allowing a restricted number of molecules and cells across the barrier. For example, white blood cells (WBC) generally do not have access to the brain, making the brain an immunoprivileged site. While protecting the brain, it impairs the effectiveness of many drugs used to treat nervous system problems.

FIGURE 8.5 *Cranial Nerves and Brainstem*

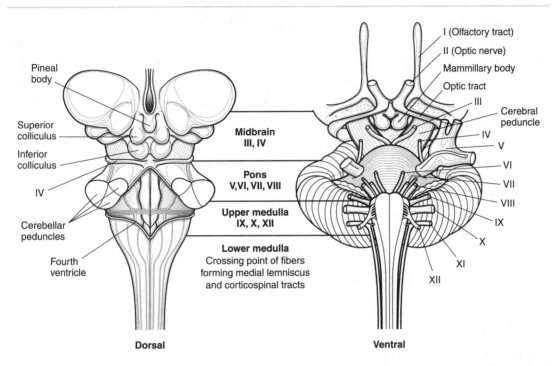

Spine

The **spine** is a flexible column formed by series of bones called **vertebrae**. There are 33 vertebrae: seven **cervical**, twelve **thoracic**, five **lumbar**, five **sacral** (fused into one), and four **coccygeal** (fused into one). The vertebrae serve multiple functions: protection of the **spinal cord**, support of the head, and assistance with spinal flexibility.

Spinal Cord

The **spinal cord** extends from the medulla to the level of the first lumbar vertebrae. It exits the cranial cavity through the **foramen magnum**. A cross-section of the spinal cord reveals **gray matter** in an **H** pattern in the central portion. It is surrounded by **white matter**. The **ascending tracts** carry specific sensory information to the higher levels of the CNS. The information comes from specialized sensory receptors in the skin, muscles, joints, viscera, and blood vessels. **Descending tracts** carry impulses from the higher levels to the lower motor neurons. The **lower motor neurons** are the final step of the nerve impulse before stimulation of skeletal muscle. **Upper motor neurons** are located in the brainstem and cerebral cores and also influence skeletal muscle movement. Damage to the upper motor neurons, sometimes seen in multiple sclerosis, may cause weakness, atrophy, hyperreflexia, or spasticity. Circulation to the spinal cord comes from three sources: **anterior spinal**, two **posterior spinal**, and branches of the descending aorta.

Peripheral Nervous System

The **peripheral nervous system** (PNS) is composed of the spinal nerves, cranial nerves, and the autonomic nervous system. The **spinal nerves** consist of 31 pairs exiting from the spinal cord. They include: eight cervical, 12 thoracic, five lumbar, five sacral, and one coccygeal. Each spinal nerve has both a sensory and a motor component for a specific area of the body. The spinal nerves are composed of a dorsal root and ventral root as they enter and exit the spinal column. The dorsal root is responsible for carrying sensory information into the spinal cord, while the ventral root is composed of motor neurons carrying signals from the upper motor neurons to the muscles.

Sensory Receptors

Sensory input is collected throughout the body by receptors of pain, temperature, touch, vibration, pressure, visceral sensation, and proprioception. This information is transmitted to the cortex, along with input from the special senses: vision, taste, smell, and hearing.

Cranial Nerves

The **cranial nerves** provide both motor and sensory innervation for the head, neck, and viscera. There are 12 cranial nerves. Anatomically they begin in and emerge from the cranium. See Figure 8.5 for more detail.

Autonomic Nervous System

The **autonomic nervous system** (ANS) has two components: **sympathetic** and **parasympathetic**. The two systems function together to maintain homeostasis of the body's internal environment. The sympathetic nervous system is responsible for the flight-fight response, such as increased heart rate, dilation of the pupils, constriction of the visceral vasculature and dilation of the vasculature, increase in the blood supply to the skeletal muscles, and decreased intestinal motility. The sympathetic and parasympathetic nervous systems act in opposition to each other.

Reflexes

A **reflex** is a response to a stimulus that occurs without conscious control. One way to classify reflexes is stretch, cutaneous, and pathologic. Muscle stretch reflexes are also called **deep tendon reflexes** (DTRs). Cutaneous reflexes are termed **superficial reflexes**. Superficial reflexes occur when noxious stimulation is applied to the skin. The response is withdrawal from the irritant. An example is contraction of the abdominal muscles when the skin is stroked. **Primitive or pathologic reflexes** are normal in infants and toddlers but should not be present in healthy adults. Presence of a pathologic reflex in an adult indicates interference

TABLE 8.2 *Cranial Nerve Function*

Nerve	Function
I. Olfactory	*Sensory:* Smell
II. Optic	*Sensory:* Sight
III. Oculomotor	*Motor:* Eye movements; contraction of iris
	Parasympathetic: Smooth muscles of eye socket
IV. Trochlear	*Motor:* Eye movement
V. Trigeminal (has 3 branches)	
Ophthalmic	*Sensory:* forehead, eye, and superior nasal cavity
Maxillary	*Sensory:* inferior nasal cavity, face, upper teeth, and superior mucosa of mouth
Mandibular	*Sensory:* jaw surfaces, lower teeth, anterior tongue, and inferior mucosa of mouth
	Motor: Muscles for chewing
VI. Abducens	*Sensory:* Eye movement
VII. Facial	*Motor:* Muscles of expression, cheek muscle
	Sensory: Taste of anterior two thirds of tongue
VIII. Vestibulocochlear (has 2 components)	
Vestibular	*Sensory:* Balance
Cochlear	*Sensory:* Hearing
IX. Glossopharyngeal	*Sensory:* Pharynx and posterior tongue (including taste)
	Motor: Superior pharyngeal muscles, swallowing
X. Vagus	*Sensory:* Viscera of chest and abdomen
	Motor: Larynx, middle and inferior pharyngeal muscles
	Parasympathetic: Heart, lungs, most of GI tract
XI. Accessory	*Motor:* Movement of neck muscles
XII. Hypoglossal	*Motor:* Movement of tongue

with the normal CNS function. The upward movement of the great toe with flaring of the pedal digits (Babinski's reflex) is an example of a pathologic reflex, indicative of upper motor neuron disease. Sensory information from the specific peripheral location is responsible for the motor impulses that return to the same peripheral location. This is called a reflex arc.

TABLE 8.3 *Sympathetic versus Parasympathetic Response*

System	Sympathetic Response	Parasympathetic Response
Neurological	Pupils dilated Heightened awareness	Pupils normal size
Cardiovascular	Increased heart rate Increased myocardial contractility Increased blood pressure	Decreased heart rate Decreased myocardial contractility
Respiratory	Increased respiratory rate Increased respiratory depth Bronchial dilation	Bronchial constriction
Gastrointestinal	Decreased gastric motility Decreased gastric secretions Increased glycogenolysis Decreased insulin production Sphincter contraction	Increased gastric motility Increased gastric secretions Sphincter dilation
Genitourinary	Decreased urine output Decreased renal blood flow	Normal urine output

Age-related Changes

As the human body ages, patients begin to experience both motor and sensory changes. Chronic diseases of the bones, muscles, or joints can have a detrimental effect on the nerves' motor function. With aging there is a decrease in both muscle bulk and nerve electrical activity. This causes diminished muscle strength and a decrease in reaction and movement time. Sensory function is diminished due to a decrease in total sensory receptors, decrease in electrical activity, and atrophy or degeneration of the taste buds, olfactory bulb, and vestibular system of the inner ear. Reflexes may diminish due to degeneration of the myelin sheath. Cognitive function continues at the same level as in younger years, unless disease impairs the brain. For example, arteriosclerosis and hypertension may lead to a cerebrovascular accident (CVA) that causes brain damage.

PHYSICAL ASSESSMENT

Assessment of the neurologic system begins with the history. The health history interview collects subjective data. The second portion is the physical examination of the neurologic system, which collects objective data. A complete neurological health history assists the nurse to identify strengths and weaknesses and determine the extent of any problems involving the nervous system. If the patient is alert, able to state his name, where he is, and what day it is, proceed with the health history. When the patient is comatose or too lethargic to cooperate, the nurse must access secondary sources, such as family or significant others.

Mental Assessment

When assessing patients with altered levels of consciousness, use the Glasgow Coma Scale (GCS). The Glasgow Coma Scale is the most widely recognized, standardized level of consciousness (LOC) assessment tool. The score is based on three categories: eye opening, verbal response, and best motor response. The best possible score is 15 and the lowest score is 3, but a score of 8 or less generally indicates a significant alteration in level of consciousness. Mental assessment should always be conducted off any sedation.

TABLE 8.4 *Cranial Nerve Assessment*

Nerve	Function	Assessment
I. Olfactory	Smell	Identify common, nonirritating substances Not usually done; unreliable in infant/child
II. Optic	Vision	Snellen or Rosenbaum Pocket Vision Screener Randomly read from a newspaper or magazine Assess visual fields using confrontation test
III. Oculomotor	Tested together	Eyelid elevation
IV. Trochlear	control eye	Pupil constriction
V. Trigeminal nerve	Ophthalmic	Corneal reflexes with puff of air
	Maxillary	Clench jaw (infant-assess sucking strength)
	Mandibular	Pin prick
VI. Abducens	muscles	Movement through 6 cardinal directions (infants will require holding of their head still)
VII. Facial nerve	Taste	Usually deferred
	Facial movement	Raise eyebrows, close eyelids, puff out cheeks, smile, and frown
VIII. Acoustic nerve	Cochlear (hearing)	Have patient listen to sounds.
	Vestibular (balance)	Walk heel to toe; walk on tip-toes; walk on heels
IX. Glossopharyngeal	Swallowing	Have patient swallow water
X. Vagus	Gag reflex	Touch back of throat with tongue blade
XI. Spinal accessory	Neck muscles	Have patient shrug shoulders and turn head against resistance *Infant:* observe side-to-side head movement
XII. Hypoglossal	Tongue muscles	Have patient open mouth, stick out tongue, and wiggle it side to side *Infant:* pinch nose and observe tongue movement.

Motor Assessment

The nerves of the motor system originate from the spinal cord and control muscle movement. The motor examination begins with the neck and proceeds from proximal (upper) to distal (lower) extremities. Major muscle groups are assessed for specific functions.

TABLE 8.5 *Major Muscle Groups of the Upper and Lower Extremities*

Level	Muscle	Action
C5, C6, C7	Serratus anterior	Movement of shoulder
C5, C6	Deltoid; supraspinatus	Abduction of shoulder
C5, C6	Biceps brachii	Flexion of elbow
C5, C6	Brachioradialis	Flexion of elbow
C7, C8	Triceps brachii	Extension of elbow
C6, C7	Extensor carpi radialis; extensor carpi ulnaris	Extension of wrist
C7, C8	Flexor carpi radialis; flexor carpi ulnaris	Flexion of wrist
C7	Extensor digitorum; extensor indicis proprius; extensor digiti minimi	Extension of fingers
C8, T1	Flexor digitorum superficialis, profundus, and lumbricalis	Flexion of fingers
T1	Dorsal interossei; abductor digiti quinti	Abduction of fingers
C8, T1	Palmar interossei	Adduction of fingers
C8, T1	Opponens pollicis	Opposition of thumb
T12, L1, L2, L3	Iliopsoas	Hip flexion
L2, L3, L4	Adductor brevis, longus, and magnus	Hip adduction
L4, L5, S1	Gluteus medius	Hip abduction
L5, S1, S2	Gluteus maximus	Hip extension
L2, L3, L4	Quadriceps	Knee extension
L5, S1, S2	Hamstrings	Knee flexion
L4, L5	Tibialis anterior; peroneus tertius; extensor digitorum longus; extensor hallucis longus	Ankle dorsiflexion
S1, S2	Gastrocnemius; soleus	Ankle plantar flexion
L4, L5	Tibialis posterior	Foot inversion
L4, S1	Peroneus longus; peroneus brevis	Foot eversion

Sensory Assessment

Evaluation of the sensory system tests the patient's ability to perceive various types of sensations. The *body areas usually assessed* are face, neck, deltoid regions, forearms, hands (top), chest, abdomen, thighs, lower legs, and feet (top). Superficial sensation is tested using various modalities: light touch, pin prick, pain, and temperature.

Deep sensation evaluates vibration, deep pressure pain, position, and discriminate fine touch.

Normally, the patient should be able to sense vibration over the bony prominences.

Instruct the patient to close his eyes when testing position sense (**propriocepetion**). Lightly grasp the patient's finger or great toe and gently move up or down. Instruct the patient to indicate verbally which direction the digit is in. Vary the direction to prevent the patient from anticipating the digit location.

When testing for **stereognosis**, ask the patient to close his eyes and place an object (coin, paper clip, key) into the patient's hand. Instruct the patient to feel the object. Ask the patient to name the object.

To test **graphesthesia**, ask the patient to close his eyes, then draw a letter, number, or shape in the patient's open hand.

Reflex Assessment

Evaluation of reflexes provides important information on the status of the central nervous system in both conscious and unconscious patients. Altered reflexes may be the earliest signs of a pathological condition. There are three categories of reflexes: deep tendon, cutaneous, and pathologic. **Deep tendon reflexes** (muscle-stretch reflexes) occur in response to a sudden stimulus (e.g., tapping with a reflex hammer). It is important to use the correct technique to elicit the specific reflex. With the muscle relaxed and the joint in neutral position and supported by the examiner, the tendon is tapped directly with the reflex hammer. Normally the muscle contracts with a quick movement of the limb or structure. Cutaneous reflexes occur in response to cutaneous sensation, such as the cremasteric reflex, where brushing on the inner upper thigh results in contraction of the cremaster muscle.

Pathological reflexes are also called primitive reflexes because they are normally seen in infants and then disappear. If these reflexes reappear, they are found in patients suffering from dementia syndromes or Parkinson's disease. Grading of pathological reflexes is documented as presence (+) is abnormal and absence (–) is normal. Examples of primitive reflexes are the Moro (startle response), stepping, rooting, sucking, tonic neck flex, plantar, palmar grasp, upgoing babinski, and gallant reflexes.

TABLE 8.6 *Pathological (Primitive) Reflexes*

Reflex	Technique
Grasp	Stimulation of palm results in a grasp
Snout	Stimulation of circumoral region results in puckering of lips
Sucking	Stimulation of lips, tongue, or palate results in sucking movement
Rooting	Stimulation of lips results in head moving toward stimulus
Palmomental	Stimulation of palm results in contraction of the chin muscles
Glabellar	Eyes blink each time the glabellar area (between eyes) is tapped Normal: Blinking stops after first few taps

TABLE 8.7 *Neurodiagnostic Studies*

Study	Purpose	Nursing Care
Lumbar puncture	Obtain CSF for analysis. Measure CSF opening pressure.	Have patient empty bladder. Position in lateral decubitis position, with back arched, knees flexed on chest, chin touching knees. Keep flat in bed for 6 to 8 hours to prevent headache. Monitor neurological status and vital signs. Encourage fluids and administer IV fluids; give analgesics PRN. Complications: headache; abscess; low back pain; meningitis; CSF leak; spinal cord puncture
Skull x-rays	Identify skull/facial fractures, tumor, cranial anomalies, bone erosion, air/fluid levels in sinuses, calcification, foreign bodies	Linear/basal fractures often missed by routine x-rays
Spine x-rays	Identify vertebral dislocation or fracture; degenerative disease; bone erosion; tumor; calcification; structural defects; injury	Prevent fracture displacement by maintaining spinal precautions.
Computed axial tomography (CT)	Identify acute vs chronic bleeding; hydrocephalus; abscess; identify tumors.	Sedation may be given. If contrast given, check for allergies and renal function. Encourage fluids post-test.

TABLE 8.7 *Neurodiagnostic Studies (continued)*

Study	Purpose	Nursing Care
Magnetic resonance imaging (MRI)	Identify strokes, tumors, trauma, seizures, edema, and herniation. Gadolinium (non-iodine contrast media) may be used.	Contraindicated in patients with iron-based (ferrous) implanted objects (artificial joints, pacemakers, bullets or metal fragments, clips/wires) Sedation may be required. Patient must lie still during test.
Magnetic resonance angiography (MRA)	Visualizes blood flow in extracranial and intracranial blood vessels. Identifies vascular lesions (stenosis, aneurysms, arteriovenous malformations).	Similar to MRI Assess boney prominences for pressure areas.
Magnetic resonance spectroscopy (MRS)	Differentiate tumor vs. abscess or infection vs. autoimmune destruction.	Similar to MRI
Functional magnetic resonance imaging (fMRI)	Functional mapping of the brain using chemical changes in response to specific tasks	Similar to MRI
Cerebral angiography (angiogram)	Visualize cerebral vasculature. Identify aneurysms, AVM, vasospasm, tumors.	Sedation may be given. Check for allergies and renal function. Post test: Maintain bed rest 6–12 hours. Maintain hydration. Monitor vital signs, assess puncture site for hematoma or bleeding, frequent neuro checks, check pedal pulses, color, sensation, and temperature of affected extremity. Complications: Anaphylaxis; seizures; stroke; thrombosis; PE; shock; aphasia; vision changes.
Digital subtraction angiography (DSA)	Same as angiogram	May be done arterially or via IV. If done arterially, nursing care is the same as angiogram. When done via IV there are fewer complications, since it is less invasive.
Positron emission tomography (PET)	Provides 3-D structure and functional view of the brain. Evaluates oxygen and glucose metabolism. Measures cerebral blood flow.	Sedation may be given. Check for allergies and renal function. Maintain hydration. Monitor vital signs; frequent neuro checks.

TABLE 8.7 *Neurodiagnostic Studies (continued)*

Study	Purpose	Nursing Care
Single-photon emission CT (SPECT)	Same as for PET scan. Uses contrast that emits gamma rays.	Same as for PET scan.
Myelogram	Visualizes spinal subarachnoid space. Detects spinal cord lesions (obstructions, compression, herniated intervertebral discs).	If done with oil-based contrast, maintain bed rest for 4–8 hours. With water-soluble contrast, elevate head of bed. Maintain hydration. Complications: Anaphylaxis, headache, nausea, vomiting, backache, neck ache, chest pain, seizures, dysrhythmias.
Electroencephalography (EEG)	Identifies areas of abnormal electrical discharge in the brain.	Withhold caffeine, tobacco, alcohol, anticonvulsants, stimulants, tranquilizers, and antidepressants 24–48 hours prior to test. Shampoo hair before and after test.
Magnetoencephalography (MEG)	Similar to EEG with addition of biomagnetometer, which detects magnetic fields generated by neural activity. Identifies location of seizure, stroke, or injury.	Similar to EEG.
Electromyography (EMG)	Nerve conduction studies. Identifies muscle disease, peripheral, neuropathies, nerve compression, nerve regeneration, muscle recovery.	May be uncomfortable. Contraindicated in patients taking anticoagulants, with bleeding disorders, or with skin infections.
Evoked potentials (EPs)	Evaluate electrical responses of brain to external stimuli. Identify spinal cord injury, tumors, neuromuscular or cerebrovascular disease, traumatic brain injury, peripheral nerve disease.	Similar to EEG.

TABLE 8.8 *Cerebrospinal Fluid Analysis*

Parameter	Normal Value	Analysis
Opening pressure	60–200 mm H_2O	<60—dehydration; blocked CSF >200—brain tumor, abscess, or cyst; subdural hematoma; hydrocephalus; cerebral edema.
Appearance	clear, colorless	*Xanthochromia* is often due to the breakdown of blood products. *Turbidity or cloudiness* is often due to increased WBC's; elevated protein levels; or infection.
RBCs (red blood cells)	none	Cell count of RBCs indicates bleeding; serial reductions in tubes sent from LP, may indicate a traumatic tap.
WBCs (white blood cells)	0–8/ L	Elevations may indicate meningitis; tumors; and multiple sclerosis.
Protein	15–45 mg/dl	Elevations with infection; tumor; hemorrhage, tumors; and multiple sclerosis.
Glucose	45–75 mg/dl	Elevations are not significant; decrease indicates infection.
Microorganisms	none	
pH	7.35	
Specific gravity	1.007	

TABLE 8.9 *Types of Evoked Potentials*

Type	Stimulus	Purpose
Visual Visual evoked potential (VEP) Pattern reversal electrical potential (PREP) Visual electrical response (VER)	Rapidly changing geometric designs or flashing lights	Locate lesion in visual pathway or visual cortex
Auditory Auditory evoked potential (AEP) Auditory brainstem evoked potential (ABEP)	Multiple clicks to each ear via earphones	Locate lesion; evaluate the central auditory pathways of the brainstem; follow the course of recovery

TABLE 8.9 *Types of Evoked Potentials (continued)*

Type	Stimulus	Purpose
Somatosensory Somatosensory brainstem evoked potential (SBEP) Somatosensory evoked potential (SEP)	Electrical stimulation of selected peripheral nerves	Differentiate lesions of the peripheral nerve from those of subcortical or cortical central sensory pathways
Carotid doppler scan	Detects atherosclerotic carotid artery disease.	No specific follow-up care is required.
Transcranial doppler (TCD)	Measures blood flow velocity of the cerebral arteries, identifies vasospasm, emboli, vascular stenosis, and brain death.	When vasospasm is identified, patient may require treatment via angiography.

PATHOLOGIES

Vascular Hemorrhage (Bleeding)

Subarachnoid hemorrhage (SAH) is bleeding into the subarachnoid space. There are multiple causes of SAH including cerebral aneurysms, arteriovenous malformations, traumatic injury to an artery, hypertensive intracranial bleeding, and hemorrhage from a brain tumor. A cerebral aneurysm is a dilation of the artery due to weakness of the middle and inner layers of the vessel wall. Most cerebral aneurysms occur at bifurcations of the large arteries at the base of the brain (circle of Willis). Aneurysms are classified as sacular or berry (ballooning of the wall with a stem-like attachment to the vessel), fusiform (usually a large atherosclerotic bulge), dissecting (bleeding into the inner layers of the arterial wall), or mycotic (infected lesion of the vessel wall).

SAH from aneurysm rupture affects approximately 30,000 Americans each year. Aneurysm rupture in childhood is rare. The incidence of SAH is greater in women and increases with age. Mortality from ruptured aneurysms is 25 percent with the majority of these patients dying within 24 hours of the initial bleeding. Significant morbidity is seen in approximately 50 percent of SAH survivors.

Presenting signs and symptoms of SAH include severe headache, brief loss of consciousness, nausea, vomiting, photophobia, focal neurologic deficits, and a stiff neck. The headache is often referred to as a "thunder clap" headache or the "worst headache of my life" by patients. Neonates may present with heart failure and children may be asymptomatic for many years. Kernig's (reflex contraction and pain in the hamstring muscles, when attempting to extend

FIGURE 8.6 *Circle of Willis*

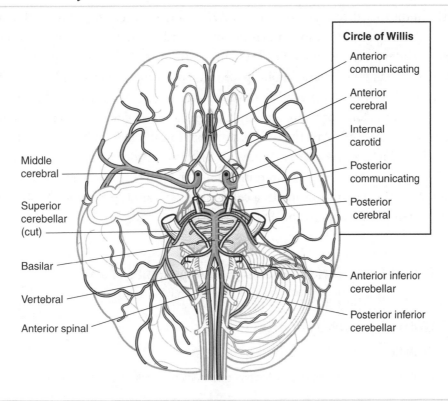

the leg after flexion) or Brudzinski's (flexion of the hips when the neck is flexed from a supine position) sign is sometimes present. These signs are seen in patients with meningeal irritation. Aneurysms are graded using several scales (Botterell, Hunt/Hess, or World Federation of Neurologic Surgeons).

Hunt/Hess Classification of SAH

Grade I: Asymptomatic or minimal headache and slight nuchal rigidity.

Grade II: Moderate to severe headache, nuchal rigidity, no neurologic deficit other than cranial nerve palsy.

Grade III: Drowsiness, confusion, or mild focal deficit.

Grade IV: Stupor, moderate-to-severe hemiparesis, possible early decerebrate rigidity, and vegetative disturbances.

Grade V: Deep coma, decerebrate rigidity, moribund appearance.

Diagnostic Studies

Diagnostic studies used for assessment of SAH include presenting signs and symptoms, computed tomography (CT) scan, lumbar puncture, and angiography. Noncontrast CT scan is the 'gold standard' for definitive SAH diagnosis. In over 90 percent of patients, CT scan demonstrates blood in the subarachnoid space when performed within 24 hours of the onset of symptoms. When the CT is negative, lumbar puncture (LP) is performed to obtain cerebral spinal fluid for color, a pressure reading, protein, and cell counts. If the LP is performed more than 5 days after the SAH, the CSF is xanthochromic (dark amber) due to breakdown of the blood products. If the CSF is cloudy, an infectious process such as bacterial meningitis is the diagnosis, not SAH. Transcranial doppler (TCD) studies are used to assess for vasospasm. After the diagnosis is made, a cerebral angiogram is performed to show the size, shape, location of the aneurysm, and any vasospasm.

Fischer Grade Scale of Radiological Appearance of SAH

Grade I: None evident

Grade II: Less than 1 mm thick

Grade III: More than 1 mm thick

Grade IV: Any thickness w/ interventricular hemorrhage or parenchymal extension

Management

Aneurysm treatment includes symptom management and either surgical or endovascular methods. Before definitive repair is attempted, symptom control may include airway management, blood pressure control, seizure control, and electrocardiogram (ECG) changes. Patients with a GCS score less than eight or patients without airway protective reflexes, should be electively intubated and mechanically ventilated. Hypertension is a common symptom prior to surgery. SAH patients should be hemodynamically monitored in the ICU. Since there is loss of cerebral autoregulation after an intracranial hemorrhage, maintaining diastolic blood pressure 120–150 mm Hg is recommended before definitive treatment. Blood pressure should not be lowered too rapidly, as this can cause cerebral ischemia. Management of hypertension may require IV sodium nitroprusside or labetalol. Seizure control should start with fosphenytoin. The most common dysrhythmias that occur after SAH are prolonged, QT interval and torsades de pointes. All of these sequelae of SAH require close monitoring of the patient's neurological status, reduction of environmental stimuli, and analgesia for pain.

Complications

Common complications of SAH are rebleeding, hydrocephalus, and vasospasm. Rebleeding of the aneurysm occurs most often 2–10 days after the initial rupture. As the clot which initially sealed the rupture site undergoes fibrinolysis, there is a risk of rebleeding. This may be accompanied by a sudden worsening of headache, severe nausea and vomiting, decrease in level of consciousness (LOC), and new focal neurological deficits. **Hydrocephalus** is the progressive dilatation of the ventricular system when the production of CSF exceeds the absorption rate. In obstructive hydrocephalus, the arachnoid villi become plugged with blood which prevents reabsorption the CSF. The patient will have a change in LOC, such as excessive drowsiness, stupor or coma. CT scan will demonstrate enlarged ventricles. Management involves insertion of a ventriculostomy to periodically drain CSF, especially when the intracranial pressure (ICP) is above the predetermined level, often 20 mm Hg. If the obstruction does not resolve, a ventriculoperitoneal shunt may be required long-term.

Cerebral vasospasm is the narrowing of a cerebral blood vessel that causes reduced blood flow distally and may cause ischemic deficits or cerebral infarction. Approximately 30 percent to 50 percent of SAH patients experience cerebral vasospasm. The patient may have a decrease in LOC, such as excessive drowsiness, focal neurological deficits (paresis/paralysis of a limb, cranial nerve deficits, and aphasia) or coma. CT scan should be done to rule out rebleeding or hydrocephalus. Management of vasospasm includes the use of nimodipine and triple H therapy (hypervolemia, hypertension, and hemodilution).

The goal of hypervolemia is to maintain a PAOP (Wedge Pressure) of 14 to 20 mm Hg and/or CVP of 10 to 12 mm Hg. The goal of hypertension is to maintain systolic blood pressure of 120 to 150 mm Hg before definitive treatment and 160 to 200 after treatment. The goal of hemodilution is to maintain a hematocrit of 30 percent to 33 percent. Nimodipine (Brand name: Nimotop) is a calcium channel blocker that is lipid soluble and therefore able to cross the blood-brain barrier. It is believed to work at the cellular level as a neuronal protector. Serial TCD studies monitor flow velocities in the cerebral vessels. When intracranial blood flow velocities greater than 100 to 120 cm/sec, this suggests vasospasm; if they are greater than 200 cm/sec, it suggests severe vasospasm.

Definitive Treatment

Surgery is indicated within 48 hours for grade I, II, or III aneurysms. Surgery is usually delayed for grades IV and V. Several surgical methods can be used: clipping, wrapping, or ligation. Clipping involves occlusion of the aneurysm neck with a ligature or metal clip. This is the most common surgical method when there is a well defined arterial neck. Wrapping the aneurysm with muscle or fibrin foam reinforces the sac. Proximal ligation of a feeding vessel is rarely done. Endovascular procedures include coiling and intravascular balloon placement.

Coiling involves placing multiple platinum coils inside the aneurysm. A clot forms around the coils and eventually the base of the aneurysm scars over and is cut off. Intravascular balloon placement involves placing a silicone microballoon into the aneurysm.

Arteriovenous Malformation

Arteriovenous malformation (AVM) is a congenital miscommunication or "tangling" of high pressure arterial flow with low pressure venous flow without the intervening capillary network. This shunting of blood causes ischemia and atrophy to the adjacent tissues. Arterial blood flow creates venous engorgement causing higher than normal pressure. Since there is no muscle layer in veins, rupture of the engorged veins occurs. AVM has three morphologic components: feeding arteries, nidus, and draining veins. The feeding arteries supply blood flow to the AVM. The nidus is the central tangle of vessels. Drainage of blood occurs via the dilated veins.

AVM hemorrhage affects approximately 300,000 people each year in the United States. AVMs are the most common cause of spontaneous hemorrhage in children with approximately 2,000 new cases per year. Mortality from AVM hemorrhage is approximately 20 percent to 60 percent. Eighty percent of symptomatic AVM patients are between the ages of 20 and 40 years. When patients present with hemorrhage, 30 percent are subarachnoid, 23 percent are intraparenchymal, 16 percent are intraventricular, and 31 percent are combined (Choi & Mohr, 2005).

Clinical Presentation

Presenting signs and symptoms of AVM include hemorrhage, seizures, headache, and progressive focal neurologic deficits. Intracranial hemorrhage is the most common initial presenting manifestation of AVM in 50 percent to 60 percent of the patients. Symptoms include sudden onset of headache, nausea/vomiting, paresis or plegia, and decreased level of consciousness. Seizures are the second most common presentation of AVM occurring in 20 percent to 25 percent of the patients. Recurrent headache that is unresponsive to the usual drug therapy, new onset of migraine-like headache, or worsening of migraine symptoms (in patients with history of migraine) may be the only manifestation seen with AVM in 15 percent of patients. Progressive focal neurological deficits symptoms depend on the specific area of the brain deprived of adequate blood supply. They may also be related to repeated small hemorrhages from the AVM (Hickey, 2008).

Diagnostic Studies

Diagnostic studies for diagnosis of AVM include CT scan, magnetic resonance imaging (MRI), magnetic resonance angiography (MRA), and four-vessel angiography. CT scan without and with contrast may reveal the bleeding site and any tissue abnormalities. MRI

TABLE 8.10 *Surgical Grading Scale for Cerebral Arteriovenous Malformations*

Category	Criteria	Point Value
Size (maximum dimension)	< 3 cm	1
	3–6 cm	2
	> 6 cm	3
Location	Noneloquent brain	0
	Eloquent brain	1
Venous drainage	Superficial only	0
	Deep	1

gives a more comprehensive analysis of the AVM and MRA examines the blood vessels instead of the brain tissue. The "gold standard" is four-vessel angiography, allowing for AVM analysis and grading of the blood flow into and out of the vessels.

Management

Before definitive repair is attempted, symptom control may include airway management, blood pressure control, seizure control and pharmacological therapy. When the patient is unable to protect her airway, she should be electively intubated and mechanically ventilated. AVM patients should be hemodynamically monitored in the ICU. Hypertension may cause rebleeding and hypotension may cause ischemia. Blood pressure should be maintained within 10 percent of prehemorrhage levels. Hypertension can be treated with labetalol (Brand name: Normodyne) or hydralazine (Brand name: Apresoline). Hypotension may require vasopressors such as phenylephrine (Brand name: Neo-Synephrine). Antiseizure medications should be given when seizures are present.

Definitive Treatment

Treatment of arteriovenous malformation includes symptom management and either surgical, radiation, endovascular methods, or conservative management. Surgery for AVM is elective and if possible is delayed as much as three weeks to stabilize the patient and allow time for the body to recover from the effects of the hemorrhage. The goals of surgery are the complete removal of the AVM (prevent further hemorrhage) and excision of the lesion without causing injury to adjacent brain tissue. If the AVM is very large (> 6 cm), embolization of large feeding vessels may be required prior to excision. Radiosurgery is the use of focused radiation beams into selected tissue with the goal of inducing an inflammatory response in the AVM walls resulting in thrombosis and obliteration of the lesion. Several types of ionizing radiation have been used to treat AVM's, including x-rays, gamma rays, and proton/helium beam radiation. Pre-treatment embolization may also be utilized. Endovascular methods (embolization) may be curative, palliative, or adjunctive to surgical excision or radiosurgery. The goal of embolization is permanent occlusion of the AVM especially when it is deep in the brain cortex or not surgically accessible. Conservative management involves lifestyle changes to decrease the chance of hemorrhage including activity restrictions, smoking cessation, and control of seizures (if present).

Traumatic Brain Injury

Trauma happens when external forces impact the body causing structural and/or physiologic alterations, or injuries. The external forces can be chemical, electrical, mechanical, radiation, or thermal forms of energy. Knowledge of the mechanism of injury helps caregivers to anticipate and predict the extent of injury. Brain injury is the leading cause of trauma-related deaths in people younger than 45 years of age and occurs twice as often in males. It is estimated that between 1.5 and 2 million traumatic brain injuries occur each year in the United States. There are approximately 50,000 deaths and significant disability is seen in 80,000 to 100,000 people per year. 300,000 brain injuries are sports-related (Bader & Littlejohns, 2004).

Etiology

Traumatic brain injury (TBI) occurs when mechanical forces are transmitted to brain tissue. These mechanisms are kinetic energy (KE) and force (F). The formula for kinetic energy is:

$$KE = \frac{M}{2} \text{ (mass divided by 2)} \times V^2 \text{ (square of the velocity)}$$

The formula for force is:

$$F = M \times A \text{ (deceleration)}$$

The impact force is determined by the force, duration, direction, and rate. There are three separate collisions that occur: vehicle hits object, victim strikes internal parts of vehicle, and soft tissue strikes the hard body surfaces. For example, an unbelted occupant in a 30 mph collision slams into the interior surfaces with the same impact as falling from a three-story building (Bader & Littlejohns, 2004).

Blunt trauma is seen in motor vehicle crashes, motorcycle crashes, pedestrian–motor vehicle crashes, bicycle injuries, falls, sports, and assaults. Blunt head trauma is caused by contact, acceleration–deceleration, and rotational forces. Contact injuries occur when an object strikes the head. The velocity of the impact determines whether the injury is restricted to the scalp or skull (low velocity) or includes the brain (high velocity). Acceleration-deceleration injuries occur when the skull strikes (or is struck by) an object. The brain is carried by force until it strikes the inside of the skull (coup injury). When the impact is strong enough, the undissipated force pitches the brain in the reverse direction, striking the opposite side of the skull (contrecoup injury). Rotational injury, often occur with acceleration-deceleration injuries, results in tearing or shearing of tissues.

Penetrating trauma injuries are caused by objects that penetrate the skull, producing significant focal damage but little acceleration-deceleration or rotational injury. The most common instruments used in penetrating trauma are guns (low/high velocity), knives, and sharp objects (knives, metal rods). With these injuries, there is deep penetration into the brain tissue and the possibility of damage to the ventricular system. A low velocity (stabbing) injury is limited to the entry tract and the greatest concern is bleeding and infection. Gunshot (high velocity) injuries cause extensive damage related to entry of bone fragments; the bullets spin irregularly, creating multiple paths and shock waves that cause extensive brain damage.

Trauma to the head may result in both primary and secondary injuries to the brain. Primary brain injury is the result of direct trauma to the brain. Secondary injury occurs as a result of injury to the brain and includes hypoxia, cerebral edema, hypertension, hypercapnia, and elevated intracranial pressure. Secondary injuries occur hours or days after the initial trauma and are a result of the body's response to the primary injury. The goal when caring for a TBI patient is to support maximum recovery from the primary brain injury and at the same time prevent, minimize, and reverse the occurrence of secondary injuries (Bader & Littlejohns, 2004).

Scalp Lacerations

The scalp has five layers which can be remembered by the pneumonic SCALP: **S**kin (dermal layer), **C**onnective tissue, **A**poneurosis (galea aponeurotica), **L**oose connective areolar tissue (subgaleal areolar space), and **P**eriosteum. The dermal layer has hair and protects the scalp from injury. Subcutaneous fascia is a tough fibrotic tissue with a vascular fatty layer that can bleed profusely when the scalp is lacerated. The galea aponeurotica is a sheet-like tendon layer that connects the frontal and occipital muscles. Below the galea is the subgaleal areolar space that contains veins that empty into the venous sinus. It is a potential area where hematomas can develop and infection can spread to the brain. The periosteum is below the subgaleal space. It is a very thin layer of tissue that can be stripped away from the skull. The extent of a scalp injury is dependent upon the object characteristics and velocity.

Scalp lacerations are common with head injury and are often associated with skull fracture. Injuries to the scalp are classified as abrasion, contusion, and laceration.

In an abrasion, the top layer of scalp is scraped away and there may be some slight bleeding. A contusion is a bruise (skin is not broken) with possible blood accumulation into the subcutaneous layer. In a laceration the scalp is torn, may bleed profusely, and suturing may be needed This is partly due to the ample blood supply received by the scalp (see below).

Arterial and Venous Anatomy of the Scalp

Arterial Blood Supply	supratrochlear, supraorbital, superficial temporal, occipital
Venous Drainage	superficial temporal, posterior auricular, occipital

Skull Fractures

Direct contact is the mechanism of skull injury. The extent of injury depends on several factors including the skull's thickness at the point of impact and the weight, velocity, and angle of impact of the intruding object. Upon impact, several actions are set in motion. The object velocity at the point of impact causes an indentation, which may be temporary or permanent. Stress waves are set in motion and radiate throughout the entire skull. When there is a high velocity impact, a depressed skull fracture with or without a dural tear and cerebral laceration may occur. With a low velocity impact, the area of indentation rebounds outward and may result in no fracture, a linear fracture, or a comminuted fracture. The fracture line extends from the point of impact toward the base of the skull.

Skull fractures are classified as linear, comminuted, depressed, open depressed, or basilar skull. **Linear** fractures are a single fracture line in the bone. In a **comminuted** fracture the bone is splintered or shattered into pieces. **Depressed** fractures occur when one or more sections of bone fragment become embedded in the brain tissue. The scalp and/or the dura may or may not be torn. The patient may require surgery to debride the wound and elevate the bone fragments. An **open depressed (compound) fracture** has openings in the scalp, dura, and bone fragments in the tissue. The patient is at greater risk for infection because the blood-brain barrier is violated. A **basilar skull fracture** is a linear fracture at the base of the skull that is associated with a dural tear. Signs and symptoms include spinal fluid and/or blood leaking from the ears or nose, raccoon's eyes (periorbital ecchymosis), and Battle's sign (bruising of the mastoid bone). The patient should be monitored for meningitis, encephalitis, and epidural hematoma.

Brain Injuries

Concussion is the mildest form of brain injury and is characterized by brief loss of consciousness (LOC). The patient complains of headache, dizziness, and possibly nausea/vomiting. Focal neurologic deficits and altered LOC usually clear in 6–12 hours. Post-concussion syndrome is common and may include short-term memory deficits, headache, cognitive difficulties, visual disturbances, lack of coordination, and lethargy. These "minor" injuries can have devastating long-term effects.

Contusions are bleeding of small vessels and necrotic brain tissue caused by acceleration-deceleration movement of the brain within the skull. Neurologic deficits may include changes in LOC, cranial nerve dysfunction, hemiparesis or hemiplegia, seizures, and intracranial hypertension. The clinical effect depends on the size, location, and related cerebral edema.

Diffuse axonal injury results from white matter shearing associated with rotational and acceleration-deceleration forces. There is disruption of the axons and neuronal pathways in the brain hemispheres, diencephalon, and brain stem. Neurologic deficits include coma, confusion, post-traumatic amnesia, and prolonged recovery. Treatment is support of vital functions and maintenance of intracranial pressure within normal parameters. Mortality rates vary between 33 and 50 percent depending on the severity of the initial injury. Many patients may survive in a vegetative state characterized by periods of wakefulness and sleep, but without observable signs of cognition.

Diagnostic studies include CT scan, MRI, and MRA. These may show brain edema, areas of small hemorrhage (severe contusion), and detection of associated injuries (carotid or vertebral dissection). EEG may show brain wave abnormalities and evoked potentials may show slowing of impulse transmission through the brainstem.

Intracranial Hemorrhage

Traumatic intracranial bleeding is a common complication of brain injury. Bleeding may begin immediately after the injury, but its presence may not become clinically apparent until enough blood accumulates to cause signs and symptoms. The time between bleeding and the appearance of clinical symptoms may be minutes to weeks, depending on the site and rate of bleeding. Hemorrhage can be a late development in a patient with a 'minor' traumatic brain injury (TBI) when there is minimal loss of consciousness. Other patients with hemorrhage may remain unconscious from the moment of injury. The types of bleeding associated with TBI are epidural hematoma, subdural hematoma, and intracerebral hemorrhage.

Epidural hematoma (extradural hematoma) is bleeding into the potential space between the lining of the skull (periosteum) and the dura mater. Epidural hematoma (EDH) is seen in 4 percent to 8 percent of all head trauma and 20 percent to 30 percent of all hematomas. Most EDHs are arterial in origin (85 percent) and are often associated with linear skull fractures that cross major blood vessels. The most frequent site is the **middle meningeal artery** located under the temporal bone. Occasionally they may be due to tearing of the dural venous sinuses. As the hematoma enlarges, the dura is gradually torn away from the skull, creating pressure on the underlying brain and causing a mass effect.

The classic description of an epidural hematoma is 'talk and die'. Patients have a brief loss of consciousness, followed be a lucid ("honeymoon") period lasting for minutes to several hours. The lucid period is followed by rapid deterioration in LOC from drowsiness to lethargy and then to coma, as mass effect and herniation develop. The most common clinical presentation is headache, vomiting, seizures, unilateral hyperreflexia, positive Babinski sign, ipsilateral occulomotor paralysis, contralateral hemiparesis/hemiplegia, and elevated ICP. Once LOC begins to deteriorate, coma occurs rapidly. Bradycardia and respiratory distress are late signs.

Diagnostic Studies

Diagnostic studies include skull and spine radiographs, CT scan of the head, and MRI. Radiographs (X-Rays) may reveal associated skull or spine fractures. CT scan will show an area of increased density and may show midline shift. Lumbar puncture is contraindicated due to elevated ICP.

Epidural hematomas require immediate surgical intervention to remove the clot. Post operative infection is usually not a concern since meninges and blood-brain barrier are intact. Prompt diagnosis and treatment prevents mortality (5 to 10 percent) from EDH.

Subdural hematoma (SDH) is bleeding between the dura mater and arachnoid layer. This is usually caused by **shearing of the cortical veins** that bridge the dura and arachnoid membrane as a result of acceleration–deceleration and rotational forces. Subdural hematoma is seen in 15 percent to 30 percent of patients with head trauma and 50 percent to 70 percent of all hematomas. It may occur with minimal trauma, when patients have a coagulation disorder or are taking anticoagulants. The majority of SDHs are seen in older patients with brain atrophy or a history of alcohol abuse. Subdural hematomas are classified based on the time interval and appearance of blood/fluid composition.

TABLE 8.11 *Subdural Hematoma Classification*

Time Interval	Blood/Fluid Composition
Acute SDH: 0 to 48 hours	Clotted blood that is hypodense is seen on CT scan.
Subacute SDH: 3 to 20 days	Clot lysis has begun, and blood products and fluids are present.
Chronic SDH: 3 weeks to months	Hemolysis of the clot draws fluid into the area, causing swelling. The SDH is hypodense on CT scan.

Clinical Presentation

Clinical presentation of SDHs varies based on classification. Acute SDHs may present gradually or with rapid deterioration of the LOC from drowsiness, slow cerebration, and confusion to coma. They may also have pupillary changes and hemiparesis/hemiplegia.

Subacute SDH symptoms are similar to acute but occur at a slower rate. Chronic SDH symptoms include headache, slow cerebration, confusion, papilledema, slowed pupillary responses, and possibly seizures. The symptoms develop gradually and may be misdiagnosed as Alzheimer's disease, 'old age,' or cerebral atrophy.

Diagnostic Studies

Diagnostic studies include skull and spine radiographs, CT scan of the head, and MRI. Radiographs (X-Rays) may reveal associated skull or spine fractures. CT scan will show an area of increased density and may show midline shift.

Management

Treatment of large hematomas requires immediate surgical intervention (craniectomy, craniotomy, or burr holes) to remove the clot. Post-operative infection is a concern since meninges and blood-brain barrier are entered to remove the clot. Patients with small SDH and minimal symptoms may be followed with close observation with serial CT scans. Once the clot liquefies, burr holes are made in the skull and the fluid is drained. A drain is placed to prevent reaccumulation of fluid in the subdural space. Elderly patients and those with a history of alcohol abuse tend to re-bleed after surgical evacuation and require careful monitoring. Prompt diagnosis and treatment prevents mortality (20 percent) from SDH.

Intracerebral hemorrhage (ICH) is bleeding into the cerebral parenchyma and may be caused by caused by trauma, tumors, bleeding disorders, anticoagulant therapy, or hypertension. When the ICH is from trauma, the injury may be due to a penetrating missile or from severe acceleration-deceleration forces that cause laceration of the deep cerebral tissues. ICH occurs in 2 to 20 percent of patients with head trauma.

Clinical Presentation

Clinical presentation of ICH varies with the area of brain involved, size of the hematoma, and rate of blood accumulation. These patients may or may not show symptoms of intracranial hypertension. Symptoms may include headache, decreasing LOC progressing to deep coma, contralateral hemiplegia, ipsilateral dilated pupil and, as ICP increases, the development of transtentorial herniation.

Diagnostic Studies

Diagnostic studies include skull and spine radiographs, CT scan of the head, and MRI. Radiographs (X-Rays) may reveal associated skull or spine fractures. CT scan will show an area of increased density and may show midline shift. MRI will show the hematoma and any associated edema.

Treatment is based on the location and extent of bleeding. Surgery rarely improves neurological outcome. Most patients are managed medically with supportive care and management of increased ICP.

Secondary Brain Injury

Secondary injury is any complicating injury occurring as a result of physiologic events related to the primary brain insult, such as ischemia, inflammation, excitotoxicity, and metabolic insults. Severe head trauma begins a cascade of ischemic and cellular level biochemical changes that can lead to neuronal injury and cell death. Some changes occur almost immediately after injury, some later. Any systemic (extracerebral) or neurological (intracerebral) complication can compromise adequate oxygen and nutrient delivery to the brain's cells, causing hypoxia or ischemia. The ischemia can begin or worsen the pathological cascade of events that leads to secondary brain injury (Bader & Littlejohns, 2004).

Ischemia is a mismatch between oxygen supply and oxygen demand. Cerebral ischemia is defined as cerebral blood flow (CBF) of less than 20 ml/100 g per minute. If oxygen demand is not matched by oxygen delivery, irreversible cellular injury begins and toxic metabolites build up in the blood. When blood flow is reduced, neurons increase their extraction of oxygen from the surrounding tissues. Inadequate blood flow to the brain and/or reduced oxygen content of the blood causes clinical manifestations. These manifestations include alterations in LOC, motor impairments, and ultimately coma. Multiple physiological stressors impact cerebral blood flow and cerebral perfusion including hypotension (due to blood loss), shock, underlying cardiovascular disease, or increased intracranial pressure. Other complications of CBF and cerebral perfusion alterations include alterations of neurotransmitter activity, glucose transport and utilization, protein synthesis, and cellular membrane stability. Prevention and management of cerebral ischemia requires maintenance of adequate blood flow and cerebral perfusion of brain tissues.

Cerebral edema is the abnormal accumulation of water in the intracellular, extracellular, or both spaces, which is associated with increased brain tissue volume. The edema usually peaks two to four days after a TBI and is associated with increased ICP. Cerebral edema is a serious complication and can be life-threatening since the increase in brain bulk puts pressure on the brain tissue, causing neurologic deficits. Severe cerebral edema can produce transtentorial herniation and progress to brainstem compression, herniation, and death. There are three types of cerebral edema: vasogenic, cytotoxic, and interstitial.

Vasogenic edema is extracellular edema of the white matter in the brain. It results from increased capillary permeability and an increase in pinocytotic vesicles in the blood-brain barrier. These alterations allow plasma-like filtrate, including large protein molecules, to leak into the extracellular space. This increases the distance that oxygen, substrates, and waste products must travel to and from cells and exerts pressure on the cells and blood vessels, compressing them and contributing to increased ICP. Vasogenic edema may be caused by trauma, infection, abscess, hypoxia, or tumor. The use of corticosteroids (dexamethasone) is effective only with brain tumors. Mannitol, an osmotic diuretic may be helpful in the acute phase. The extent of cerebral edema can be minimized by controlling oxygenation, ventilation, and blood pressure.

Cytotoxic edema is an increase of fluid in the neurons, glial, and endothelial cells as a result of ATP-dependent sodium-potassium pump failure. Fluid and sodium accumulate within the cells, leading to diffuse brain swelling involving both gray and white matter of the brain. Cytotoxic edema is associated with hypoxic or anoxic episodes (cardiac arrest, asphyxiation), water intoxication, hyponatremia, and syndrome of inappropriate antidiuretic hormone (SIADH) secretion. Corticosteroids (dexamethasone) are not effective in treating cytotoxic edema. Osmotic diuretics may be beneficial in the acute stage when hypoosmolarity is present.

Interstitial edema is caused by a buildup of CSF pressure within the ventricular system forcing CSF into the periventricular white matter. It is associated with acute or subacute hydrocephalus and benign intracranial hypertension (pseudotumor cerebri). Hydrocephalus may be communicating (non-obstructive) or non-communicating (obstructive). Communicating hydrocephalus is due to a defect in the absorption of CSF at the arachnoid villi or sagittal sinus. Non-communicating is caused by a blockage of CSF at or above the fourth ventricle. Corticosteroids and osmotic diuretics are not effective. A decrease in CSF production occurs with the administration of acetazolamide (Brand name: Diamox). Treatment includes temporary drainage of CSF via a ventriculostomy until the condition corrects itself or surgical placement of a shunt.

Cellular excitotoxicity occurs when the traumatic brain injury causes a massive depolarization of the brain cells. There is a rapid increase in excitatory neurotransmitter release (glutamate, aspartate,) that changes the normal ionic gradients of the neuronal membranes, glial cells, and cerebral vascular endothelial cells. This change begins a chain of disruption of crucial cellular processes. Aerobic metabolism and production of adenosine triphosphate (ATP) stops quickly, reducing the energy stores of the affected cells. Potassium leaves the cells, allowing calcium, sodium, and water to enter the damaged cells, resulting in edema.

Intracranial pressure is the force normally exerted by the CSF that circulates around the brain, spinal cord, and cerebral ventricles. The normal range of ICP varies in different age groups:

- Newborns: 0.7–1.5 mm Hg

- Infants: 1.5–6 mm Hg

- Children: 3–7.5 mm Hg

- Adults: 0 to 10 mm Hg (15 mm Hg is considered the upper limit of normal)

When patients have cerebral trauma or other neurological disorders, the normal homeostatic mechanisms may be disrupted, causing a sustained elevated ICP that may result in death. The intracranial space has three components: brain (80 percent), CSF (10 percent), and blood (10 percent). Essential to the understanding of the pathophysiology of ICP is the Monro-Kellie hypothesis. The hypothesis is based on these principles:

- The brain is enclosed within a rigid box.

- Cerebral blood volume is constant.

- Outflow of venous blood equals the incoming arterial blood flow.

The **Monro-Kellie hypothesis** states that if the volume of one component increases, a reciprocal decrease in the volume of one or both of the others must occur or an increase in ICP will result. This hypothesis applies only when the skull is fused (closed). Infants and very young children with non-fused skulls have the ability to expand in response to increased ICP.

Autoregulation of cerebral blood flow (CBF) includes multiple compensatory mechanisms that maintain the intracranial volume in homeostasis including CSF displacement from the subarachnoid space and ventricles via the foramen magnum to the spinal subarachnoid space and via the optic foramen to the basal subarachnoid cisterns; compression of the low pressure dural sinuses; decreased production of CSF; and vasoconstriction of the cerebral blood vessels, but the amount of displacement is limited. Once the compensatory mechanisms are exceeded, the ICP increases and intracranial hypertension is the result. Mean arterial pressure (MAP) of 50 to 150 mm Hg does not change CBF when autoregulation is present. With intracranial hypertension, CBF becomes dependent on the perfusion pressure. **Intracranial hypertension** is a sustained elevated intracranial pressure (ICP) of 20 mm Hg or higher.

Cerebral blood flow varies with changes in cerebral perfusion and constriction or dilatation of the cerebrovascular vessels. Normal cerebral blood flow is:

- Neonates—varies based on percent of circulating fetal hemoglobin

- Children—105 ml per 100 g per minute

- Adults—50 ml per 100 g per minute

The brain comprises two percent of body weight but it requires 15 percent to 20 percent of the total cardiac output and 15 percent to 20 percent of oxygen consumed at rest.

Systemic Factors That Alter CBF

Increase	Decrease
Hypercapnia	Hypocapnia
Hypoxemia	Hyperoxemia
Decreased blood viscosity	Increased blood viscosity
Hyperthermia	Hypothermia
Vasodilators	Vasopressors
	Intracranial hypertension

Intracranial Pressure Monitoring

Intracranial pressure monitoring is the standard of care in the ICU and is the most significant factor in determining the morbidity and mortality of neurosurgical patients (Bader & Littlejohns, 2004). There are four sites used for monitoring ICP: the intraventricular space, the epidural space, the subarachnoid space, and the parenchyma. When the **intraventricular** space is used, a catheter is inserted into the anterior or occipital horns of the lateral ventricle. The use of a three-way stopcock allows both ICP monitoring by a pressure transducer and drainage of CSF as needed. This method is also called ventriculostomy. Advantages of this method are that it allows direct measurement of ICP and instillation of medications or contrast media for diagnostic studies. Disadvantages include increased risk of infection (two to five percent), hemorrhage, CSF loss, midline shifting, and increased cerebral edema.

The **epidural** sensor method uses a fiber-optic sensing device inserted via a burr hole into the epidural space between the skull and the dura mater. Advantages are that the sensor is easier to insert, less invasive, and generates a lower infection rate (less than one percent). Disadvantages are that it is unable to drain excess CSF and that pressure readings are higher than other methods.

When a **subarachnoid** screw or bolt is used, the device is inserted into the subarachnoid space through a burr hole and connected to an external transducer. Advantages include easier insertion method than with a ventriculostomy, it is a direct measurement of ICP, there is no penetration into the brain, and the risk for infection is low (one to two percent). Disadvantages are CSF drainage is not possible, it requires frequent recalibration, the device may become occluded with debris (clots, tissue) causing inaccurate measurements, and it is more easily dislodged than a catheter.

In the **intraparenchymal** method, a fiber-optic-tipped probe is inserted through a burr hole and placed 1 cm into the brain tissue, and then connected to an external monitor providing waveforms for evaluation.

Advantages are that it is easy to insert, head position has no effect on readings, and placement is not dependent on ventricular size or position. Disadvantages include CSF drainage is not possible, it cannot be re-zeroed once it is in place, the probe is fragile and easily bent, broken, or kinked, and there is an increased risk of intracerebral bleeding and infection.

ICP Waveform Monitoring

Monitoring systems allow the ICU nurse to observe the ICP waveform pattern. The ICP waveform is similar to an arterial hemodynamic waveform. A normal ICP waveform has three defined peaks of decreasing height, identified as P_1, P_2, and P_3. P_1 is an upward spike called a systolic or percussion wave, which represents the blood being ejected from the heart. Extreme alterations in blood pressure produce changes in P_1. P_2 is a second upward spike called the tidal wave; it is more variable, ends on the dicrotic notch, and is indicative of brain compliance. When P_2 is equal to or higher than P_1, decreased compliance exists and can be helpful in predicting the risk for increases in ICP. P_3 follows the dicrotic notch and represents closure of the aortic valve.

Abnormal ICP waveforms include A waves, B waves, and C waves. A waves (plateau waves) are the most clinically significant for the patient with already consistently elevated ICP readings of 20 mm Hg or higher. It is a sudden, transient increase in ICP to levels of 50 to 100 mm Hg and last for 5 to 20 minutes before starting a rapid return to the level of or below the baseline ICP. An A wave is pathologic and requires immediate treatment. B waves are sharp, rhythmic oscillations with a sawtooth appearance that occur 30 seconds to 2 minutes with pressures as high as 50 mm Hg. They are related to changes in CBF and may serve as a warning of the potential risk for increased ICP and impaired brain compliance. C waves are rapid, rhythmic oscillations that are related to systemic arterial pressure. They occur every four to eight minutes at normal ICP levels.

Herniation Syndromes

Herniation is defined as the displacement of brain structures due to increased ICP, causing a sequence of neurologic signs and symptoms related to compression of brain structures and compromised cerebral blood flow. There are four types of brain herniation syndromes caused by expanding mass lesions: cingulate, central, uncal, and tonsillar (infratentorial). In cingulate herniation the brain squeezes under the falx cerebri. The brainstem herniates caudally in central herniation. In uncal herniation the uncus and the hippocampal gyrus herniate into the tentorial notch. The cerebellar tonsils herniate through the foramen magnum in tonsillar herniation.

Cingulate Herniation

In cingulate herniation (most common), the innermost part of the frontal lobe is forced under part of the falx cerebri (the dura mater at the top of the head between the two hemispheres of the brain). Cingulate herniation can be caused when one hemisphere swells and pushes the cingulate gyrus by the falx cerebri. This does not put as much pressure on the brainstem as the other types of herniation, but it may interfere with blood vessels in the frontal lobes that are close to the site of injury (anterior cerebral artery), or it may progress to central herniation. Interference with the blood supply can cause dangerous increases in ICP that can lead to more dangerous forms of herniation. Symptoms for cingulate herniation are not well defined. Usually occurring in addition to uncal herniation, cingulate herniation may present with abnormal posturing and coma. Cingulate herniation is believed to be a precursor to other types of herniation.

Central Herniation

In central herniation (transtentorial herniation), the diencephalon and parts of the temporal lobes of both of the cerebral hemispheres are squeezed through a notch in the tentorium. Downward herniation can stretch branches of the basilar artery, causing it to tear and bleed. The result is usually fatal.

Uncal Herniation

In uncal herniation, the innermost part of the temporal lobe, the uncus, can be squeezed so much that it goes by the tentorium and puts pressure on the brainstem. The tentorium is a structure within the skull formed by the dura mater. Tissue may be stripped from the cerebral cortex in a process called decortication. The uncus can squeeze the third cranial nerve, which controls parasympathetic input to the eye on the side of the affected nerve. This interrupts the parasympathetic neural transmission, causing the pupil of the affected eye to dilate and fail to constrict in response to light as it should. A dilated unresponsive pupil is an important sign of increased intracranial pressure. Cranial arteries may be compressed during the herniation. Compression of the posterior cerebral artery may result in loss of the contralateral visual field. This type of herniation can also damage the brain stem, causing lethargy, slow heart rate, respiratory abnormalities, and pupil dilation. Uncal herniation may advance to central herniation.

Tonsillar Herniation

In tonsillar herniation (downward cerebellar herniation), the cerebellar tonsils move downward through the foramen magnum, possibly causing compression of the lower brainstem and upper cervical spinal cord as they pass through the foramen magnum. Increased pressure on the brainstem can result in dysfunction of the centers in the brain responsible for controlling respiratory and cardiac function.

Complications

The patient may become paralyzed on the same side as the lesion causing the pressure or on the side opposite the lesion. Increased pressure on the midbrain, which contains the reticular activating network that regulates consciousness, will result in coma. Damage to the cardio-respiratory centers in the medulla will cause respiratory and cardiac arrest.

Spinal Cord Injury

Spinal cord injury (SCI) results from excessive force being exerted on the vertebral column. SCI is most often due to acceleration-deceleration forces that result in hyperflexion, hyperextension, deformation, axial loading, excessive rotation and penetrating injuries. **Hyperflexion** produces compression of the cord, vertebral body, and intervertebral discs and tearing of the posterior muscles and ligaments. **Hyperextension** causes fractures of the posterior vertebral elements and tearing of the longitudinal ligaments. A mild form of hyperextension causes a whiplash injury. **Deformation** occurs when the spinal column and the supporting structures are altered to accommodate abnormal movements. **Axial loading** (also known as vertical compression) results when a vertical force is exerted on the spinal column. The most common axial loading injuries are from diving accidents or falling from a height and landing on the feet or buttocks. Excessive rotation occurs when the head is turned beyond the normal range on the horizontal axis. **Penetrating injury** can be caused by a knife, bullet, or any other object that penetrates the spinal cord.

The annual incidence of SCI in the United States has been estimated to be approximately 10,000 to 15,000. The number of people living with SCI is estimated to be 180,000 to 200,000. Over half of the injuries occur in people 16 to 30 years old, and greater than 80 percent are male. Cervical injury is rare in children. The most common causes of SCI are motor vehicle crashes, falls, sports injuries, missile injuries, and diving accidents. Spinal cord injury and traumatic brain injury are often seen together and SCI should be considered a possibility when the patient is unconscious.

Spinal cord injury can be devastating since the loss of body function also means the loss of independence. The loss of function may be temporary or permanent, depending on the type of injury. The injury may be complete or incomplete. Complete transection of the spinal cord results in flaccid paralysis and total loss of motor and sensory function below the level of the injury. Incomplete SCI results from partial transection of the spinal cord. With an incomplete lesion, some of the spinal tracts may be intact and loss of sensory and motor function will depend on the level of injury and type of incomplete injury.

There are five syndromes associated with incomplete injury: central cord syndrome, anterior cord syndrome, Brown-Séquard syndrome, posterior cord syndrome, and cauda equina syndrome.

Central cord syndrome usually occurs in the cervical area from hyperextension injury, very small hemorrhages, and edema. This syndrome presents with upper extremity weakness greater than lower extremity weakness. Recovery depends of resolution of the edema as soon as possible. If the spinal tracts are intact, loss of function will be less. **Anterior cord syndrome** may be due to acute disc herniation or hyperflexion associated with vertebral fractures. This results in motor paralysis and decreased pain and temperature sensation below the level of the injury. Touch, vibration, position, and motion sensation are not affected. Surgical decompression may be necessary to remove bone fragments. **Brown-Séquard syndrome** (lateral cord syndrome) is often caused by penetrating injuries or ruptured discs that transect half of the spinal cord. There is motor paralysis and loss of vibration and position sense on the ipsilateral (same side) as the injury. Contralateral (opposite side) loss of pain and temperature sense occurs. **Posterior cord syndrome** is due to cervical hyperextension causing compression of the posterior portion. There is loss of position sense (proprioception) but motor function and pain and temperature sense is salvaged. **Cauda equina syndrome** results from injuries below L1-2 with compression of cauda equina. Motor, sensory, bowel bladder and sexual dysfunction may vary. Better prognosis for recovery than spinal cord injury.

The same principles of cellular response to injury seen with head injury also apply to spinal cord injury (primary and secondary injury). Treatment goals are the same: minimize secondary injury and prevent complications. Secondary damage to the spinal cord can occur in response to hypovolemic shock (hypoperfusion of the spinal cord). The immediate signs and symptoms of complete SCI are flaccid paralysis, loss of all spinal reflexes, loss of all sensory function, loss of autonomic function below the level of the injury, and bowel and bladder dysfunction.

The physical destruction and ischemia caused by the primary injury triggers multiple secondary processes that exacerbate the spinal cord damage over hours to weeks post injury. These secondary processes include spinal shock, neurogenic shock, orthostatic hypotension, and respiratory insufficiency. **Spinal shock** is the loss of all neurological function below the level of injury during the acute phase and includes bradycardia and hypotension. The spinal shock may last for four to six weeks and require blood pressure support. Recovery from spinal shock is a gradual process. The flaccidity is slowly replaced with spasticity and hyperreflexia. The earliest indicator of the end of spinal shock is the return of the perianal reflexes. **Neurogenic shock** results from the loss of sympathetic input to the systemic vasculature of the heart and decreased peripheral resistance. The loss of sympathetic outflow causes the vasodilation of the vascular beds, bradycardia from the suppression of the cardiac accelerator reflex, loss of temperature control, and inability to sweat below the level of injury. The presence of both bradycardia and hypotension differentiates this type of shock from hypovolemic shock. **Orthostatic hypotension** is a rapid drop in blood pressure when the vertical position is assumed. Inadequate blood supply to the brain causes syncope. Orthostatic hypotension is seen in patients who have been supine in bed for long periods of time, in postoperative lumbar sympathectomy patients, and new SCI related to neurogenic shock. Just raising the head of the bed in a new quadriplegic patient can result in a drastic lowering of the blood pressure. Blood pressure usually returns to pre-injury level in one to two weeks. **Respiratory insufficiency** is seen in cervical injuries. Since innervation of the diaphragm comes from C-1 to C-4 level, high cervical injuries will require intubation and mechanical ventilation. An SCI below C-4 may require respiratory support.

Prehospital Management

The prehospital management of SCIs is critical to the patient's long-term outcome. Until proven otherwise, all trauma patients with mechanism of injury for potential SCI should be immobilized at scene with rigid collar and supportive blocks on a backboard with straps. Advanced Trauma Life Support (ATLS) guidelines should be followed. Basic management at the injury site includes:

- Rapid assessment at the site to determine the extent of the injury

- Immobilization and stabilization of the head and neck to prevent injury extension

- Safe removal of the patient from the vehicle or injury site

- Stabilization and control of any life-threatening injuries

- Triage to the appropriate facility

- Rapid and safe transport

The rescue personnel must be well trained since improper handling of a minor spinal fracture can turn it into a major, irreversible SCI.

In the emergency department (ED), a report of the prehospital management and a history of the injury are rapidly collected. The ED staff's focus is on rapid stabilization and assessment. Since hypoxia, hypotension, or hypertension can contribute to secondary injury and other life-threatening complications, attention to the ABC's (airway, breathing, circulation) is the first step in ED management. The primary survey includes assessment of airway patency, adequate ventilation, and adequate circulation. Prevention of hypoxemia may require supplemental oxygen or intubation and mechanical ventilation. Oxygen saturation should be maintained at 100 percent. If the patient shows signs of hypotension, bradycardia, and hypothermia (neurogenic shock), treatment must be initiated immediately to provide hemodynamic stability. After the primary survey, a neurological assessment should be obtained which includes spinal cord function, an approximation of the level of injury, and evaluation for traumatic brain injury. Assessment includes motor, sensory, reflexes, and bowel/bladder function. The ASIA scale is used to rate the impairment classification of the SCI.

American Spinal Injury Association (ASIA) Impairment Scale

A = Complete. No sensory or motor function is preserved in sacral S4–S5.

B = Incomplete. Sensory function is preserved below level of injury preserved (includes sacral S4–S5), but no motor function.

C = Incomplete. Motor function below level of injury preserved, at least half of key muscles have < motor grade 3.

D = Incomplete. Motor function below level of injury preserved, more than half of key muscles have > motor grade 3.

E = Normal. Motor and sensory function is normal.

Diagnostic Studies

X-ray films are used for the initial evaluation of the spine. Plain radiographs assess the integrity and alignment of the vertebrae and spacing of the bones and joints. Lateral films detect vertebral fractures in 60 percent to 80 percent of patients with spinal injury, evaluate the anterior-posterior (AP) diameter of the spinal canal, alignment of the spine, height and shape of the vertebral bodies and disc spaces, joint spacing, the atlas/axis complex, and any prevertebral soft tissue swelling. AP views evaluate the interpedicular distance, the spinous process alignment, the shape and thickness of the pedicles, and the presence of lesions or soft tissue masses. Evaluation of the cervical spine may require special positioning, such as odontoid (open mouth) for evaluation of C-1 and C-2 integrity; swimmer's view for patients with short, thick necks; and flexion-extension views to identify instability (subluxations) of the spine, when it is moved from the neutral position.

CT scan three-dimensional imaging is helpful for operative planning. MRI provides improved detail of soft tissue such as the spinal cord, ligaments, and discs. Angiography or MRA can assist in the identification of vascular injuries associated with cervical spine injury (carotid or vertebral arteries). Spinal somatosensory evoked potentials (SSEPs) measure the functional integrity of the ascending (sensory) pathways.

Early Management

Research studies have shown that using high-dose intravenous (IV) methylprednisolone within 8 hours of the initial injury improves motor and sensory outcome for both complete and incomplete SCIs. Only treatment with methylprednisolone has shown effectiveness in the acute phase of SCI. The treatment protocol is as follows: 30 mg/kg bolus is given over 15 minutes; wait 45 minutes; then begin a continuous infusion of 5.4 mg/kg for 23 hours. The infusion should continue even during surgery, if possible. The improvement in neurological function occurs due to the reduction of edema at the injury site, reduction of leukocytes, a decrease in free fatty acid production, and inhibition of phospholipids breakdown which improves blood flow to the spinal cord and alters the inflammatory response, thus avoiding secondary injury.

After initial stabilization, serial neurological assessment, and early steroid treatment in the ED, the patient will most likely be admitted to the intensive care unit (ICU). In the ICU the patient may require mechanical ventilation with supplemental oxygen, IV fluids, continuous cardiac monitoring, and an indwelling urinary catheter, a nasogastric tube, antiembolism stockings (TEDs), and sequential compression devices. Invasive monitoring with an arterial line and pulmonary catheter may be necessary. After resuscitation measures are complete, treatment decisions are considered and the patient is continuously monitored for potential complications.

Complications

Complications of SCI include hypertension, hypotension, autonomic dysreflexia, and bowel and bladder dysfunction. Blood pressure should be maintained within normal limits. Avoid systolic blood pressure less than 90 mm Hg or greater than 190 mm Hg. Maintain mean arterial pressure (MAP) 85–90 mm Hg for 7 days post injury. Autonomic dysreflexia is due to the uninhibited sympathetic response to noxious stimuli and is seen in SCI at T-6 or above. Clinical manifestations of autonomic dysreflexia include hypertension, headache, chills, flushing, diaphoresis, bradycardia, nausea, piloerection (goose bumps), nasal congestion, blurred vision, anxiety, and apprehension. This is a medical emergency. Treatment involves finding the cause and managing it:

- Check for bladder distention.
- Check for bowel distention, constipation.
- Check for skin breakdown, wrinkled sheets.
- Elevate head of the bed 90°.
- Place legs in a dependent position.
- Remove constricting clothing.
- Make sure patient is positioned with spine in alignment.
- Treat hypertension.

Definitive Treatment

The primary treatment goal in management of SCI is to optimize outcomes by preserving or improving neurological function. Treatment is accomplished by neural decompression, spinal realignment, and stabilization through either surgical or nonsurgical approach. Surgery may be done on an emergency basis if neurological deterioration is apparent on serial assessments. Stabilization is needed to prevent new or further extension of neurological damage. Management depends on the type of SCI, associated injuries, and any patient co-morbidities. The surgical procedure used most frequently for stabilization is a decompression laminectomy. It may or may not include instrumentation or fusion.

Nonsurgical cervical stabilization of fractures or dislocations may be accomplished by the use of traction. The traction reduces pain by separating and aligning the injured vertebrae and by reducing or eliminating muscle spasms. The halo vest system offers many advantages: easy access to the neck for diagnostic procedures or surgery; early mobilization and ambulation; limits rotation, flexion, extension, and lateral bending of cervical spine (C1-4); and most are MRI compatible. Pin care for patients using a halo vest include: cleanse with H_2O_2 (hydrogen peroxide) twice a day; no ointments or antiseptics for routine care; "clicking" sound may indicate loose pin; infected pin sites should be changed; and never lift or turn by metal frame. Skin care for patients using a halo vest include: using warm, damp towel (wrung out); pulling folded towel back and forth under vest; and not using soap, lotion, or powder under the vest.

Nonsurgical thoracic and lumbar stabilization of fractures or dislocations also involves immobilization using various braces or orthotics, such as thoracic lumbar sacral orthotic (TLSO) brace; a canvas corset; or a Jewett brace. The TLSO brace is an external motion control device that limits flexion and extension, but not rotation or lateral bending. It is applied by logrolling, with patient supine in bed. The patient wears a cotton t-shirt without wrinkles and the nurse must assess the skin for pressure areas.

Infections

Infections of the central nervous system include meningitis, encephalitis, intracranial abscess, and Guillian-Barré syndrome. **Meningitis** (bacterial, fungal, viral) is an inflammatory process of the meninges and CSF within the subarachnoid space. There is a very high incidence of meningitis in young children, especially those younger than 1 year. The infecting organism multiplies rapidly stimulating inflammatory cytokine (interleukin-1[IL-1], tumor necrosis factor [TNF]) release. Blood brain barrier permeability is altered allowing PMNs into the brain. These events cause formation of purulent exudate that obstructs CSF flow, vasogenic edema, and increased ICP. Early and aggressive diagnosis and treatment helps to prevent the development of complications. Presenting signs and symptoms may include progressively worsening headache, fever, nausea, vomiting, photophobia, nuchal rigidity, positive Kernig's and Brudzinski's sign, altered LOC, and seizures. Diagnosis is usually determined by clinical examination and lumbar puncture.

The CSF is cloudy or xanthochromic and shows elevated pressure, elevated protein, decreased glucose, and the presence of WBCs. CT scan of the head may show hydrocephalus or diffuse enhancement in severe cases. Management includes symptom control, patient isolation (meningococcal), and administration of appropriate anti-infectious agents. Nursing care includes monitoring for LOC changes, maintenance of low stimulation environment, and medication administration.

Encephalitis is inflammation of brain tissue usually caused by a virus (most common), fungus, bacteria, or parasite. Incidence is highest in children younger than 10 years of age, then it decreases and is constant until about 40 years of age, when it decreases further. It is most common in the immunosuppressed. Acute encephalitis is usually caused by a virus such as herpes simplex, Epstein-Barr, equine, and arbovirus. Arbovirus and equine virus (transmitted by ticks and mosquitoes) include West Nile, malaria, Eastern equine, Western equine, and St. Louis varieties. Presenting signs and symptoms may include progressively worsening headache, fever, nausea, vomiting, photophobia, nuchal rigidity, positive Kernig's and Brudzinski's sign, altered LOC, and seizures. Diagnosis and management is the same as for meningitis.

Intracranial abscesses are pockets of infection in the brain tissue caused by infection outside the brain that is carried to the brain by the bloodstream. The most common abscess sites are the cerebrum, epidural, and subdural spaces. Presenting signs and symptoms may include fever, lethargy, focal neurologic deficits, speech and motor deficits, and seizures. Diagnosis is made using CT scanning and lumbar puncture. Medical management includes both intravenous and intrathecal antibiotics, after the infecting agent is identified. Surgical excision and drainage may be requires to remove as much purulent drainage as possible. Nursing care includes monitoring for LOC changes, maintenance of low stimulation environment, and medication administration. If the patient requires surgery, the head of the bed should be elevated 30 degrees to facilitate venous drainage.

Guillian-Barré syndrome is an inflammatory process of the nervous system characterized by demyelination of the peripheral nerves. Incidence of Guillian-Barré syndrome (GBS) is 1 to 2 per 100,000 people in the United States. It affects all ages, races, and genders equally. A flu-like illness, one to three weeks prior to symptoms, has been implicated in 60 to 70 percent of GBS cases. The syndrome is thought to be autoimmune, triggered by the infectious event. Macrophages attack normal myelin, producing demyelination of the axons. Presenting signs and symptoms include acute onset of bilateral lower extremity muscle weakness that ascends rapidly upward; tingling; hypoactive or absent deep tendon reflexes (DTR's); cranial nerve deficits; impaired respiratory muscle function that can progress to respiratory failure; and autonomic nervous system dysfunction.

Surgical Procedures

Neurosurgical procedures include craniotomy, craniectomy, cranioplasty, and burr holes.

Craniotomy is surgical opening of the skill to allow for access to brain tissue. There are three types of craniotomies: supratentorial, infratentorial, and transsphenoidal. Supratentorial approach is just above the tentorium and is used to access the cerebral hemispheres (frontal, parietal, temporal, occipital). This approach is used to:

- remove intracranial tumors, hematomas, abscesses, or seizure foci.
- clip or ligate aneurysm or AVMs in the anterior circulation.
- placement of ventricular draining shunts (venous, pleural, peritoneal).
- debridement of fragments or necrotic tissue; elevate and realign bone fragments.

Infratentorial approach is below tentorium in the posterior fossa and is used to access the brain stem (midbrain, pons, medulla) and cerebellum. This approach is used for removal of cerebellar tumors and hemorrhages, acoustic neuromas, brainstem tumors, cranial nerve tumors, and abscesses. The transsphenoidal approach is frequently used to remove pituitary tumors or to control pain associated with metastatic cancer.

Craniectomy is excision of a portion of the skull without replacement and may be used for decompression after cerebral debulking or removal of bone fragments from a skull fracture.

Cranioplasty is the repair of skull using synthetic material. **Burr holes** are small holes drilled through the skull allowing access to the underlying structures. They are frequently used for evacuation of epidural or subdural hematomas, insertion of an intraventricular catheter for CSF drainage, or insertion of ICP monitoring device.

Complications of cranial surgery may include intracranial hypertension, brain ischemia or infarction, hemorrhage, CSF leak, CNS infection, seizures, fluid and electrolyte imbalance, hydrocephalus, deep vein thrombosis, or stress ulcers. Most neurosurgery patients are admitted to an ICU for close observation and extensive physiological monitoring. Patients will have a turban-style head dressing covering the incision and require frequent monitoring for bleeding or CSF drainage. After the dressing is removed the incision is monitored for redness, drainage, or signs of wound infection. Frequent neurologic assessments are needed to identify and prevent possible complications. Medication administration is needed to control conditions that may increase the cerebral metabolic rate including anticonvulsants; analgesics; antipyretics; sedation; and muscle paralytics or barbiturates if indicated. Maintain CPP of 60 to 100 mm Hg by preventing and treating hypertension or hypotension. DVT and stress ulcer prophylaxis should be ordered by physicians as per ICU protocols.

Seizures

A **seizure** is a sudden, uncontrolled discharge of electricity in the brain. Seizures are frequently a symptom of an underlying pathology. Seizures secondary to systemic or metabolic pathology are not considered epilepsy if the seizures stop when the pathology is resolved. A **convulsion** is the abnormal motor response or jerking movements that occur during a seizure. About 2.5 million people in the United States have epilepsy with an increase of approximately 180,000 new patients each year.

Etiology

Seizure generation has two components: a seizure focus and the neuronal connections to that focus. The seizure focus is a group of hyperexcitable neurons. The area of the brain that is connected to the focus will determine the seizure manifestations. For example, a slow-growing brain tumor near the frontal lobe will eventually cause a seizure to occur. The seizure focus is near the motor cortex, adjacent to the increasing tumor mass. When the hyperexcitable focus discharges, it is transmitted to the motor strip and a clonic seizure is the result.

Causes of seizures include CNS infections, inborn errors of metabolism, congenital malformations, acquired metabolic disorders, and structural lesions. Acquired metabolic disorders such as hypoglycemia, uremia, and electrolyte and acid-base disturbances may complicate care and cause seizures in TBI, SCI, stroke, and cranial surgery patients.

Clinical Manifestations

The clinical manifestations of a seizure are determined by the site of the disturbance (focus). Phases of a seizure include **prodromal phase**, **aural phase**, **ictal phase**, and **postictal phase**. The prodromal phase is the signs or activity before the seizure. For example, headache or feeling depressed: The aural phase is a sensation or warning which the patient remembers. An aura can be visual, auditory, gustatory, or visceral in nature. For example, an odor or flashing lights: The ictal phase is the actual seizure, while the postictal phase is the period immediately following the seizure. During this phase the patient is usually confused, disoriented, and does not remember the seizure. If left alone, the patient may sleep deeply for several hours. A seizure may include some or all of the phases.

Additional clinical manifestations may include **automatisms**, **clonus**, **autonomic symptoms**, or **Todd's paralysis**. Automatisms are coordinated involuntary motor activities that occur during the seizure. Examples include lip smacking, chewing, fidgeting, and pacing. Clonus is the descriptive term for the pattern of spasm with muscle rigidity followed by muscle relaxation. Autonomic symptoms occur in response to stimulation of the autonomic nervous system. These symptoms include pallor, sweating, epigastric discomfort, flushing, piloerection, or dilation of pupils. Todd's paralysis is a temporary, focal weakness or paralysis following a seizure, which can last up to 24 hours.

Types of Seizures

Seizures are divided into two major classes: generalized and partial. Generalized seizures originate in all of the regions of the brain cortex. There is no aura or warning, but there is loss of consciousness. The seizure may last for a few seconds or several minutes.

- Absence seizures usually occur during childhood and last 5–10 seconds. If the seizure lasts for more than 10 seconds, there may be automatisms such as eye blinking or lip smacking. They frequently occur in clusters and can occur dozens or even hundreds of times per day. The electroencephalogram (EEG) will show a 3-Hz (cycles per minute) spike and wave pattern, unique to this type of seizure.

- Atypical absence seizures usually begin before age five and are associated with mental retardation and a tendency for multiple seizure types. They last longer and are associated with muscle spasms.

- Myoclonic seizures are characterized by sudden, brief arm muscle contractions. Consciousness is usually not impaired.

- Clonic seizures demonstrate rhythmic, repetitive clonic movements of the arms, neck, and face. These movements are bilateral and symmetric.

- Tonic-clonic (formerly called grand mal) seizures are the most common type of generalized seizure. The seizure will progress through all of the seizure phases and last two to three minutes. Because of the suddenness of this type of seizure, injuries such as limb fractures, tongue biting, and head trauma can occur. These seizures can occur any time of the day or night, whether the patient is awake or not. Seizure frequency is highly variable.

- Atonic seizures (drop attacks) are a sudden loss of muscle control, usually the legs, that results in falling to the floor, increasing the possibility of injury.

- Partial seizures begin in a specific brain region and consciousness is usually not impaired. The clinical manifestations depend on the region of the brain where the seizure focus starts. There may be an aura or warning signs.

- Simple partial seizures are when consciousness is not lost. Depending on the seizure focus, there may be motor, sensory, autonomic, or higher level cognitive clinical manifestations.

- Complex partial seizures are the most common type of epileptic seizure in adults. Consciousness and awareness of surroundings is lost. Automatisms may occur. The seizure typically lasts one to three minutes.

Status Epilepticus

Status epilepticus is defined as either continuous seizures lasting more than five minutes or two or more different seizures with incomplete recovery of consciousness between them. The most common cause of status epilepticus is abruptly stopping of antiepileptic drugs (AEDs). Clinically status epilepticus can present with tonic, clonic, or tonic-clinic movements. It is a medical emergency since it is often accompanied by respiratory distress brought on by hypoxia or anoxia. Morbidity and mortality for status epilepticus is 20 percent. Subclinical status epilepticus is seen with partial seizures but can only be verified by EEG. It is estimated that between 50,000 and 100,000 patients experience status epilepticus each year in the United States.

During status epilepticus, cerebral metabolism is increased. Initially compensatory mechanisms increase CBF and metabolism, increase autonomic activity with catecholamine release, and cause cardiovascular changes. These changes can lead to hyperglycemia, hypertension, increased cardiac output, increased central venous pressure, tachycardia, increased salivation, sweating, hyperpyrexia, vomiting and incontinence. Hyperglycemia is due to the increased release of epinephrine and activation of hepatic gluconeogenesis. Hypertension is caused by the increased CBF in response to the increased metabolic demands for oxygen and glucose. Tachycardia is the result of the increased cardiac output. Hyperpyrexia is due to the excessive muscle activity and increased catecholamine release. Anaerobic muscle metabolism causes lactic acidosis. The elevated catecholamines and lactic acidosis promote cardiac dysrhythmias, and autonomic dysfunction causes excessive sweating and vomiting leading to dehydration and electrolyte disturbances.

When metabolic demands can no longer be met, decompensation occurs. This causes decreased CBF, systemic hypotension, increased ICP, and failure of cerebral autoregulation. The patient develops both metabolic and respiratory acidosis due to the hypoxia, hypoglycemia from depleted energy stores, hyponatremia, and hyper or hypokalemia. Lack of oxygen and glucose stimulates the production and release of glutamate, changing the electrical balance and causing calcium influx and the development of oxygen free-radicals. These changes make the brain cells electrically unstable and cause cellular injury. As the seizure activity continues, the patient may develop pulmonary edema, cardiac dysrhythmias, rhabdomyolysis, damage to striated muscle fibers, and acute intravascular coagulation. Prompt diagnosis and treatment are imperative since the duration of the seizure is a good predictor of outcomes.

Management

Status epilepticus (SE) is a medical emergency associated with significant morbidity and mortality (20 percent). Initial management includes providing the standard ABCs of life support, administering medications, finding and treating the underlying cause, and preventing and treating any complications. Establishing a patent airway with adequate ventilation is the first priority of treatment. This may require insertion of an artificial airway or intubation if the mouth cannot be opened. Oxygen supplementation or mechanical ventilation may be required. Protection from injury is the next priority. Loosening of constrictive clothing, turning the patient on his side, padding of immediate area, and not restraining the patient's movements will minimize or prevent injury. Medications need to be given to stop the seizure activity, if possible. For adults, the first choice is lorazepam (Brand name: Ativan) or diazepam (Brand name: Valium) for stopping the seizure. In children and neonates, the drug of first choice is phenobarbital (Brand name: Luminal), because it rapidly and efficiently enters the CSF and has minimal adverse side effects. Then, medications to prevent seizure recurrence include phenytoin (Brand name: Dilantin), fosphenytoin (Brand name: Cerebyx), or phenobarbital (Brand name: Luminal). Other agents used for refractory SE are pentobarbital (Brand name: Nembutal), midazolam (Brand name: Versed), and propofol (Brand name: Diprivan). Close monitoring for hypotension and respiratory distress are necessary until seizure activity has ended. Once SE is terminated, diagnostic studies will be ordered to determine the underlying cause of the seizure activity.

Seizure Diagnostic Studies

- CT scan or MRI of the brain (rule out tumors, hemorrhage)

- Routine laboratory studies: (CBC; electrolytes; LFTs, toxicology screen)

- Skull X-rays (to rule out fractures, bone erosion, or separated sutures)

- EEG: (if no seizure activity on standard test, may require 24 hour continuous test)

- Other: PET scan; SPECT scan

(CBC = complete blood count; CT = computed tomography; LFTs = liver function tests EEG = electroencephalography; MRI = magnetic resonance imaging; PET = positron emission tomography; SPECT = single proton emission computerized tomography)

Stroke

Cerebrovascular accident (CVA) is commonly known as stroke or "brain attack." Stroke is the third leading cause of death (160,000 per year) and the leading cause of adult disability in the United States. There are 750,000 new or recurrent strokes each year (NSA, 2007). There are two major types of stroke: hemorrhagic and ischemic. **Hemorrhagic stroke** is caused by a blood vessel that breaks and bleeds into the brain. Fifteen percent of strokes are hemorrhagic but account for more than 30 percent of all stroke deaths. **Ischemic stroke** is caused by a blood clot that blocks or plugs a blood vessel in the brain. Almost 85 percent of all strokes are ischemic. Transient ischemic attacks (TIAs) occur when the blood supply to the brain is briefly interrupted.

Etiology

Stroke is characterized by the onset of neurological deficits due to decreased oxygen supply causing cellular changes leading to the destruction of neural tissue and brain damage. Ischemic strokes (80 percent) are caused by either a thrombus or an embolus. A thrombus (blood clot) may develop secondary to atherosclerotic plaque blocking blood flow and stimulating platelet aggregation or hypercoagulable states (cancer, polycythemia). Emboli are small clot or plaque particles travel distally and lodge in small blood vessels. Risk factors for emboli include atrial fibrillation, coronary artery disease, bacterial endocarditis, valvular heart disease, deep, vein thrombosis, and air/fat embolism. A hemorrhagic stroke (20 percent) occurs when a cerebral blood vessel ruptures and blood leaks into the brain tissue. The major risk factor for hemorrhagic stroke is poorly controlled, long-standing hypertension. The most common sites of hemorrhagic stroke are basal ganglia (50 percent), thalamus (30 percent), cerebellum (10 percent), and pons (10 percent).

Pathophysiology

Stroke is the sudden development of focal neurological deficits caused by interruption of blood flow to brain tissue. Since the brain cannot store glucose or oxygen, it is dependent on a constant supply of these nutrients. Once cerebral blood flow is insufficient to maintain neuronal activity, ischemic injury occurs. The severity of neuronal injury in ischemic tissue is proportional to the reduced cerebral blood flow. In the infarction core area, brain tissue deprived of blood and oxygen dies. The area surrounding this core is known as the ischemic penumbra. The neurons of the ischemic penumbra become electrically silent but remain potentially viable for several hours. If the ischemia is not reversed, irreversible damage occurs. Severe brain tissue ischemia initiates a cascade of metabolic events, including increased lactic acid production, release of glutamate, and ATP depletion. In addition, sodium and calcium enter the cells, cytotoxic edema develops, and mitochondrial death occurs.

Clinical Manifestations

Symptoms of stroke are sudden: numbness or weakness of the face, arm or leg (especially on one side of the body); confusion, trouble speaking or understanding speech; trouble seeing in one or both eyes; trouble walking, dizziness, loss of balance or coordination; or severe headache with no known cause.

Diagnostic Studies

When stroke is suspected, prompt (within three hours of symptom onset) accurate diagnosis and treatment are necessary to minimize brain tissue damage. Diagnosis includes a medical history and a physical examination including neurological examination to evaluate the level of consciousness, sensation, and function (visual, motor, language) and determine the cause, location, and extent of the stroke. A noncontrast CT scan is performed as soon

TABLE 8.12 *Acute Ischemic Stroke Criteria for rtPA Administration*

Exclusion Criteria	Inclusion Criteria
Seizure at stroke onset	Stroke symptom onset < 3 hours
Symptoms suggestive of SAH	Clinical diagnosis of ischemic stroke
Stroke or serious TBI within 3 months	Neuro deficit using NIH stroke scale
Major surgery/serious bodily trauma < 2 weeks	Older than 18 years
History of a prior ICH	CT scan indicates ischemic stroke
Intracranial neoplasm	SBP <185 mm Hg; DBP < 110 mm Hg
Arteriovenous malformation or aneurysm	Glucose >50mg/dL; < 400 mg/dL
GI or urinary tract hemorrhage within 21 days	
Arterial or lumbar puncture within 1 week	
Concomitant oral anticoagulant (INR > 1.7)	

as possible. CT scanning is widely available, requires 15 minutes or less to complete, can be evaluated quickly, and differentiates between ischemic and hemorrhagic stroke. Treatment for ischemic stroke can begin to rapidly save brain tissue. Laboratory tests commonly ordered include complete blood count (CBC), electrolytes, renal panel, coagulation panel, liver function studies, and others depending on presenting symptoms.

Treatment

Emergency department treatment of acute ischemic stroke includes assessment for conditions that mimic stroke, thrombolytic therapy, and treatment of complications. Acute stroke therapies try to stop a stroke while it is happening by quickly dissolving the blood clot causing an ischemic stroke or by stopping the bleeding of a hemorrhagic stroke. Hemorrhagic stroke treatment and management was discussed with brain injuries. Other conditions requiring rapid evaluation are hypoglycemia, toxic or metabolic disorders, migraines, brain tumors, and seizures. Thrombolytic therapy (rtPA) is the most common treatment for ischemic stroke in selected patients. Treatment must be completed within three hours of symptom onset and patients must meet inclusion/exclusion criteria. Giving rtPA more than three hours after symptom onset has not been shown to be beneficial. Before starting rtPA, two peripheral IV catheters are inserted and all invasive procedures completed. The rtPA dose is 0.9 mg/kg up to a maximum of 90 mg with 10 percent of the total dose given as a bolus over one to two minutes followed by the remaining 90 percent over 60 minutes. All antithrombotics are withheld for 24 hours to prevent bleeding complications.

Post Treatment Management

After initial treatment in the ED, the patient will be admitted to the intensive care unit (ICU) for frequent monitoring of complication either from the stroke or treatment. There is an increased risk of conversion from an ischemic stroke to a hemorrhagic stroke. Vital signs and neurologic checks are done every 15 to 30 minutes for 6 to 12 hours. Neurological deterioration needs to be communicated immediately and the patient prepared for a STAT CT scan to rule out hemorrhage. Blood pressure monitoring and management varies depending on treatment modalities, and the patient may require vasoactive medications. The cerebral edema that is a result of the ischemia may require invasive monitoring or even surgery. Blood glucose levels require close monitoring and management to prevent hyperglycemia. Secondary complications include decreased airway maintenance, risk for aspiration, decreased level of consciousness, cranial nerve deficits, and deep vein thrombus.

Pediatric and Neonatal Neurological Abnormalities

Congenital Neurological Abnormalities

All of the congenital neurological disorders are called neural tube defects (NTDs). Neural tube defects include spina bifida malformations, Arnold-Chiari malformation, and anencephaly. Spina bifida malformations fall into three categories: spina bifida occulta, myelomeningocele, and meningocele. The most common location of the malformations is the lumbar and sacral areas of the spinal cord. Myelomeningocele is the most significant form, leading to disability in most affected individuals. The terms spina bifida and myelomeningocele are usually used interchangeably. In spina bifida there is incomplete closure of the embryonic neural tube, resulting in an incompletely formed spinal cord. Additionally, the vertebrae overlying the open portion of the spinal cord do not fully form and remain unfused and open. This allows the abnormal portion of the spinal cord to protrude through the opening in the bones. There may or may not be a fluid-filled sac surrounding the open spinal cord.

Spina bifida occulta is one of the mildest forms, although the degree of disability can vary depending upon the location of the lesion. In occulta there is no opening of the back, but the outer part of some of the vertebrae are not completely closed. The split in the vertebrae is so small that the spinal cord does not protrude. The skin at the site of the lesion may be normal, it may have some hair growing from it, a dimple in the skin, a lipoma, a dermal sinus or a birthmark. Many people do not even know they have it or symptoms do not appear until later in life. Most children and adults with this condition experience problems with bowel and bladder control since the nerves which control these functions originate at the lowest part of the spinal cord. This may result in incontinence from neurogenic bladder. The amount of functional impairment depends on the extent of the neural tube defect and the associated neural tissue.

Many people with spina bifida will have an associated abnormality of the cerebellum, called the Arnold-Chiari malformation. In affected individuals the back portion of the brain is displaced from the back of the skull down into the upper neck. In approximately 90 percent of the people with myelomeningocele, hydrocephalus will also occur because the displaced cerebellum interferes with the normal flow of cerebrospinal fluid.

Diagnosis may occur during maternal screening for neural tube defects, during the 16th and 18th weeks of gestation, using serum alpha-fetoprotein (AFP) levels. When the neural tube is not closed, AFP leaks into the amniotic fluid and increases the level in the maternal blood. Elevated AFP levels must be confirmed using ultrasound. Infants born with spina bifida require spinal x-rays to identify the exact level of the deformity and rule out lesions at other levels. CT scan or MRI is done to visualize the ventricular system and brainstem.

Surgical closure of the protruding sac is done to preserve all neural tissue, provide a closed skin barrier, and control progressive hydrocephalus. The surgery is done as soon after birth as possible. Intrauterine surgery for spina bifida has been performed and the safety and efficacy of this procedure is currently being investigated. To reduce and/or prevent hydrocephalus, a ventricular shunt may be surgically inserted to provide a continuous drain for the cerebrospinal fluid produced in the brain. These shunts usually drain into the abdomen. Nursing management includes monitoring vital signs, healing of incisions, laboratory studies, and neuro status. Other nursing interventions include providing nutrition, administering medications, offering emotional support, and maintaining a safe environment.

Anencephaly is a condition in which the portion of the neural tube, which will become the cerebrum, does not close resulting in the absence of a major portion of the brain, skull, and scalp. Children with this disorder are born without a forebrain, the largest part of the brain consisting mainly of the cerebral hemispheres (responsible for higher level cognitive functioning). The remaining brain tissue is often exposed—not covered by bone or skin. Infants born with anencephaly are usually blind, deaf, unconscious, and unable to feel pain. Although some individuals with anencephaly may be born with a rudimentary brainstem, which controls autonomic and regulatory function, the lack of a functioning cerebrum is usually thought of as ruling out the possibility of ever gaining consciousness. Reflex actions such as breathing and responses to sound or touch may occur.

Anencephaly can often be diagnosed before birth using maternal AFP screening and fetal ultrasound. There is no cure or standard treatment for anencephaly and the prognosis for affected individuals is poor. Most anencephalic babies do not survive birth, accounting for 55 percent of non-aborted cases. If the infant is not stillborn, then he or she will usually die within a few hours or days after birth from cardiorespiratory arrest. In almost all cases anencephalic infants are not aggressively resuscitated since there is no chance of the infant ever achieving a conscious existence. Instead, the usual clinical practice is to offer hydration, nutrition and comfort measures and to "let nature take its course." Artificial ventilation, surgery, and drug therapy are usually regarded as futile efforts.

Congenital Infections

The more common viruses linked to congenital infections include the cytomegalovirus (CMV), herpes, rubella (German measles), parvovirus, varicella (chickenpox), and enteroviruses. Congenital infections can adversely affect the unborn fetus or newborn infant. They are generally caused by viruses that may be picked up by the baby at any time during the pregnancy up to and including the time of delivery. The viruses initially infect the mother who subsequently may pass it to the baby either directly through the placenta or at the time of delivery as the baby passes through the birth canal. Mothers generally do not feel sick with the viruses. Sometimes they have flu-like symptoms. Even if the mother is known to have a viral illness during her pregnancy, her immune system may prevent the virus from infecting the fetus or newborn infant. Pre-pregnancy or routine prenatal screening to determine the presence or susceptibility to some of these infections can enable appropriate management to prevent adverse fetal outcomes.

Calcifications in the brain associated with brain damage may be seen with CMV infections. The brain grows poorly and the head subsequently appears small (microcephaly). Hydrocephalus ("water on the brain") and groin hernias may also occur. Diabetes mellitus and heart problems can be seen with congenital rubella infections. Recurrent eye and skin infections are typical for herpes. Infants with congenital infections may suffer particular damage to the developing brain and sensory organs. The subsequent effects of the infection

TABLE 8.13

Test	Purpose	Action
Rubella IgG	Determine rubella susceptibility	If negative, give MMR before conception or post-partum.
Hepatitis B Surface antigen	Determine chronic carriers	If positive, administer hepatitis B immune globulin and vaccine to infant at birth (prevents carriage in 95%).
Syphilis	Detect active infection	If reactive, treat with penicillin and consult a specialist.
HIV antibody	Should be offered to all pregnant women so that measures can be taken to reduce vertical transmission	If positive, antiretroviral treatment for both mother and infant reduces vertical transmission rates significantly. Refer HIV specialist.

are quite diverse, resulting in a broad range of developmental outcomes. Hearing loss is the most common developmental disability, especially from CMV and rubella infections. It may be present at birth or develop later in childhood and be progressive. Hearing loss may be difficult to detect in infancy. Visual impairments are common, especially with herpes and rubella infections. The impairments result from the development of cataracts or from actual destruction of the tissues of the eye. Mild to severe brain damage may occur, resulting in various degrees of mental retardation, learning and behavioral disorders, and autism. Special education is frequently required.

Shaken Baby Syndrome

Shaken baby syndrome (SBS) is a form of child abuse that is believed to occur when an abuser violently shakes an infant or small child, creating a whiplash-type motion that causes acceleration-deceleration injuries. The injury is estimated to affect between 1,200 and 1,600 children every year in the United States. A remarkable feature of SBS is the typical lack of external evidence of trauma. It is a major cause of mortality in infants, is often fatal, and can produce lifelong disability from neurological damage. Up to half of deaths related to child abuse are reportedly due to shaken baby syndrome. As many as a third of infant victims with SBS die from their injuries.

The signs associated with SBS include retinal hemorrhages, petechiae on the body or face, multiple fractures of the long bones, and subdural hematomas. Additional effects include diffuse axonal injury, oxygen deprivation and swelling of the brain, which can raise intracranial pressure and damage delicate brain tissue. Long-term problems resulting from SBS include learning disabilities, seizure disorders, speech disability, hydrocephalus, behavioral problems, cerebral palsy, and visual disorders. Prevention is similar to the prevention of child abuse in general.

Neuromuscular Disorders

Muscular dystrophy (MD) refers to a group of genetic, hereditary muscle diseases that cause progressive muscle weakness. Muscular dystrophies are characterized by progressive skeletal muscle weakness, defects in muscle proteins, and the death of muscle cells and tissue. Most types of MD are multi-system disorders with manifestations in body systems including the heart, gastrointestinal and nervous systems, endocrine glands, skin, eyes and other organs.

Presenting symptoms include: progressive muscular wasting (weakness), poor balance, frequent falls, walking difficulties, waddling gait, calf pain, muscle contractures, respiratory difficulty, drooping eyelids (ptosis), gonadal atrophy, scoliosis (curvature of the spine), and an inability to walk. Some types of MD can affect the heart, causing cardiomyopathy or arrhythmias.

The diagnosis of muscular dystrophy is based on the results of a muscle biopsy. In some cases, a DNA blood test may be all that is needed. The prognosis for people with muscular dystrophy varies according to the type and progression of the disorder. Some cases may be mild and progress very slowly over a normal lifespan, while others produce severe muscle weakness, functional disability, and loss of the ability to walk. Some children with muscular dystrophy die in infancy while others live into adulthood with only moderate disability. The muscles affected vary, but can be around the pelvis, shoulder, face or elsewhere. Muscular dystrophy can affect adults, but the more severe forms tend to occur in early childhood.

There is no specific treatment for any of the forms of muscular dystrophy. Physical therapy to prevent contractures, orthopedic appliances used for support, and corrective orthopedic surgery may be needed to improve the quality of life in some cases. The myotonia (delayed relaxation of a muscle after a strong contraction) may be treated with medications such as quinine, phenytoin, or mexiletine but no actual long-term treatment has been found.

Werdnigg-Hoffman Disease

Werdnigg-Hoffman disease is an autosomal recessive neuromuscular disease that affects the lower motor neurons only. It is evident before birth or within the first few months of life. There may be a reduction in fetal movement in the final months of pregnancy. Affected children never sit or stand unassisted and will require respiratory support to survive before the age of two years. Symptoms include tongue fasciculations; hypotonia in legs, arms, rib, chest and bulbar muscles (infant lies in a frog-leg position, i.e., hips abducted & knees flexed); flaccid quadriplegia; respiratory difficulties; poor feeding; weak cry, and areflexive extremities.

Diagnosis is made using EMG, showing fibrillation and muscle denervation and serum creatinine kinase (normal or increased). Treatment is symptomatic and supportive and includes treating pneumonia, curvature of the spine and respiratory infections, if present. For individuals who survive early childhood, assistive technology can be vital to providing access to work and entertainment. Genetic counseling is imperative.

Space-occupying Lesions

Brain tumors are due to an abnormal proliferation of the central nervous system (CNS) cells, producing a space-occupying lesion. Most brain tumors develop from the glial cells that support the neurons by providing protection, structural support, and nutrition. These cells are astrocytes, ependymal cells, oligodendroglia, and microglia.

TABLE 8.14 *Brain Tumor Classification*

Location	Cell Type	Descriptors
Infratentorial		
Brainstem	glioma	malignant
Cerebellum	astrocytoma	malignant
Medulla	medulloblastoma	malignant
Ventricles	ependymoma	benign
Supratentorial		
Cerebrum	glioma	malignant
Optic chiasm	glioma	malignant
Midline	craniophyngioma	malignant
Pineal gland	astrocytoma	malignant

Brain tumor symptoms vary greatly based on location, growth rate, age, and developmental stage of the child. Generally symptoms include increased ICP (most common), headache, impaired balance and coordination, ataxia, nystagmus, and cranial nerve defects. Diagnostic studies may include CT or MRI scans, serum human chorionic gonadotropin (hCG) and alpha-fetoprotein (AFP) levels, CSF polyamines, and brain biopsy. Medical management may include surgery, radiation, or chemotherapy. Nursing management includes monitoring vital signs, ICP, healing of incisions, laboratory studies, and neuro status. Other nursing interventions include providing nutrition, administering medications, offering emotional support, and maintaining a safe environment.

Spinal Fusion

Scoliosis is a lateral curvature of the spine greater than 10 degrees. There are three types of scoliosis: congenital, neuromuscular, and idiopathic. Pathologic changes start in the soft tissues, shortening the curve. Changes in the vertebrae are a result of unequal forces applied to the growth plates. Growth spurts increase the curve. A large curve may compromise breathing and can be physically disabling.

Physical signs of scoliosis can include a 'hump' on one side of the back when the patient bends forward, a sideways curve to the spine, uneven shoulders, and uneven hips. Diagnostic studies include serial x-rays and pulmonary function tests to monitor curve progression. Treatment includes electrical stimulation, bracing, and surgery.

Spinal fusion is the most common treatment for scoliosis. It is a safe and effective treatment for the condition. Spinal fusion involves attaching rods to the spine and using a bone graft. They are attached above and below the curved part of the spine by wires and screws. These rods will help to straighten the spine. A bone graft is used to fuse the spine. The bone from the graft heals over the rods and acts as "cement" that fuses the spine together. The part of the spine that has not been fused will still be flexible, and allow nearly normal movement. Nursing management involves postoperative management includes pain management, fluid and electrolyte status, monitor for infection, and provide a safe environment.

The Gastrointestinal System

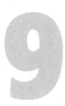

OVERVIEW OF THE GASTROINTESTINAL SYSTEM

The gastrointestinal system (GI) is basically composed of a long tube that extends from the mouth to the anus and accessory organs of digestion (the liver, gallbladder, and pancreas). The primary purpose of the GI system is to break down ingested food and provide the body with nutrients, while eliminating waste. The gastrointestinal wall is composed of four layers: serosa, muscularis, submucosa, and mucosa. The outer connective tissue layer, called the serosa, secretes mucous to prevent friction with visceral organs of the abdomen. The muscalaris is a muscular layer that provides the rhythmic contraction needed to break down food. The submucosa contains connective tissue, elastic fibers, blood vessels, lymphatic vessels, and the enteric autonomic nervous system. The innermost layer, the mucosa, absorbs nutrients and fluids and receives the majority of the blood supply. In the small intestine this innermost layer is referred to as the microvilli. In times of critical illness the mucosa may erode due to trauma, hypoperfusion, stress, medications, or surgery. The erosion may lead to bleeding or infection.

Components

The organs that make up the GI tract are the mouth, esophagus, stomach, small intestine, large intestine, rectum, and anus. Accessory organs assisting with digestion are the liver, gallbladder, and pancreas.

Primary Functions

The functions of the digestive system are ingestion and propulsion of food, secretion of digestive juices, mechanical and chemical digestion, absorption of digested food, and the elimination of waste products through bowel movements. The accessory organs secrete substances necessary for digestion to occur. Secretions from the liver, gallbladder, and pancreas are delivered to the second portion of the duodenum through ducts. The liver produces bile that is stored between meals in the gallbladder. The bile is released in response to ingestion of fats. The pancreas releases enzymes that assist in digestion of carbohydrates, proteins, and fats.

FIGURE 9.1 *Human Digestive Tract*

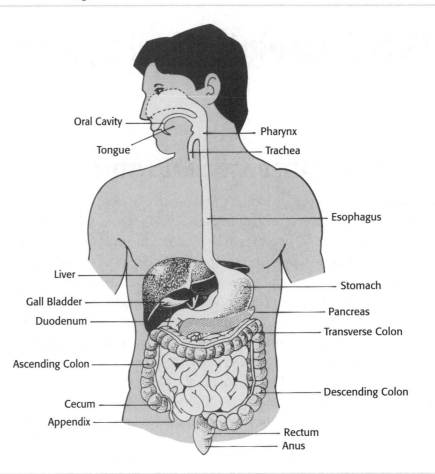

ANATOMY AND PHYSIOLOGY

Organs of the Gastrointestinal Tract

- **Mouth:** Food is chewed and mixed with saliva in the mouth. Salivary glands secrete salivary amylase, which digests carbohydrates to disaccharides. Saliva production is controlled by the sympathetic and parasympathetic nervous system but not controlled by hormones. The pH of saliva is 7.4, which helps to neutralize acids and prevent tooth decay. Saliva production is about 1,000 milliliters in 24 hours.

- **Esophagus:** The upper third of the esophagus has striated *voluntary* muscle, the middle third has striated and smooth muscle, and the lower third has only smooth muscle. The upper third is fully voluntary, where the contractions of the middle and lower third of the esophagus are involuntary. The vagus nerve innervates the esophagus. Swallowing occurs in the esophagus as food is propelled to the stomach. The peristaltic action of sequential contraction and relaxation is mediated by the swallowing center in the brain. Sphincters at the upper and lower end of the esophagus prevent regurgitation.

- **Stomach:** Food is stored in the stomach during eating as digestive enzymes partially digest and move the partially digested food called chyme into the duodenum. The upper sphincter of the stomach between the stomach and esophagus is called the cardiac sphincter, also known as the gastroesophageal (GE) junction. The lower sphincter is known as the pyloric sphincter, which relaxes to expel food into the duodenum. The stomach is divided into the fundus, body, and antrum. The stomach is relatively sterile of bacteria due to acid secretion. The contents of the stomach are acidic secondary to the presence of hydrochloric acid (HCl). Hydrochloric acid is secreted by the parietal cells in the stomach and involves acetylcholine, gastrin, and histamine. HCl secretion can be blocked by certain medications histamine receptor (H2-blockers) and proton-pump inhibitors (PPIs) such as famotidine and omeprazole, respectively. The main digestive enzyme in the stomach is pepsin and is secreted by the chief cells of the stomach. Pepsin is originally secreted as a zymogen (pepsinogen), which is an inactive form of the enzyme. When the pepsinogen is exposed to the acidic lumen of the stomach, the HCl cleaves the pepsinogen into the active enzyme. Gastric ulcers may involve a gram-negative bacteria, Helicobacter pylori, that damages the gastric mucosa. Some medications like aspirin and ibuprofen can damage the gastric mucosa and cause ulcerations. The stomach also synthesizes intrinsic factor, which is necessary for the absorption of vitamin B12 in the ileum of the small intestine.

- **Small Intestine:** The small intestine is about 20 feet long consisting of three segments: the duodenum, jejunum, and ileum. The ileocecal valve controls the flow of digested food from the ileum into the large intestine and prevents reflux into the small intestine. Major nutrients are absorbed by the small intestine villi and microvilli that cover numerous intestinal folds, creating a mucosal surface known as the brush border. The brush border contains enzymes that break down disaccharides and dipeptides, because by the time the chime reaches the small intestine, enzymes from other parts of the GI tract have broken down the nutrients to the level of dissacharides and dipeptides, but these cannot be absorbed. The dissacharidases (e.g., maltase and lactase) and dipeptidases need to break down these molecules to monosaccharides (e.g., glucose) and amino acids in order for them to be absorbed.

- **Large Intestine:** The large intestine contains mucous-secreting goblet cells and is about six feet long consisting of the cecum, appendix, colon (ascending, transverse, descending, and sigmoid), rectum, and anus. Water reabsorption is the primary function of the large intestine. The large intestine is sterile at birth but becomes colonized with Escherichia coli, Clostridium welchii, and Streptococcus bacteria within a few hours. Intestinal bacteria help to metabolize bile salts and synthesize vitamins and drugs.

Accessory Organs

- **Liver:** The liver is the largest organ in the body, located under the right diaphragm in the right upper quadrant. The liver secretes bile, excretes bilirubin, metabolizes fats, serves to detoxify drugs (e.g., Tylenol and narcotics) in the body, convert glucagons to glucose during times of fasting, store vitamins and nutrients, synthesize the majority of the proteins in the body that maintain the oncotic pressure (e.g., albumin), synthesize the majority of clotting factors that are dependent on vitamin K, and metabolize ammonia (a breakdown product of protein metabolism in the GI tract) to urea.

- **Gallbladder:** Located under the liver in the right upper quadrant. The gallbladder holds about 90 milliliters of bile. Within 30 minutes of eating fat, bile is secreted into the duodenum from the gallbladder via the action of a hormone called Cholecystokinin (CCK).

- **Pancreas:** Located behind the stomach with its head in the curve of the duodenum and its tail touching the spleen in the left upper quadrant. The exocrine (secretion into ducts, external to the vascular system) pancreas secretes enzymes and alkaline fluids that assist with digestion. The endocrine (secretion into the blood) pancreas secretes insulin and glucagon.

NURSING ASSESSMENT

History

Gather information about past and present symptoms. A thorough history can assist with diagnosis and treatment. Many people with GI disturbances have a functional disorder with no anatomic abnormality. Elicit information about appetite, nausea, vomiting, bowel elimination, and pain. Ask about any previous abdominal surgeries or changes in weight. A weight gain of 2 pounds or 1 kg is equal to 1 liter of fluid. Include family history of colon cancer, ulcer disease, or inflammatory bowel disorders. Include social history of any tobacco, drug, or alcohol use along with work or family stress. Facilitation or open-ended questions should be used to help the patient report symptoms through spontaneous associations.

Physical Assessment

Height, weight, frame size, and body mass index (BMI) are measures to provide information about nutritional status and body mass. To determine BMI, divide the patient's weight in kilograms by the height in meters squared. Desirable BMI range is 20–25, obesity is greater than 30, and underweight is less than 17.5. Assess the mouth for symmetry, color, and hydration status. Palpate the patient's lips, gingivae, and buccal mucosa. Inspect for any loose teeth or masses. Direct physical assessment of the abdomen begins by observation of the skin and inspection. Note any asymmetry, scars, or bruising. Ask the patient to take a deep breath and hold it to determine contour and palpate organs of the abdominal cavity. A bluish periumbilical discoloration, *Cullen's sign,* suggests intraabdominal bleeding. Bruising in the lower abdomen and flank area, *Grey-Turner's sign,* indicates retroperitoneal hemorrhage. Recent striae are pink or blue, but Cushing's disease striae remain purple. Scars could indicate possible abdominal adhesions. Inspect the umbilical cord of newborns for two arteries and one vein.

Auscultate bowel sounds and vascular sounds for one to two minutes or more. Loud bowel sounds known as borborygmi ("growling stomach") indicate hunger. High pitched bowel sounds may indicate intestinal fluid or air under pressure as with an intestinal obstruction. Decreased or absent bowel sounds indicate obstruction or paralytic ileus. Auscultate with the bell of the stethoscope for any bruits or venous hums.

Percussion is used to assess the size of the organs and presence of fluid (ascites) or air. Tympany is the most common sound due to air in the stomach and intestine. Dullness is heard over organs and solid masses. A distended bladder produces dullness above the symphysis pubis. Mark the liver span after percussion upward along the midclavicular line of the left upper quadrant. A span of more than 2–3 cm below the costal margin indicates an enlarged liver or downward displacement from the lungs as with emphysema. Percuss downward over the lungs on the right to determine the upper border of the liver and mark it with a pen. The upper border is usually at the 5th–7th intercostals space. A larger span indicates liver enlargement. Usual liver span is 6–12 cm, but this is dependent on the size of the patient. Percuss the spleen at the midaxillary line of the left upper quadrant.

Palpation with the palm or bimanual (one hand on the other) is used to detect muscle spasm, masses, fluid, and any tenderness. Rigidity or board-like hardness is indicative of peritonitis. Attempt to palpate the gallbladder below the liver margin. A healthy gallbladder will not be palpable. If there is gallbladder disease the patient may halt inspiration due to pain—Murphy's sign. The spleen is usually not palpable. The right kidney is more frequently palpable than the left. Aortic pulsations may be palpated to the left of the midline and should be in the anterior direction. A prominent pulsation indicates aortic aneurym. Bladder distension can be felt as a smooth, round, tense mass above the pubic bone. Abdominal reflexes can be elicited by stroking the abdomen. Rebound tenderness (Blumberg sign) is pain with sudden removal of the hand after deep palpation and indicates peritonitis.

TABLE 9.1 *Laboratory and Diagnostic Studies*

Laboratory Studies	Description	Interpretation/ Nursing Responsibilities
Liver function tests (LFTs) Aspartate Aminotranspeptidase (AST formally SGOT) Normal result = <40 units/L Alanine Transaminase (ALT formally SGPT) Normal result = <40 units/ L Lactate dehydrogenase enzyme (LDH) Normal result = 100–330 units/L	Elevations indicate liver disease (hepatitis) or damage to cardiac muscle.	Drugs may increase liver enzymes due to hepatocellular damage. Obtain a list of medications the patient is taking.
Total Bilirubin Normal result = <1.9 mg/dl Direct Bilirubin (conjugated) Normal result = <0.3 mg/dl Neonate = <0.6 mg/dl Infant = <0.2 mg/dl Indirect bilirubin (unconjugated) Normal result = <1.9 mg/dl Infants < 1 day = <5.2 mg/dl Infants 1–2 days = <7.6 mg/dl Infants 3–5 days = <11.1 mg/dl Infants >1 month = <1.9 mg/dl	Bilirubin is a breakdown product of hemoglobin. Used to assess hepatobiliary disease. Direct bilirubin is primarily used as a marker for hepatobiliary obstruction. These tests describe the ability of the liver to conjugate bilirubin.	Elevated in obstructive jaundice.
Urinary bilirubin Normal result = negative Urine Urobilinogen Normal result = <17 mcmol/L Fecal Urobilinogen Normal result = 30–220 mg/100g of stool	Colorless degradation product of bilirubin found in urine and feces. The absence of urobilinogen in urine in a jaundiced patient indicates complete biliary obstruction.	Decreased fecal urobilinogen will cause clay-colored stools.
Alkaline prosphatase Normal result = 44–147 units/L	Found in liver, biliary tract, bone, intestine, and placenta.	Elevated in gallbladder disease.
Prothrombin time (PT) Normal result = 11–13 seconds	Indicator of the liver's ability to manufacture coagulation factors.	May be altered in liver disease and biliary obstruction.
Albumin Normal result = 3.4–5.4 g/dl	Plasma-binding protein synthesized by the liver.	Low in liver disease.

TABLE 9.1 *Laboratory and Diagnostic Studies (continued)*

Laboratory Studies	Description	Interpretation/ Nursing Responsibilities
Acute hepatitis panel		
Hepatitis A antibody (anti-HAV) Normal result = negative	IgM antibodies detect acute hepatitis A infection within 1 week. Persist for 6 months. IgG develops 4 weeks after IgM and persists for years.	
Hepatitis B, antigen and antibody (HbeAg, HbeAb, HbcAb, HbsAb, HbsAg) Normal result = negative	IgM antibodies against hepatitis B virus core detected 6–8 weeks after acute hepatitis B infection. IgG antibodies usually indicate acute or previous exposure.	
Hepatitis C antibody (anti- HCV) Normal result = negative	Indicates past or present infection with hepatitis C.	
Hepatitis D (delta agent)	Hepatitis B delta agent is only seen in co-infected HBsAg-positive patients.	
Pancreatic enzymes		Elevated in pancreatitis.
Amylase Normal result = 23–140 units/L	Enzyme that degrades carbohydrates.	
Lipase Normal result = <160 units/L	Enzyme that degrades fatty acids. Remains elevated 7–10 days after acute pancreatitis.	

Diagnostic Studies	Description	Interpretation
Radiology	X-rays can penetrate dense tissues. Contrast of radi-opaque substance may be used to visualize upper and lower bowel.	Air appears black, bone appears white, and soft tissue appears gray. Contraindicated in pregnancy. Gather information about allergies to contrast media, iodine, or shellfish.
Angiography	X-ray of vascular beds.	
Ultrasound	Visual inspection of soft tissues by using sound waves.	Bowel cleansing or clear liquids may be ordered prior to test.
Computed tomography (CT)	Noninvasive x-ray producing cross-sectional images.	Requires patient to lie still. May require sedation.

TABLE 9.1 *Laboratory and Diagnostic Studies (continued)*

Diagnostic Studies	Description	Interpretation
Endoscopy	Uses fiberoptic instrument to visualize internal organs and tissues.	Biopsy may be taken.
Magnetic resonance imaging (MRI)	Uses magnetic imaging sources without radiation.	Assure patient has no metal implants or jewelry on prior to test.
Biopsy	Invasive procedure resulting in collection of tissues.	

ALTERATIONS OF THE GASTROINTESTINAL SYSTEM

Acute Abdominal Trauma

Abdominal trauma accounts for 15 percent of trauma deaths. Intra-abdominal trauma may involve more than one organ system injury. Rib fracture may result in laceration or penetration of abdominal organs. The liver is the most commonly injured organ in abdominal trauma.

Common Causes

Half of all cases of acute abdominal trauma are due to motor vehicle accidents (MVAs). Head and chest injuries may accompany abdominal injuries. Penetrating injuries can occur from guns or knives. Blunt trauma can occur as a result of a fall or contact sports. Wearing seat belts could decrease abdominal trauma during accidents. Shearing, crushing, or compressing forces may rupture the bowel or other abdominal organs. Perforation of the stomach or bowel may lead to peritonitis and sepsis.

Clinical Manifestations

- Injuries to the **diaphragm**—decreased breath sounds or acute chest pain.
- Injuries to the **esophagus**—pain at the site of perforation, fever, difficulty or pain with swallowing, or cervical tenderness.
- Injury to the **stomach**—epigastric pain or tenderness, signs of peritonitis, or bloody gastric drainage.
- Injury to the **liver**—persistent hypotension (due to massive hemorrhage) despite adequate fluid resuscitation and guarding over the right upper quadrant are indicative of liver injury.
- Injury to the **spleen**—hypotension (due to massive hemorrhage), tachycardia, shortness of breath.

- Injury to the **pancreas**—epigastric pain , nausea, vomiting, ileus.

- Injury to **small intestine**—mild abdominal pain, peritoneal irritation, fever, jaundice, intestinal obstruction ileus.

- Injury to **large intestine**—pain, muscle rigidity, blood on rectal exam.

Management

Initial management of abdominal trauma follows the ABCs of resuscitation. Titrate intravenous fluids to maintain a systolic pressure of 100 mm Hg. Life-threatening injuries require immediate treatment and stabilization. Infusion of blood products may be needed. The patient is kept NPO if surgical intervention is anticipated. Assess and provide adequate pain control. Emotional support for the patient and family are key nursing interventions. Careful assessment by the nurse is vital as the patient is prepared for surgery. More teaching will be required postoperatively. Discharge teaching may involve wound and/or ostomy care.

Acute GI Hemorrhage

Gastrointestinal bleeding is a common critical care problem. Both upper and lower GI bleeds can be arterial in origin, depending on the etiology. Upper GI bleeds may present with hematemesis, nausea, and melena. They generally will present in patients with hepatic cirrhosis because of dilation of esophageal varices. If the bleeding is brisk, then instead of melena those with upper GI bleeds may present with bright red blood per rectum. Lower GI bleeds may be arterial in origin, particularly if there is an arterio-venous malformation (AVM). About 80 percent of GI hemorrhage stops without intervention, but recurrent bleeding can become a life-threatening emergency.

Common Causes

The most frequent cause of GI bleeding is peptic ulcers. Other common causes are ruptured esophageal or gastric varices, ruptured esophageal ulcers, malignancy, esophageal perforation, and tears of the esophageal mucosa. Chronic gastritis and bulimia can erode the gastric mucosa. Certain non-steroidal anti-inflammatory medications (NSAIDS) like ibuprofen, naprozen, and aspirin can also affect. Anticoagulants may predispose patients to GI bleed when patients are supratherapeutic on their dosage. Any previous history of GI bleed should be determined.

Clinical Manifestations

Suspect an upper GI bleed if the patient presents with abdominal or chest pain, nausea, bloody or coffee ground emesis, vomiting, dark tarry stools, occult blood, or change in level of consciousness.

Management

Tests that the physician will likely order may include CBC, chemistry panel, activated partial thromboplastin time, protime (with INR), hepatic enzyme panel (total bilirubin, direct bilirubin, alkaline phosphatase, gamma glutamyl transferase, AST, ALT, total protein, and albumin), amylase, lipase, blood type, and crossmatch. Focus on restoring circulating volume and preventing complications of hypovolemia by inserting two large bore intravenous access lines. Position the patient to prevent aspiration with the head of the bed elevated and turn the patient to his side. Give supplemental oxygen and monitor the cardiac rhythm. Anticipate further treatment of insertion of nasogastric tube, administration of vitamin K or vasoactive medication (e.g., vasopressin or norepinephrine). Insert an indwelling catheter and administer pain medication. If bleeding is from esophageal varicies then sclerotherapy or balloon tamponade with Sengstaken-Blakmore tube may be indicated, as determined by the treating medical team. Generally, octreotide will be initiated on the first confirmed evidence of a GI bleed. This medication decreases the splanchnic blood flow, thereby helping decrease the amount of blood lost. Patients should also be started on a proton pump inhibitor twice a day. Other medications that may be used, but are not first line, are antacids and sucralfate. Patient will require bed rest and, possibly, modification of their diets. Small meals at frequent intervals help to avoid stimulation of gastric acid that occurs when the stomach is empty. Bland low-fiber foods are suggested, although there is no direct evidence to suggest that these are superior to other diets. However, avoidance of alcohol, caffeine, and tobacco may decrease discomfort. Identification and elimination of stressors are important teaching components for the nurse when a patient has peptic ulcer disease.

As with many GI disturbances, nutritional support may be needed in the form of a total enteral nutrition (TEN) by way of a gastrostomy or jejunostomy tube. When the patient cannot be fed orally or by tube, then total parenteral nutrition (TPN) or peripheral venous nutrition (PVN) may be indicated. Clinical indications for TPN or PVN are malabsorptive syndromes like short-bowel syndrome, motility disorders like ileus, intestinal obstruction, perioperative nutrition for severe malnutrition, and low-flow states. The goal of supplemental nutriotion is to meet nutritional requirements.

Bowel Infarction, Obstruction, Perforation

Blockage of the GI tract can occur at any level from the esophagus to the intestine. Obstruction of the small intestine is a common surgical complication due to adhesions from scar tissue in post operative patients.

Common Causes

Esophageal obstruction is primarily the result of neoplasm. Risk factors are heavy alcohol intake and smoking. Intestinal obstruction can occur due to tumors, adhesions, or foreign bodies. Occlusion of blood supply to the mesentery results in tissue death and cellular death of the bowel. Other causes of obstruction are Schatzki ring, achalasia, esophageal spasm, or fibrosis from Crohn's disease (less common). If not treated for a long period of time, the patient may experience weight loss and possibly even visceral perforation, as the intraluminal pressure increases beyond the capacity of the intestine. Multiple medications, like anticholinergics and opioids, can reduce gastric motility leading to a paralytic ileus. Any handling of the bowel during surgery can result in the postoperative complication of paralytic ileus, as well.

Clinical Manifestations

Esophageal manifestations are usually asymptomatic until the malignancy is large enough to cause problems with swallowing. Signs and symptoms of malnutrition occur as a result of decrease intake. Intestinal obstruction results in increased bacterial growth due to trapped fluid. Vomiting is present if the obstruction is above the jejunum. Distention occurs with lower GI obstruction. Pain and abdominal cramping increase as peristaltic action attempts to move the obstruction. Signs and symptoms of hypovolemia may result. Electrolyte and chemistry studies reveal inflammation with elevations in BUN, creatinine, sodium, and serum amylase. Leukocytosis is common with WBC elevation from 15,000–25,000.

Management

On evidence of obstruction or GI bleed, patients should be made NPO, a naso-gatric tube (NGT) should be placed to intermittent suction, laboratory tests should be ordered as indicated above, and plain abdominal films should be obtained in the supine upright and decubitus positions to look for free air. If there is evidence of free air or complete small bowel obstruction, surgical exploration and correction may be necessary. Maintenance of support with fluids and electrolyte balance may be necessary until the obstruction is resolved. A pulmonary artery catheter may be inserted to determine fluid needs. An indwelling foley catheter is inserted to measure hourly output. Broad-spectrum antibiotics may be given if peritonitis develops. Continual nursing assessment is needed and pain management. Teaching and patient support are key nursing interventions.

GI Surgeries

Types of gastrointestinal procedures vary depending on the patient problem. Patients with obstruction, cancer, trauma, or hemorrhage may require surgical interventions. Approximately 10 to 50 percent of patients who have undergone GI surgery experience some form of dumping syndrome postoperatively. Nutritional deficiencies may result in the inability of the GI tract to absorb needed vitamins and minerals. Total gastrectomy results in a lack of intrinsic factor absorption, thus requiring B12 injections for life to prevent pernicious anemia.

Gastric Surgeries

- **Total gastrectomy:** complete excision of the stomach with esophageal-jejunal anastomosis
- **Subtotal or partial gastrectomy:** a portion of the stomach is removed
  - Billroth I procedure: gastric remnant anastomosed to the duodenum
  - Billroth II procedure: gastric remnant anastomosed to the jejunum
- **Gastrostomy:** rectangular stomach flap created into abdominal stoma, used for intermittent tube feedings

Hernia Surgeries

- **Herniorrhaphy:** surgical repair of a hernia with suturing of the abdominal wall
- **Hernioplasty:** reconstructive hernia repair with mesh for reinforcement

Bowel Surgeries

- **Appendectomy:** excision of the vermiform appendix
- **Bowel resection:** segmental excision of small and/or large bowel with varied approaches

Laparoscopic Surgeries

- Cholecystectomies and appendectomies are routinely done through laparoscopy.
- Advantages include reduction of postoperative pain and shorter hospital stay.
- Contraindications include obesity, internal adhesions, and bowel obstruction with distention.

Preoperative Care

Nursing care involves helping explain all diagnostic tests and procedures to the patient to promote cooperation and relaxation. Proper patient education will help ensure that the patient is prepared for the type of surgery, as well as postoperative care, including insertion of IV, patient-controlled analgesia pump, NG tube, surgical drains, incision, and ostomy care. The patient should be instructed in measures that will help prevent postoperative complications, such as pulmonary toilet and splinting incision. IV fluids or TPN may be ordered before surgery to improve nutritional status. Strict monitoring of the inputs and outputs is routine and should be done. Preoperative laboratory studies are obtained. Bowel cleansing may be ordered or modifications in diet. Antibiotics are given preoperatively to prevent bacterial growth in the colon. An ostomy nurse may be consulted if the patient is scheduled for an ostomy. The patient, if not already NPO, will be kept NPO after midnight the night before surgery. Medications may be withheld to keep the GI tract clear. Encourage communication with the significant other and family to promote support postoperatively.

Postoperative Management

Physical assessment is completed once per shift or more often if needed. Vital signs are monitored for signs of infection and shock (fever, hypotension, and tachycardia). Intake and output are strictly monitored. Output from drains is collected and analyzed for abnormal amounts or signs of infection and/or bleeding. Nursing assessment of abdominal incisions is needed often to check for abnormal bleeding, odor, or dehiscence. Unstable patients may have open incisions or wound vacuums in place. Post-operative nursing assessment should include routine evaluation of the abdomen for increased pain, distension, rigidity, nausea, or vomiting. You should expect diminished bowel sounds immediately postoperatively, but these should return upon passing of flatus or feces. If there is a fecal odor to the vomitus, it may indicate obstruction. Laboratory values are primarily monitored for any electrolyte imbalances. If the NG tube is left in place, then the nurse should check NG tube for placement and irrigate as needed with 30 ml of normal saline every two hours as needed, but this should be approved by the treating medical team, as there may be contraindications to immediate gastric fluid administration. If there are large amounts of NG output then intravenouse fluid replacement may be needed. Antiembolism stockings and foot movement such as Ted hose and sequential compression devices may be used to prevent stasis of venous blood in legs. Turning, coughing, and deep breathing are used with incentive spirometry every two hours to serve as pulmonary toilet and help prevent atlectasis and post-operative pneumonia. Pain control is paramount in postoperative care following GI surgery and early ambulation. Dressings are changed daily or as needed using aseptic technique. The patient's diet may be advanced by the primary medical team after the NG tube is removed and the presence of bowel sounds has been verified. Progression goes from ice chips, sips of water, clear liquids, full liquids, and then soft or regular foods. Dietary education and ostomy teaching (if relevant) should be reinforced by the nursing staff. It may take three months to a year before a patient can eat normally. Possible complications of gastric surgeries include marginal ulcers where gastric acids come in contact with the operative site or anastomosis, hemorrhage, reflux, gastric dilation, or nutritional problems. Dumping syndrome is most common after the Billroth II procedure and gastric bypass operations. Management of dumping syndrome involves decreasing the amount of food taken at one time and maintaining low-carbohydrate, high-protein, dry diet. Lying down after meals and avoidance of fluids one hour before, with, or two hours after eating helps to decrease dumping syndrome.

Hepatic Failure

Loss of function of the liver can be a slow progression or a sudden acute problem. Every organ in the body is affected by the liver failure. Damage to the liver cells occurs directly from liver disease or indirectly from obstruction of bile flow or hepatic circulation. Parenchymal cells respond to noxious agents by replacing glycogen with lipids, thereby producing fatty infiltration and cell death. Cell regeneration can occur if the disease process is not too toxic or the liver may become fibrotic, as seen with cirrhosis. Cirrhosis leads to portal hypertension, ascites, hepatorenal syndrome, and encephalopathy. The complications of cirrhosis occur mainly due to alteration in the blood flow through the liver and portal circulation. Portal hypertension can occur from increased resistance within the venous system as with cirrhosis or rarely from other causes that may increased blood flow like arterial-portal venous fistulas from infection or neoplasm. The spleen may become enlarged due to congestion within the portal system.

Common Causes

The most common causes of **acute liver failure** are viral hepatitis and drug-induced liver injury. Causes of **chronic liver failure** are cirrhosis, chronic cholestatic disease, chronic viral hepatitis, excessive alcohol intake, malnutrition, diabetes mellitus, alpha1-antitrypsin deficiency, Wilson's disease, hemochromatosis, repeated toxin exposure, and malignant disease such as carcinoma and cholangiocarcinoma.

Types of viral hepatitis are hepatitis A, hepatitis B, hepatitis C, hepatitis D, hepatitis E, hepatitis G, and cytomegalovirus (primarily in immunosuppressedor transplant patients). Hepatitis A and E are known as infectious hepatitis and are the result of poor sanitation; hence, they are transmitted by fecal–oral route. The difference is that Hepatitis A is found in situations of food handling that are unsanitary, where Hepatitis E is a water-borne virus affecting mostly young adults. On the other hand, hepatitis B is spread through close contact with blood and body fluids of infected individuals. Health care workers are at high risk for acquiring this form of hepatitis because of contact with the blood of carriers. Hepatitis D, if present, is found in the presence of hepatitis B, but note that hepatitis B infection can occur without hepatitis D. Hepatitis C accounts for most post-transfusion hepatitis infections and is also associated with IV drug use. Hepatitis C and G are spread by close contact with the blood or body fluids of infected individuals, similar to hepatitis B.

Clinical Manifestations

Manifestations of hepatic failure including hepatitis are systemic and vary greatly. The early phases of hepatic failure include weight loss from nausea and vomiting that may, in some cases, proceed to acute life-threatening liver failure. Listed below are some clinical manifestations of hepatic failure.

- **General:** decreased weight, muscle wasting, malnourishment, malaise, and fatigue

- **Cardiovascular:** increased cardiac output and heart rate, systolic ejection murmur, bounding pulses, decreased blood pressure, dysrhythmias, and peripheral edema

- **Immune:** leucopenia, splenomegaly, thrombocytopenia

- **Skin:** jaundice, palmar erythema, hair loss, pruritus and dry skin, bruising and spider angiomas

- **Endocrine:** peripheral edema, increased weight, moon face and striae, testicular atrophy, gynecomastia, decreased libido, impotence, hypoglycemia

- **Gastrointestinal:** anorexia, nausea, steatorrhea, hyperlipidemia, melana or clay-colored stools, epistaxis, and gingival bleeding

- **Neurologic:** hepatic encephalopathy, sensory disturbances, foot drop, ptosis, nystagmus

- **Renal:** deceased renal blood flow and urine output, dark foamy urine, increased urine osmolality

- **Pulmonary:** diaphragm elevation, dyspnea, decreased oxygen saturation

Management

Management focuses on supporting liver function until it can regenerate while protecting the other body systems from failure. Priorities include maintaining circulating volume, stabilizing hemodynamics, providing nutritional support, and controlling ammonia levels to prevent encephalopathy. Patients with acute liver failure supported in an intensive care unit have increased survival rates. Deterioration of handwriting is an early manifestation of hepatic encephalopathy due to asterixis. Nursing assessment of patients who are irritable or drowsy may include having the patient write her name each shift to observe for subtle early changes. Cerebral edema develops in 80 percent of the patients with encephalopathy. Patients who

TABLE 9.2 *Stages of Hepatic Encephalopathy*

Stage 1	Fatigue, restlessness, irritability, decreased intellectual performance, decreased attention span, decreased short-term memory, personality changes, sleep pattern reversal
Stage 2	Deterioration of handwriting, asterixis, drowsiness, confusion, lethargy, fetor hepaticus
Stage 3	Severe confusion, inability to follow commands, deep somnolence but arousable
Stage 4	Coma, unresponsive to pain, decorticate or decerebrate posturing

develop cerebral edema require intracranial pressure monitoring. The medical team may perform a therapeutic paracentesis to provide temporary relief from pressure on the diaphragm and/or abdominal distention. Patients with ascites are usually limited to two grams of sodium per day and restricted to no more than 1.5 L of fluid intake per day. Lactulose reduces the pH of the intestine and helps decrease ammonia levels. Oral or enteric feedings are generally withheld during the acute phase. Patients with liver failure are often hypoantremic and hypokalemic. The nature of the hyponatremia is hypovolemic and should be treated with fluid restriction as stated above. However, the hypokalemia should be corrected in these patients aggressively, since is a factor of the liver failure, as well as diuretic treatment administered for the ascites. Liver transplant may be indicated for patients with irreversible liver disease, if they meet certain criteria. Histamine receptor (H2) antagonists are given to decrease gastric secretions and prevent gastric ulcers. Thiamine is given to reduce neuropathies. Vitamin K is given to promote production of coagulation factors and prothrombin to help prevent bleeding tendencies. Sedative and acetaminophen are avoided because of poor metabolism and increased toxicity to the liver. Aspirin is avoided because of decreased platelet aggregation.

Pancreatitis

Pancreatitis is an inflammatory disease process resulting in autodigestion of the pancreas by its own enzymes. The pancreatic enzymes, lipase, trypsin, chymotrypsin, and amylase are activated for reasons that are unclear. The pancreas becomes necrotic and severe pain results. The patient is at risk for shock and sepsis. Mortality can be 50 percent or higher. Chronic pancreatitis results in permanent damage. Acute pancreatitis is an attack of a previously normal pancreas where permanent damage to the pancreas does not occur. In necrotizing pancreatitis, the most severe form, necrosis of the pancreas and hemorrhage can occur with shock, multiorgan failure, and death.

Common Causes

Alcohol and biliary disease, specifically gallstones, are associated with acute pancreatitis. Biliary disease is the most common cause of acute pancreatitis in nonalcoholic patients. Another cause of pancreatitis is use of certain drugs like thiazide diuretics, furosemide, steroids, and transplant medications. Hypertriglyceridemia, hypercalcemia, infection, and trauma are other known causes of pancreatitis. As many as 20 percent of patients with pancreatitis have no known cause but are thought to have biliary sludge.

Clinical Manifestations

Patients present with a broad range of symptoms from asymptomatic to agonizing pain. Abdominal pain is the most common symptom and may be constant. Nausea and vomiting are common and there may be foul smelling diarrhea, due to the lack of fat digestion. If hemorrhage occurs there will be ecchymosis in the flank region (Grey Turner's sign) and ecchymosis in the periumbilical area (Cullen's sign). Tissue damage and inflammation lead to release of chemicals that make the capillaries more permeable leading to fluid shifts of as much as 6 liter of fluid into the interstitial compartment. Patients with pancreatitis may develop fevers, especially if they experience the complication of an abscess or pseudocyst. Hypovolemia may result with manifestations of dry mouth, low blood pressure, tachycardia, and decreased urine. Vasodilation, myocardial depression, and hypovolemia lead to shock and tissue death. Decreased renal perfusion results in acute kidney injury, formerly known as acute renal failure. Respiratory depression is the leading cause of death in acute pancreatitis.

Laboratory levels of amylase are elevated in pancreatitis within 2–12 hours after onset of the disease. However, elevated amylase levels have a lower specificity for the diagnosis of pancreatitis, compared to elevated lipase levels. Where amylase levels may return to normal within a week, lipase levels rise and remain elevated longer. In some patients, triglyceride and blood sugar levels are elevated. Hypokalemia and hypomagnesemia contribute to the hypotension that already exists. Hypocalcemia is common and patients may exhibit bronchospasm, tetany, cardiac dysrhythmias, positive Chvostek's sign and positive Trousseau's sign.

CT and abdominal ultrasound are diagnostic tests used to diagnose pancreatitis. Some facilities measure C-reactive protein (CRP), but this is rather non-specific because CRP is an acute phase reactant and may be elevated for a large number of reasons. An increase level above 150 mg/L 48 hours after symptom onset indicates severe acute pancreatitis.

Management

The management of pancreatitis revolves around the following: make the patient NPO, administer intravenous fluids, pain control with opiods (theoretically hydromorphone carries less risks than morphine in pancreatitis), NG tube to intermittent suction. Meperidine (Demerol) is frowned upon for pain control in pancreatitis patients) and is less effective than hydromorphone and morphine. Morphine is believed to be less safe than hydromorphone because it carries the potential to cause a spasm of the sphincter of Oddi, causing additional injury to the pancreas. Comprehensive critical nursing is required for patients with severe pancreatitis. Urine output should be monitored and interventions taken to manage the volume replacement. Urine output should be at least 0.5–1 ml/kg per hour. Fluid replacement is with crystalloids like lactated ringers or normal saline. Daily weights help to reflect overall fluid balance. Respiratory insufficiency is the most common complication of acute pancreatitis. Mechanical ventilation with positive end-expiratory pressure (PEEP) and pleural taps may be needed to relieve respiratory depression. TPN may not be useful for patients unless they have been NPO for three to five or more days. Enteral feeding may be used when the tube is placed in the jejunum. Further, there may be added benefit to the patient if H2 blockers are administered intravenously. Antibiotics are used seldom and then only when an infection is identified or if necrotizing pancreatitis if evident on radiographic imaging. The medical team may also consider the use of antibiotics if the patient clinically appears to be infected clinically (e.g., fevers, leukocytosis, hypotension). Blood transfusions may be needed in hemorrhagic pancreatitis. Some patients require surgical intervention to treat complications of acute pancreatitis. Anxiety and facing problems with alcohol are addressed by providing supportive nursing discussions with encouragement to seek support groups such as Alcoholics Anonymous. The critical care RN may also be instrumental in initiating consults to social work to help the patient identify resources that he may utilize to seek outpatient support.

Gastroesophageal Reflux (GERD)

Gastroesophageal reflux is caused by a backward flow of contents from the stomach into the esophagus. Inappropriate relaxation of the lower esophageal sphincter occurs for unknown reasons resulting in heartburn. If reflux occurs often it results in breakdown of the esophageal lining and may lead to premalignant tissue formation (Barret's Esophagus) or adenocarcinoma. The scarring of the esophagus leads to stricture/fibrosis and dysphagia (difficulty swallowing).

Common Causes

Many patients with gastroesophageal reflux (GERD) have hiatal hernias. Reflux esophagitis exposes the esophageal mucosa to the acidic gastric contents that gradually erode the esophageal tissue. Some patients have delayed emptying of the stomach and obesity which causes pressure on the lower esophageal sphincter. Certain foods and medications are associated with GERD. For example, fatty foods, peppermint, alcohol, and caffeine can increase the frequency and/or severity of GERD. Medications and drugs such as nicotine, beta-adrenergic blockers, nitrates, theophylline, and anticholinergic drugs may have similar effects because they lower tone and contractility of the lower esophageal sphincter. GERD can occur at any age but is most common in people over 50 years of age.

Clinical Manifestations

The history is almost diagnostic for GERD. Patient may complain of retrosternal aching or burning typically after large meals, worsened by lying flat or bending over. Regurgitation of fluid or food particles may predispose the patient to recurrent pneumonia or bronchospasm. Pain or difficulty swallowing may be accompanied by chest heaviness and pressure radiating to the jaw or shoulders. Due to the association with distress on eating, patients may complain of a "burning feeling" in their chest or chest pain, as well as weight loss. Since GERD can be described as chest pain, the symptoms may overlap with those of ACS. Hence, do not simply assume heartburn history is GERD, as it may be a manifestation of ACS, the likewise is also true.

Management

Diagnostic tests are needed in atypical or severe cases. The gold standard is esophageal manometry with pH monitoring in the lower esophagus. Endoscopy or CT of chest may also be done, but are of limited value in the context of manometry and pH monitoring.

TABLE 9.3 *Acid-Controlling Agents*

	Antacids	H2 Antagonists	Proton Pump Inhibitors	Other
Mechanism of Action	Neutralizes gastric acid	Blocks histamine by binding on surface of parietal cells	Blocks all gastric secretion	Mucosal protective agent that provides protective barrier over active stress ulcerations by binding to the base of the area
Interactions	Several drug interactions if given at the same time as other medications due to changes in the pH of the stomach to a more alkaline enviroment	May inhibit the action of certain drugs that require acidic GI environments for gastric absorption like ketoconazole	May increase levels of certain drugs like diazepam and phenytoin	Impairs absorption of certain drugs like tetracycline
Side Effects and Adverse Effects	Magnesium containing-diarrhea Aluminum and Calcium containing-constipation	Headache, confusion, diarrhea, increased liver function tests, creatinine, flushing, urticaria, thrombocytopenia	Same as H2 antagonists	Constipation, nausea and dry mouth
Major Drugs in Category	**Aluminum-containing** • Aluminum carbonate (Amphojel) **Magnesium-containing** • Milk of Magnesia • Gaviscon **Calcium-containing** • Tums **Combination** • Maalox • Mylanta	• Cimetidine (Tagamet) • Famotidine (Pepcid) • Nizatidine (Axid) • Ranitidine (Zantac)	• Lansoprazole (Prevacid) • Omeprazole (Prilosec) • Rabeprazole (Aciphex) • Pantoprazole (Protonix) • Esomeprazole (Nexium)	• Sucralfate (Carafate) • Misoprostol (Cytotec)

Nursing measures involve encouraging the patient to eat multiple small meals per day of low fat foods. If obesity is present, weight loss is helpful for symptoms. Smoking cessation is suggested. Teach patients to avoid food for three hours prior to sleep and rest with the head upright following meals and during sleep. It is also useful to teach patients to not strain when defecating and to limit fats and carbohydrates in their diets. Antacids and especially PPIs are helpful in controlling symptoms. Surgical procedures involving wrapping the esophagus with the fundus of the stomach (Nissen Fundoplication) are used for patients whose GERD is not relieved with medications.

Pediatric and Neonatal Gastrointestinal Abnormalities

Intussusception

Intussusception occurs when one portion of the intestine prolapses and telescopes into the segment distal. It is a frequent cause of intestinal obstruction in children. The most common site is the ileocecal valve after some disturbance in gut motility from medication, virus infection, or an unknown cause. Inflammation from the walls rubbing together leads to edema and decreased blood flow which may result in necrosis, perforation, hemorrhage, and peritonitis.

Onset of intussusception is abrupt with acute abdominal pain, vomiting, and passage of red currant jelly stools (blood and mucus). A palpable mass may be felt in the upper right quadrant or mid-upper abdomen. Diagnosis is made after x-ray, ultrasound, or barium enema. Nursing management focuses on relieving fluid and electrolyte imbalances. Usually a barium enema will not only be diagnostic, but also therapeutic and surgery can generally be avoided in most cases of intussusception. Similar to pancreatitis, patients are maintained NPO, receive intravenous fluids, pain control, and, if indicated, NG tube with intermittent suction. Vital sign assessment and abdominal assessment are done at least every four hours.

Necrotizing Enterocolitis

Necrotizing enterocolitis is a potentially life-threatening inflammatory disease of the intestinal tract that occurs most often in premature infants and low-birth-weight infants five to seven days after feedings are begun. Most often the terminal ileum and colon are affected. Several things, including intestinal ischemia, bacterial or viral infection, or immaturity of the GI tract, can cause necrotizing enterocolitis. Initially the baby has problems with feeding (gastric residuals, vomiting, irritability, and abdominal distention). Bloody diarrhea develops due to the hemorrhage in the bowel. Signs of sepsis (hypothermia or hyperthermia, jaundice, respiratory distress, hepatomegaly, abdominal distention, anorexia, vomiting, and lethargy) follow as the child deteriorates. The bowel is dilated and free fluid is evident in the peritoneum on x-ray. Laboratory studies show anemia, leukopenia, leukocytosis, thrombocytopenia, electrolyte imbalance, and metabolic or respiratory acidosis. Blood cultures may be positive for bacteria.

Early recognition and treatment minimize bowel loss. Assess for feeding intolerance by measuring checking residuals after feeding and abdominal circumference serially. Feedings progress slowly in preterm infants, by 2 to 8 ml/kg/day. Human milk has been shown to protect against the disease.

Treatment consists of discontinuation of enteral feedings and placement of an orogastric tube to prevent gastric distention. Intravenous fluids, TPN, and antibiotics are given. Surgical placement of an ostomy may be needed if the bowel is necrotic or perforated. Strict enteric precautions are used to prevent the spread of infection to other premature infants. Nursing care of the infant requires holding and cuddling the infant who is NPO, and offering a pacifier to meet sucking needs. Cholestasis (disruption of bile flow) is the most common problem of survivors of necrotizing enterocolitis. It occurs about two weeks after TPN is initiated.

Hirschprung's

Hirschprung disease is also known as congenital aganglionic megacolon. The congenital anomaly results in decreased motility and mechanical obstruction of the intestine. Males are more affected than females and a familial pattern is demonstrated. The disease may occur along with other congenital syndromes. Symptoms include failure to pass meconium, refusal to suck, distention, and bile vomitus. If left untreated, complete obstruction leads to respiratory distress and shock. In older children the symptoms include abdominal pain, progressive distention, delayed growth and failure to gain weight with a history of alternating diarrhea and constipation. Stools may be normal or have a ribbonlike appearance.

Diagnosis is made from the history as well as anorectal manometry (reaction of the anal sphincter to distention of the rectum), barium and x-ray studies, and colonic biopsy (revealing absence of autonomic parasympathetic ganglion cells in the colon). The rectum is small in size and does not contain stool.

Treatment involves surgical removal of the aganglionic bowel and sometime creation of a temporary colostomy. Enterocolitis may occur after surgery. Treatment may include total parenteral nutrition and a lactose-free diet.

Biliary Atresia

Biliary atresia occurs with pathological closure or absence of the hepatic or common bile ducts leading to cholestasis, fibrosis, and cirrhosis. It is the most common cause of liver disease leading to the need for liver transplant. Initially the newborn is asymptomatic, then bilirubin levels increase, abdominal distention, hepatomegaly, and splenomegaly develop. The infant bruises easily and has prolonged bleeding times. Stools are white, malodorous, and puttylike due to the presence of fat in the stool (steatorrhea). Maldigestion of fat leads to malbsorption of fat soluble vitamins (A, D, E, and K). Urine is bile or tea-colored. Without treatment, nutritional deficiencies lead to death.

Laboratory findings show elevated bilirubin levels, elevated serum aminotransferase and alkaline phosphatase, prolonged prothrombin time, and increased ammonia levels. Nursing care involves emotional support for and explanations to parents. As the disease progresses the child is irritable due to build up of toxins and intense itching of skin. Tepid baths with gentle patting to dry skin may help relieve the itching. Post transplant care involves immunosuppressant medications and close monitoring for vascular complications.

Hyperbilirubinemia

Jaundice (yellowing of skin) is the most common finding in the newborn. It develops due to deposits of yellow pigment bilirubin in the tissues. Normally the placenta clears fetal uncon-jugated bilirubin (indirect) in utero unless an abnormal hemolytic anemia occurs. After birth the infant's liver must conjugate bilirubin (convert lipid-soluble pigment into water-soluble pigment). Half of all newborn and about 80 percent of preterm infants develop physiologic jaundice within 24 hours after birth. Unconjugated bilirubin levels in cord blood is approxi-mately 2 mg/dl at birth. Between days 3–4 after birth the level rises to 5–6 mg/dl and then begins to decease until it is not visible after 10 days.

Should bilirubin continue to increase then hyperbilirubinemia rises, crossing the blood-brain barrier and damaging brain cells. This kernicterus or bilirubin encephalopathy causes permanent neurologic damage if left untreated. The classic case of hyperbilirubinemia is most commonly found with Rh and ABO blood group incompatibility but can be treated successfully with phototherapy and exchange transfusions. Early discharge and discharge before the mother's milk comes in leads to dehydration and hyperbilirubinemia.

Newborns of women with type O blood or Rh negative blood should be carefully assessed for jaundice and serum bilirubin levels checked. Serum bilirubin levels rising more than 0.2 mg/dl/hour or 5 mg/dl/day are cause for concern. A positive Coomb's test determines whether jaundice is due to Rh or ABO incompatability. Infant's with a positive direct Coomb's test are at increased risk for jaundice.

No matter the cause of hyperbilirubinemia, the management is directed toward relieving the anemia, removing maternal antibodies and sensitizing erythrocytes, increasing serum albu-min levels, reducing serum bilirubin levels, and minimizing the consequences of elevated bilirubin levels. Hemolytic disease may be treated with phototherapy, exchange transfusion, and drug therapy. Suspect hemolytic disease in the placenta is enlarged. Loose stools and increased urine output occur during phototherapy from increased bilirubin excretion.

Erythroblastosis fetalis occurs when an Rh negative mother is pregnant with an Rh positive child and the maternal antibodies cross the placenta. Because of the use of immune globulin (RhoGAM), the incidence is decreasing.

Hydrops fetalis is the most severe form of erythroblastosis fetalis. This occurs when mater-nal antibodies attach to the Rh site and destroy fetal red blood cells. Severe anemia, cardio-megaly, hepasplenomegaly, and multiorgan failure result.

The Renal System

10

The renal portion of the critical care nursing certification exam is approximately five percent of the total number of questions. The renal system can be described as a complex filtering system which serves a variety of functions within the human body to assist in homeostasis. The primary organs of the renal system are the kidneys. In addition to these organs, there is a system serving as the collective mechanism for urine, which is the byproduct of the filtration of the blood. The ureters, urinary bladder and urethra are the components of the urinary collection system. The homeostatic functions include maintaining fluid and electrolyte balance, removal of metabolic wastes, regulation of blood pressure, acid-base balance, and synthesis of red blood vessels. The purpose of this chapter is to review renal anatomy and physiology, normal renal function, and conditions which impact renal function such as acute and chronic renal failure, acute tubular necrosis, renal trauma, and electrolyte disturbances, and to describe nursing implications of these conditions and the nursing interventions which should be implemented to improve patient outcomes in the critically ill patient. A clear understanding of the basic anatomy and physiology of the renal system is necessary to apply more advanced concepts in the critically ill patient with renal disorders.

ANATOMY OF THE RENAL SYSTEM

There are two terms to describe the anatomy within the renal system and specifically the kidneys: **macroscopic** and **microscopic**. The macroscopic anatomy is that which can be visualized by inspection with the naked eye, while microscopic is that which requires specialized equipment such as a microscope.

Macroscopic Anatomy

The kidneys are two matching organs which are similar in shape to a bean which is flattened on one side. The typical size of a normal kidney is 4" in length, 2 to 2½" in breadth, and 1" in thickness. The weight of a kidney is an adult male is 4½ to 6 ounces and 4 to 5½ ounces in an adult female. The location of the kidneys within the abdominal cavity is retroperitoneal, one on each side of the vertebral column at approximately the 12th thoracic vertebrae at the upper edge and the 3rd lumbar vertebrae at the lower edge. Typically, the right kidney is slightly lower than the left due to the liver encumbrances. The location is significant in cases of renal trauma, as it is often determines the most predominate type of traumatic injury.

The shaping of the kidneys along the external border is convex and directed outward and upward, while along the internal border is concave, directed forward and slightly downward. Superiorly, the kidneys are directed inward and upward and can be described in this area as thick and rounded. Inferiorly they are directed outward and downward and in this area are smaller and thinner. As the microscopic anatomy is described, the differences in shaping will be explained through the description of the functional units within the kidneys. The kidneys are protected by the skeletal structures of the rib cage anteriorly and posteriorly. Fibrous tissues in the renal fascia form a smooth covering to protect the organs.

Within the kidneys there are two distinct layers of anatomical structures, specifically, the **cortex** and the **medulla**. The *cortex* is the outermost portion and contains the microscopic anatomical structures of the glomeruli, proximal tubules, cortical portions of the loops of Henle, distal tubules, and the cortical collecting ducts. The *medulla* is the innermost portion and contains the medullary portions of the loops of Henle and collecting ducts. Visually, the appearance of the medulla of the kidneys is one of multiple pyramids (approximately 6–10) which are formed by the collecting ducts. These pyramids taper to join together and form the *minor calyx*, which in turn join together to form the *major calyx*. The renal pelvis is formed by the funneling of the major calyx and function to direct urine into the ureters. The capacity of the collecting system is only 5 to 10 millimeters and, therefore, functionally is primarily one of a conduit or channel to drain urine.

Microscopic Anatomy

The functional microscopic anatomical structure within the kidney is the **nephron**. There are an estimated one million nephrons within each kidney. Structurally, there are both cortical and juxtamedullary nephrons whose function is based on their location within the kidneys. Nephrons in the cortex make up approximately 85 percent of the total nephrons. The components of the *nephron* are the glomerulus, afferent and efferent arterioles, Bowman's capsule, proximal and distal tubules, collecting ducts, and loops of Henle. The kidneys will continue to function even with destruction of thousands of nephrons from diseases or other conditions which cause damage.

The **glomerulus** serves as the first structure within the nephron and functions as a high pressure capillary bed to filter the blood. The *afferent arteriole* brings blood to the glomerulus at a higher pressure than the exiting *efferent arteriole*. This variation in gradient allows for *filtration* to occur. Within the glomerulus is the basement membrane, which is semipermeable and does not allow larger particles such as albumin, protein, or red blood cells

FIGURE 10.1 *Microscopic Anatomy of the Nephron*

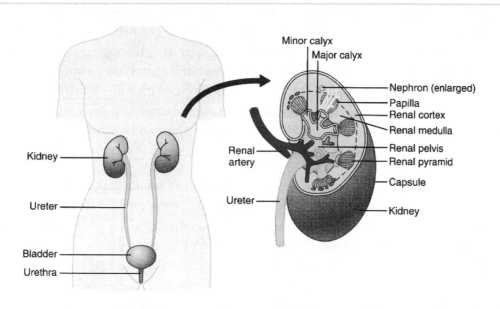

to enter the filtrate. If these are seen in the filtrate, there is likely damage to the membrane. Other factors which impact the filtration of molecules include electrical charge, protein binding, and molecular shape.

The glomerulus is surrounded by a membranous layer of epitheal cells which is called **Bowman's capsule**. This capsule serves as a holding space for the filtrate until it moves into the proximal convoluted tubule.

The **proximal tubule** is the initial component of the tubular system which also includes the loop of Henle, distal tubule, and collecting tubule. The main purpose of the tubular system is reabsorption of the key solutes such as glucose, amino acids, and bicarbonate. Additionally, water and electrolytes including potassium, sodium and calcium are reabsorbed after being filtered by the glomerulus. Osmolality of the filtrate is adjusted by the proximal tubules through the process of reabsorption of solutes. The hyperosmolar filtrate becomes isoosmotic upon exiting the proximal tubule. The kidneys filter nearly 200 liters of fluid in a 24-hour period. It is recognized that this amount of filtrate, if excreted and not reabsorbed in its majority, would completely deplete the body of all water and electrolytes. The nephrons have the primary purpose of separating that which must be conserved and that which must be excreted.

The **loop of Henle** has three segments named for their position in the loop. These are the *thin descending loop*, the *thin ascending loop*, and the *thick ascending loop*. The cortical and juxtamedullary nephrons vary in the length of the loops of Henle within their structure. Shorter nephrons are located in the cortical nephrons and have excretion and regulatory functions. The longer nephrons located in the juxtamedullary nephrons serve to concentrate and dilute the urine. The permeability within these loops is what determines whether water or solutes such as urea, sodium, potassium, and calcium are reabsorbed and at what point. The thinner descending loop is more permeable to water and, therefore, urea and sodium are not reabsorbed there. This causes the isoosmotic filtrate to become hyperosmotic as it moves into the thin ascending and thick ascending loops. Within the ascending loop, the filtrate becomes more dilute. The membrane of the thick ascending loop is impermeable to water, thus the reabsorption of electrolytes such as potassium, sodium, calcium, and bircarbonate occurs. This causes the filtrate to become hypoosmotic.

The next entry point for the filtrate is the **distal convoluted tubule** at the cortex of the kidney. At the termination of the thick descending limbs of the loop of Henle is found the specialized cells called the **macula densa cells**. These cells are a component of the **juxtamedullary apparatus** and serve to assist in regulation of blood pressure. Sodium, potassium, and chloride are reabsorbed in the first section of the distal tubule, while this section is impermeable to water and urea. The later section regulates all these solutes based on hormonal, acid-base, and electrolyte balance. The late distal tubule reabsorbs sodium and water, and excretes potassium. ADH (antidiuretic hormone) assists in the regulation of water and solutes in the late distal tubule which changes the osmolality of the filtrate.

The final section of the nephron is the **collecting tubule**. These tubules are located initially in the cortex and extend through the medulla and empty into the papilla. Predominantly the function of the collecting tubules is to transport sodium, potassium, hydrogen and bicarbonate and acidification of the urine. This is done by specialized cells called *principle and intercalated cells*. ADH and aldosterone also play a critical part in water reabsorption and the dilution/concentration of urine and produce compensatory vasoconstriction in the nonessential vasculature and conservation of sodium and water within the distal convoluted tubule.

Renal Vasculature

Despite their size, the kidneys receive approximately 20 to 25 percent of the resting cardiac output. These organs are the only ones within the human body which have an arteriole-capillary-arteriole blood flow system at the microscopic level. Additionally, another distinguishing factor regarding the renal vasculature is that there are *two capillary beds*, the glomerular and the peritubular capillary beds, separated by an efferent arteriole. The capillary bed itself is more porous and creates a size and charge barrier to prevent larger molecules such as albumin to pass which is unlike systemic capillaries.

The renal vasculature begins as the renal artery branches off the aorta and enters the kidney near the hilar region. This artery begins to branch into three smaller vessels—**interlobar, arcuate, interlobular**—which provide circulation to the renal cortex and medulla.

FIGURE 10.2 *Renal Vasculature and Microcirculation*

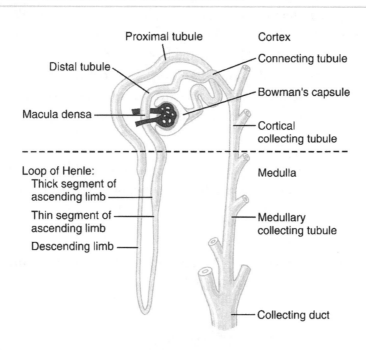

The afferent arterioles emerge from the interlobular arteries which extend from the renal artery to the cortex. These arterioles form the capillary bed of the glomerulus. The efferent arterioles serve as the exit system for the blood flow from the glomerular capillary bed. As above, this is different from other organs vasculature where there is an arteriole-capillary-venule system. The arteriole-capillary-arteriole structure allows for the maintenance of intercapillary pressure regulation which allows movement of the fluid out of the capillary bed. The efferent arterioles form the second capillary bed which is called the peritubular capillaries.

The kidneys have the ability to regulate *hydrostatic pressure* within the capillary system by adjusting the resistance of the afferent and efferent arterioles, and in turn, changing the rates of filtration, reabsorption, or both to provide homeostasis in the body.

PHYSIOLOGY OF THE RENAL SYSTEM

Glomerular Filtration, Reabsorption, Secretion and Excretion

One of the key functions of the renal system is called glomerular filtration. This process is essentially the formation of urine. The rate of filtration of the kidneys is affected by many factors within the human body such as changes in blood pressure, tone of the arteriole system, dehydration, and obstructions of the drainage of urine. As a rule most adults filter approximately 180 liters/day or 125 milliliters (ml)/min. From this filtrate, urine is formed and excreted at rate of 1–2 liters/day, or 40–80 ml/hour. Oliguria is defined as urine output less than 400 ml./day. Normally, the filtrate will have a specific gravity of 1.010 and be protein-free and plasma-like in characteristics. Abnormally, if there are deficiencies in the permeability of the membranes within the filtering system, the filtrate will have protein, electrolytes, or glucose, which may change the specific gravity and the concentration of urine.

The process of filtration occurs due to a change in hydrostatic pressure within the glomerulus and the colloid osmotic pressure (oncotic pressure of the plasma proteins in the blood supply).

FIGURE 10.3 *Fundamentals of Pressure Variations and 1) Excretion 2) Filtration 3) Reabsorption and 4) Secretion*

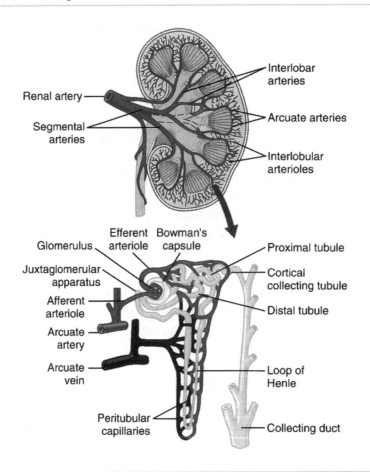

Typically the hydrostatic pressure within the glomerulus is higher than the osmotic colloid pressure and the Bowman's capsule pressure which creates a *pressure gradient* favoring filtration. The glomerular filtration rate (GFR) is used to clinically assess the patient's renal function in addition to the blood urea nitrogen (BUN) and creatinine (Cr) levels. The formula for calculation of GFR and creatinine clearance is as follows:

$$\textbf{GFR} = (Ux \times V)/Px$$

where:

x = substance freely filtered through the glomerulus and not secreted or reabsorbed by the tubules

P = plasma concentration of x

V = urine flow rate in ml/min

U = urine concentration of x

As above, the normal estimated GFR in an adult is 180 liters/day.

$$\textbf{Creatinine clearance (ml/min) for adult male [CrCl]} = \frac{(140\text{-age}) \times \text{actual weight in kg}}{72 \times \text{serum creatinine (mg/dL)}}$$

For women the estimated **CrCl** above is multiplied by 0.85. Normal **CrCl** is 90–140 ml/min for men and 80–125 ml/min for women.

The significance of both of these figures is in the effectiveness of the renal system with regard to filtration, reabsorption, secretion, and excretion. Initially blood enters the glomerulus at a pressure of approximately 50 mm/Hg. The tissue pressure or pressure within the capillary bed is lower at –10 mm/Hg while the plasma oncotic pressure is also lower at –25 mm/Hg.

The glomerular capillary membrane filters several hundred times as much water and solutes than a normal body capillary membrane and is still able to prevent larger molecules such as proteins from filtration. This property is based on the permeability and thickness of the basement membrane. The basement membrane of the glomerulus also is *negatively charged* which prevents large negatively charged molecules from being filtered. Without this barrier some proteins such as albumin would be able to pass through the membrane.

The resultant filtrate is stored in the Bowman's capsule temporarily until the process of reabsorption takes place by the tubular system within the nephrons of the kidneys. This process takes the 180 liters of filtrate and reabsorbs the necessary solutes and water back into the blood supply by the peritubular capillaries. The reabsorption takes place through both *passive* and *active* transport of water and solutes.

FIGURE 10.4 *Filtration by the Glomerular Capillaries*

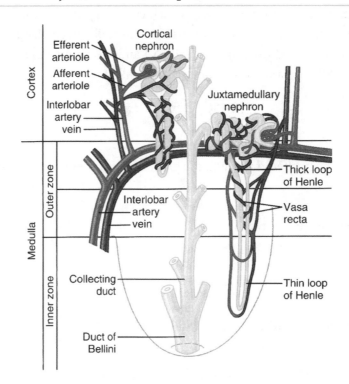

Passive/Active Transport, Diffusion, and Osmosis

Passive transport occurs through the pressure gradient created by the hydrostatic pressure and changes in solute concentrations. Passive transport, as the name implies, does not require active energy to support. The two primary processes which occur in passive transport are diffusion and osmosis. **Diffusion** is defined as the spontaneous movement of molecules across a *semi-permeable membrane* from higher concentrations of the compound to lower concentrations of the compound. Reabsorption of water from the filtrate produces a higher concentration on the tubular side resulting in a movement of molecules. One example of this is as water is reabsorbed by the tubules, the concentration within the tubules increases. As a result molecules such as urea will move from the tubules to the plasma to balance the concentrations.

Osmosis is the other form of *passive transport* and involves the movement of water from an area of lower solute concentration to higher solute concentration. Alternatively, it can be described as the diffusion of water. The most common solute which changes the balance of concentration is sodium. If the concentration of sodium within the tubular system is higher, then water will move from the capillary bed to the tubules to balance the concentrations.

Active transport is as its name implies, and requires energy to help move substances such as glucose, amino acids, calcium, phosphate, potassium and sodium across the semi-permeable tubular membrane. Adenosine triphosphate (ATP) is the source of energy for this process. The reabsorption is achieved by the use of transport molecules in the tubular membrane of the nephron that are designed to move these molecules from the tubules to the capillaries and, finally, back to the venous circulation. There are specific thresholds for these carriers which can prevent the molecules from being reabsorbed and subsequently excreted in the urine or causing a change in metabolic state, e.g., with bicarbonate causing a metabolic acidosis or glucose causing a glycosuria. Because there is a high degree of energy required in this transport, the process is very susceptible to hypovolemia and low perfusion states as well.

Secretion and Excretion

Another function of the kidneys is the **secretion** of substances from the peritubular capillaries to the tubules. This is referred to as *counter transport* and involves the exchange of substances across the membranes either through passive or active transport. Typically, these are regulated by the needs of the body such as hyper- or hypo-kalemia states. Drugs may also be secreted in this fashion.

Excretion refers to the elimination of wastes within the renal system. There is a selective filtration from the circulation system by the kidneys of substances such as urea and creatinine which are byproducts of protein metabolism. Other substances which are excreted from the body via the renal system include drug metabolism byproducts, bilirubin, and metabolic acids. These substances may significantly change the characteristics of the urine, such as color or pH. Two lab values which consistently are used to measure the performance of the renal system (filtration/reabsorption/secretion) are blood urea nitrogen (BUN) and creatinine (Cr). An increase in these values can be indicative of conditions such as a catabolic state or renal failure.

In summary, the components of the nephrons and their functions are as follows:

- **Proximal tubules:** reabsorption of sodium, chloride, bicarbonate, glucose, hydrogen, phosphates, and calcium

- **Loop of Henle:** concentration and dilution of urine

- **Distal convoluted tubule:** water reabsorption directly via ADH (vasopressin) control and indirectly via aldosterone (which causes reabsoprtion of sodium in the collecting duct)

Hormonal Regulation of Blood Pressure

When the patient's arterial blood pressure falls, the kidneys attempt to maintain circulating blood volume through the regulation of fluid balance and retention of water and alteration in the peripheral vascular resistance. This is done by the initiation of the rennin-angiotensin-aldosterone cascade.

Within the **juxtaglomerular apparatus**, where the distal tubule contact the afferent arteriole, there are specialized cells called the **macula densa**. These cells sense changes in blood flow and send messages to the arterioles to control the blood flow through constriction or dilation. Without this regulation, blood flow to the kidneys will be reduced in a low volume state. Additionally, a mean arterial pressure (MAP) less than 60 mm/hg for greater than 40 minutes can cause renal ischemia which, in turn can lead to acute tubular necrosis (ATN) or acute renal insufficiency. It is critically important to preserve renal blood flow and oxygenation to prevent nephron damage in the kidney. Therefore, if the patient's own protective mechanisms are unable to respond to these insults, the critical care RN must intervene in a timely manner to protect renal function.

FIGURE 10.5 *Renin-Angiotensin-Aldosterone Cascade*

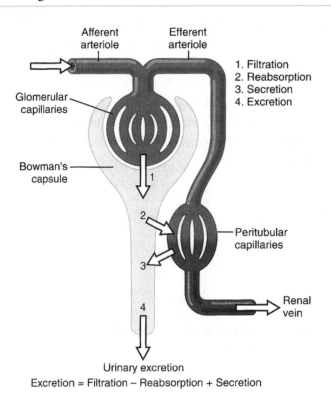

Urinary excretion
Excretion = Filtration − Reabsorption + Secretion

Electrolyte Regulation

The kidneys regulate electrolytes within the body through the filtration, reabsorption, and secretion process. Some of the electrolytes considered essential to the physiology of the body include potassium, sodium, calcium, magnesium, phosphorus, and bicarbonate. The redistribution of these electrolytes is crucial to organ function. For example, hyperkalemia can cause cardiac abnormalities including cardiac arrest if the levels are elevated. The body also requires a homeostasis of electrolytes to assure acid-base balance.

As with most electrolytes, the serum potassium value is actually only a small portion of the body's stores since most potassium in the body is located intracellular. The normal serum level of potassium is 3.5 to 5.0 mg/dL, depending on the laboratory standards of the testing lab. Despite the fact that the potassium remains primarily intracellular, changes in the extracellular serum levels can accurately predict changes which are occurring intracellularly. Additionally, since both potassium and sodium are cations, there is a constant competition both intracellularly and extracellularly to remain in balance to protect electrical neutrality at the cell membrane.

Potassium levels are maintained through both diffusion and active transport across the cell membrane. There are many factors which can influence the distribution of potassium. These may include insulin storage and use, aldosterone secretion, catecholamine secretion, acid-base abnormalities, cell destruction, strenuous exercise, and fluid osmolarity. Potassium moves out of the cell through diffusion, 65 percent of which is reabsorbed under normal conditions via active transport at the level of proximal tubule and another 25 to 30 percent at the loop of Henle. The day-to-day excretion of potassium occurs in the late distal and cortical collecting tubules, based on the body's needs for metabolism. The gastrointestinal tract does excrete a small amount of potassium in fecal material; however, the primary controller of potassium levels within the body is the kidney. Some of the functions of potassium are enzyme activity associated with protein and carbohydrate metabolism for energy production, aiding nerve impulse conduction and muscle contraction, and maintenance of intracellular osmolality.

The most abundant electrolyte within the body is sodium. It is primarily extracellular, in contrast to potassium—which is mostly intracellular. Sodium controls most of the regulation of body water which is retained or excreted by the kidneys. The other primary function of sodium is the transmission of nerve impulses via the active transport mechanism called the "sodium/potassium pump" which occurs at the cellular level. Another secondary function of sodium is the regulation of acid-base balance in the body as it combines with chloride or bicarbonate. The normal value of serum sodium is 135 to 145 mEq/L. Sodium, similar to potassium, is primarily reabsorbed by the proximal tubules and the loop of Henle. The renin-angiotensin-aldosterone system discussed earlier in the chapter explains the process of water retention and the role three organs: the kidneys (renin secretion), adrenal glands (aldosterone secretion), and the posterior pituitary gland (ADH secretion) play to effectively manage the fluid level in the body. Thirst also plays a role in maintaining a normal hydration state in the body. The thirst center is located in the anterior hypothalamus and when an individual becomes dehydrated, the neuronal cells cause the sensation of thirst.

Overall, **calcium** is the electrolyte which is most plentiful in the body, with approximately 99 percent stored in the bones. However, calcium is very important to several other functions in the body. These include maintaining the internal integrity of the cell, influencing myocardial contractility, cardiac action potential, neuromuscular activity, cell permeability, coagulation of blood, and strength of bones and teeth. The remaining one percent of calcium that serves to carry on these additional functions is located in the extracellular fluid. Mobilization of calcium normally stored in the bone, during extracellular depletion states, requires parathyroid hormone (PTH) to stimulate tubular reabsorption. Secondarily, PTH stimulates phosphate excretion which serves as an exchange for calcium. Calcium in the intravascular space is either protein bound or circulating in an ionized state. Calcium is measured in both as ionized calcium and total calcium as the data can be deceptive when the patient has elevated or decreased albumin levels. Ionized calcium may be bound to the albumin and give a false lower serum ionized calcium blood level. When albumin falls, the ionized calcium is freed and creates a rise in the serum ionized calcium level. When this occurs, calcitonin, secreted by the thyroid, will attempt to return the ionized calcium back to the bone, and yet another inaccurate reflection of the true availability of ionized calcium. The normal serum calcium level is 8.5 to 10.5 mg/dL. A change of 1 gm/dL of serum albumin will result in a serum calcium change of 0.8 mg/dL, which is the reason why all calcium measurements should be done in conjunction with serum albumin. Calcium uptake is dependent upon several factors including levels of phosphorus, magnesium and vitamin D, as well as, PTH and calcitonin in the body.

Similar to calcium and magnesium, **phosphorus** is primarily stored in the bone and with very little circulating serum levels. The normal phosphorus level is 2.5 to 4.5 mg/dL. Approximately 75 percent of the body's total phosphorus is stored in the bone. The remaining amount is located intracellular. Intake of phosphorus rich foods such as milk, poultry, fish, and red meat can significantly impact the phosphorus level in the serum. This is due to the fact that the primary absorption of phosphorus occurs in the gastrointestinal tract, but its excretion takes place in the kidney. This occurs in the distal convoluted tubules. Phosphorus functions to form ATP, which is the functional component in the production of energy for the cell. Active transport cannot occur without ATP. Additional functions of phosphorus include stabilization of the cell membrane, acid-base balance, oxygen delivery at the level of tissues, and bone strength. Within the renal filtrate phosphorus combines with other ions, sodium and hydrogen, to produce sodium diphosphate ($NaHPO_4$), then later disassociates into the individual components for reabsorption. There is a significant converse relationship between phosphorus and calcium. When one electrolyte is elevated the other is depleted and vice versa. This complex process involves several other functions including PTH secretion, vitamin D use, and reabsorption and secretion in the renal tubules. This is also an important concept when further discussion takes place regarding conditions of the renal system and symptomotology associated with them.

Magnesium is another electrolyte which is regulated by the kidney, but primarily stored in the bone and absorbed in the gastrointestinal tract. Approximately 60 percent of the magnesium in the body is stored in the bone stores, and only 1 percent is in the extracellular fluid, while the balance is in the intracellular fluid. Normal magnesium levels are 1.2 to 2.1 mEq/L. There is a competitive absorption in the gastrointestinal tract for both magnesium and calcium with the preference for whichever electrolyte is in the higher concentration there. Magnesium is critical for the functioning of the intracellular carriers that transport both sodium and potassium across the cell membrane, and therefore help to balance stores. The effect of a depleted magnesium level is a release of potassium to the extracellular fluid, in turn causing the kidneys to excrete potassium to prevent hypokalemia. The other functions of magnesium include enhancing coronary blood flow in acute myocardial infarction patients, improving ventricular function while decreasing mortality rates, transmission of CNS (central nervous system) messages, maintaining neuromuscular activity, and in the metabolism of proteins and nucleic acids.

Chloride is one of the few electrolytes which is found most commonly in combination with another cation such as sodium or potassium. If the chloride levels are below or above normal levels of 97 to 110 mEq/L, most likely this is due to an imbalance of the other cation or in acid-base balance. Because of chloride's relationship with sodium, this electrolyte plays an important role in balance of serum osmolality and water as well. The competitive nature of chloride and bicarbonate for the sodium cation, can also impact acid-base balance through excretion during acidosis and reabsorption during alkalosis. Most of us get our intake of chloride through intake of everyday table salt. Finally, chloride combines with hydrogen produced in the stomach and gastric secretions to form hydrochloric acid. Other functions of the chloride anion involve oxygenation of red blood cells by the release of hydrogen and bicarbonate from carbonic acid within the red blood cells. Hydrogen binds with the hemoglobin molecule while bicarbonate leaves the intracellular space in exchange with chloride. This movement allows carbon dioxide in the form of bicarbonate to move to the lungs for excretion.

The final solute for consideration in this section is **bicarbonate**. Bicarbonate is an anion, a negatively charged ion, as it is held in the extracellular fluid. The function of bicarbonate is primarily that of acid-base balance, although it is not the sole controller. The normal serum level of bicarbonate is 24 to 28 mEq/L. The two components which assist in the control of acid-base balance are bicarbonate and carbonic acid, and should exist in a ratio of 1 mEq/L of carbonic acid to 20 mEq/L of bicarbonate. Thus, the normal levels of carbonic acid are 1.2 to 2.4 mEq/L. Balance between these two substances is regulated by the kidney through reabsorption and excretion, based on the concentration of hydrogen ions.

The regulation of the electrolytes discussed in this section is a critical function of the kidneys. Many functions within the body, such as respiration, acid-base balance, cardiac activity, etc., are dependent upon levels of these electrolytes in both the intracellular and extracellular spaces. The other physiological functions of the kidneys will be discussed in the following sections.

Excretion of Waste Products

The major waste products excreted by the kidneys are in the form of **BUN, uric acid,** and **creatinine** (Cr). This is done through *selective filtration* of the products from the blood as it circulates through the renal vasculature. These products are primarily byproducts of protein metabolism. Other substances such as bilirubin, drug byproducts, ammonium chloride and over 200 additional metabolic waste products are eliminated from the body by the kidneys.

Urea and Creatinine

Physicians typically use these two lab measurements to do a preliminary assessment of renal function. Creatinine and BUN are byproducts of protein metabolism and are reabsorbed and excreted within the nephron. **BUN** is a byproduct of the breakdown of ammonia within the liver. The serum BUN level can be affected by other factors such as GFR, inadequate metabolism of protein such as in catabolic states, medications, and diet intake of protein. If the kidney is unable to filter adequately, BUN levels will become elevated, which may be an indication of acute tubular necrosis (ATN) or renal insufficiency. It is generally not used as a diagnostic tool in isolation, but rather in conjunction with the Cr level, the patient's overall clinical presentation, and other related values such as urine output and other electrolyte levels. An elevation in the BUN, which does not have a similar rise in the creatinine, is often indicative of other conditions such as dehydration, low renal perfusion state, or increased breakdown of protein as in a catabolic state. The normal BUN ranges from 9 to 20 mg/dL. In general, the BUN to creatinine ratio is less than 20:1. Ratio that is 20:1 or greater is indicative of a prenal acute renal insufficiency, such as dehydration or fluid loss state.

Creatinine is a byproduct of muscle metabolism. Serum creatinine can be a strong indicator of renal function. Normally, creatinine is *completely filtered* by the kidneys so an elevation in the blood can be directly related to kidney impairment. It is also directly related to GFR. Normal creatinine is 0.7 to 1.5 mg/dL.

Acid-Base Balance

A combination of regulation of hydrogen ions and maintenance of fluid balance in the body within the renal system assists in maintaining a state of homeostasis in acid-base balance. Other organs participate in this regulation of acid-base balance including the lungs and buffers within the body such as in the blood. The lungs can respond to acid-base changes in a much more rapid fashion than the kidneys. Thus, the lungs are able respond to critical or emergent situations, while the kidneys function to maintain the balance on a more day-to-day basis.

The kidneys regulate acid-base balance through the *reabsorption of bicarbonate and secretion of hydrogen.* The reabsorption of bicarbonate takes place primarily in the proximal tubule, but also occurs in the distal tubules. Secretion of hydrogen occurs passively in the proximal tubule and actively in the distal tubule. Both occur with the exchange of sodium ions. Bicarbonate is synthesized in the distal tubule by excreting hydrogen in the urine at the same time that the sodium and bicarbonate is delivered to the extracellular fluid. As above, this occurs through ionization of carbonic acid. Buffering also takes place with the combination of ammonia (NH_3^+) and phosphate (HPO_4^{-2}) before excretion without lowering the pH and the molecules are transported to the tubular filtrate and excreted in the urine.

In an acidotic state, the kidney will increase hydrogen ion secretion in the distal tubule, while all bicarbonate is reabsorbed by the proximal tubule. In akalemia the opposite occurs with decreasing hydrogen ion secretion, while bicarbonate is excreted, causing the urine to become more alkaline.

Fluid and Water Regulation

One of the most important physiological functions of the kidneys is the regulation of fluid and water to help maintain homeostasis in the body. Without this regulatory effect there could potentially be two totally diverse fluid states: fluid overload or severe dehydration.

To begin the discussion of this regulatory effect, the concept of *fluid compartmentalization* must be explained. Within the body there are two distinct compartments: the intracellular and the extracellular. Between these two compartments are membranes which serve to separate the two spaces and filter both fluids and solutes. These membranes are semi-permeable. The semi-permeable membrane has openings which allow molecules of specific sizes or weights and prevents movement of other molecules. The specificity of the membrane permeability is based on its location in the body. Within the extracellular space there are also two subcompartments: the *intravascular* and the *interstitial* compartments. About 40 percent of the patient's body weight is in the intercellular space. Five percent is in the intravascular space and the rest (15 percent) is in the extracellular spaces of the tissues (remember that 60 percent of the body weight is composed of water).

The composition of the fluids within these compartments varies slightly. Movement of the molecules must occur simultaneously with the fluids within the spaces. The *intercellular space* is primarily electrolytes such as sodium, potassium, magnesium, etc., water, and proteinate. The *extracellular space* includes organic acids, phosphates, and similar substances.

FIGURE 10.6 *Basic Renal-body Fluid Regulation Mechanism of Blood Volume, Extracellular Fluid, and Arterial Pressure*

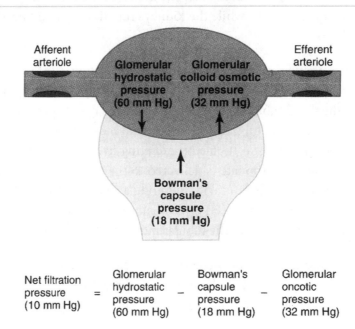

| Net filtration pressure (10 mm Hg) | = | Glomerular hydrostatic pressure (60 mm Hg) | − | Bowman's capsule pressure (18 mm Hg) | − | Glomerular oncotic pressure (32 mm Hg) |

The substances disassociate into ions either positively or negatively charged when dissolved in water. Movement of electrolytes within the nephron has been discussed earlier in the chapter. One factor that impacts fluid movement is the dissolution of these electrolytes in water and the creation of ions which are either negatively or positively charged. The electrical charges influence the movement through the semipermeable membranes and the maintenance of homeostasis.

In discussing fluid movement between these spaces, it is also important to understand the concepts of isotonic, hypertonic, and hypotonic. These terms describe the differences between concentrations of solutions on two sides of a membrane. The term "isotonic" refers to a state when the concentrations on both sides of the membrane are the same. "Hypertonic" refers to when the concentration of the solution outside the cell has a higher concentration of solutes than the solution inside the cell. Finally, "hypotonic" refers to when the concentration of the solution outside the cell has a lower concentration of solutes than the solution inside the cell The key to understanding these terms is that, in medicine, these terms refer to the solute concentration of the solution outside the cell; hence, when you have a hypertonic state, the solution outside the cell is more concentrated. These concepts are important in helping understand the movement of water between compartments. The measurement of this concentration or the number of particles in a solution is called osmolality.

In an isotonic solution, water will remain constant on both sides of the membranes because the concentrations of solutes on both sides of the membrane are equal and there is no osmotic gradient. Infusing hypertonic solutions, such as 3% saline, into the body will result in a fluid shift from inside the cells and into the extracellular space, causing a withering of the cell itself. Infusions of this nature may be of some value if the goal is getting fluid to move from the cells and into the intravascular space and bolstering blood pressure due to elevation of blood volume. Using hypotonic solutions would have the reverse effect, causing fluid to shift from the extracellular compartment to the intracellular compartment.

Using the above concepts and the fact that hydrostatic pressures force blood through the vasculature of the renal system, one can hypothesize a solute gradient is used in the process of secretion, filtration, and reabsorption in the nephron. Water movement is typically a function of the concentration of plasma proteins in the intravascular space and the solute content of both the extracellular and intracellular fluids. A decrease in plasma protein will cause the fluid to move into the interstitial space causing interstitial edema. In reverse, an increase in the plasma proteins would cause the movement of fluid from the interstitial space into the intravascular space. In hypotensive states, the body may try to preserve volume by pulling fluid from the cells into the intravascular space, though at a risk of depleting the cells of fluids which are needed for normal function.

Antidiuretic Hormone (ADH)

ADH, also known as vasopressin, is a hormone secreted by the anterior pituitary gland in response to the need to regulate the extracellular fluid balance. The secretion of ADH by the pituitary gland results in the stimulation of water reabsorption by the distal tubules and collecting ducts. The effect of this is an increase in the volume of extracellular fluid and excretion of hypertonic (cocnetrated) urine. There are stimulants for the release of ADH, one of which is physical or emotional stress. Intracellular dehydration will also stimulate the sensation of thirst, which in turn encourages the individual to drink fluids to return the body to the appropriate water balance. If the body is unable to compensate for the loss in this manner, ADH release will be stimulated by an increase in serum osmolality. As above, this causes the kidneys, specifically the distal tubules, to reabsorb water. When the serum osmolality is corrected, ADH secretion will be inhibited. ADH secretion is also inhibited during water intoxification.

FIGURE 10.7 *ADH Feedback Mechanism and Regulation of Extracellular Fluid*

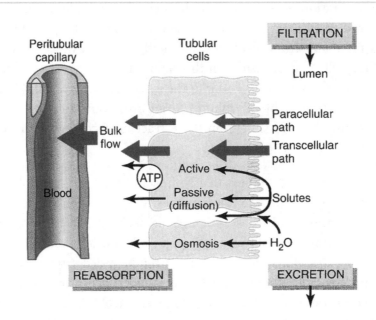

KEY COMPONENTS OF THE NURSING ASSESSMENT RELATED TO THE RENAL SYSTEM

Patient History

A complete patient history with discussion of the patient's chief complaint and reason for presentation should be done on admission. This should include onset and length of symptoms and any factors which influence the symptoms. Symptoms which may be indicative of renal dysfunction include: *dyspnea, edema, itching, dry or scaly skin, weakness, fatigue, nausea, and metallic taste in mouth.* Medication history, both prescribed and over-the-counter, is important and must include recent antibiotic therapy, contrast media that may have been administered during diagnostic procedures or non-steroidal anti-inflammatory drugs. All of these medications have the potential of causing renal dysfunction. Any recent injuries or strenuous exercise should also be investigated, as these have the potential of causing rhabdomolysis. Rhabdomolysis can be the result of muscle damage and the release of myoglobin into the bloodstream which can block structures of the kidneys. The patient should be questioned regarding any recent weight gain which may indicate water overload and potential renal dysfunction. Excessive nausea and vomiting or loss of appetite caused by changes in taste may indicate uremia. A family history is also helpful to ascertain if there are similar symptoms in relatives which may help to identify the condition. The history should be taken simultaneously while completing the physical exam in critically ill patients. Illnesses which may be of significance in the family history are hypertension, diabetes, renal diseases such as polycystic kidneys, heart failure, or headaches.

The Physical Examination

An *initial set of vital signs* should be completed in addition to an admission weight. These should be compared to the patient's normal values. *Orthostatic blood pressures* will assist in identification of dehydration and should be done if the patient can tolerate having these obtained. If possible, a central line should be inserted and will provide information to the patient's fluid status with the measurement of a central venous pressure (CVP). The CVP is indicative of the right atrial filling pressure and is a measurement of preload of the right ventricle.

The initial assessment should begin with the inspection for *signs of bleeding* such as in the flank or abdomen which may be indicative of renal trauma. The nurse should observe for *signs of volume depletion or overload* which might include poor skin turgor, swollen extremities, distended neck veins (done initially while the patient is flat, then at a 45 to 90 degree angle), peripheral vein distention, and dry oral cavity. Measurements in the degree of edema need to be consistent with 1+ indicating minimal pitting and 4+ indicating severe pitting edema. Edema should be noted to be peripheral or extended to larger areas such as the sacrum in a reclining patient.

Heart and lung sounds should be auscultated. Any cardiac murmur or arterial bruit auscultated (carotid or renal artery) may be indicative of fluid overload or stenosis. The most common murmur heard in a patient with fluid overload is the 4th heart sound (S_4). Also auscultation for a pericardial friction rub should be done. Uremia may cause pericarditis. Any extra lung sounds such as rales are probably indicative of fluid overload. The patient should be observed for *dyspnea or tachypnea*.

The physician may add to the physical assessment with the palpation of kidneys where masses or unusual shaping of the kidney would be noted. Percussion is used to detect pain or air, fluid, or solid accumulation particularly in the retroperitoneal area which could be indicative of infection or traumatic injury.

Other *hemodynamic monitoring* devices may be used to gather additional information. This may include an arterial line, pulmonary artery or SVO_2 catheter. In the majority of cases the mean arterial pressure and central venous pressure are sufficient to provide adequate information in patients with real or potential renal disorders. The pulmonary artery catheter is used if the patient has comorbidities such as cardiovascular disorders, while the SVO_2 is helpful in patients with possible sepsis. Patients in the critical care unit should always have careful intake and output monitored.

Diagnostic Testing

The two most familiar diagnostic tests done in patients with renal dysfunction are **BUN and creatinine levels**. These two serum tests when used in conjunction will give the practitioner excellent information about renal function. However, these tests are not used in isolation and other serum testing should include the standard chemistry panel with the **major electrolytes, osmolality, albumin, hemoglobin** and **hematocrit**. The calculation of the **anion gap**, which looks at the difference between measurable cations (sodium and potassium) and anions (chloride and bicarbonate) will provide information regarding acid-base balance, especially since renal failure can manifest as a metabolic acidosis.

Additional testing should include a **standard urinalysis** and if indicated, a urine culture. A random urine specimen can also be collected for a **urine osmolality**, sodium, potassium, urea, and Cr. The urinalysis will perform a screening for the presence of blood, glucose, and protein. An abnormal urinalysis for any of these components should be followed up with a repeat urinalysis and further testing as indicated. This will provide information regarding the ability of the kidneys to reabsorb solutes or if there is tubular damage resulting in hematuria.

In addition to serum testing, radiological testing should be completed to ascertain if there is mechanical, vascular, or traumatic injury to the renal system. Imaging tests which may be ordered by the physician include a flat film of the kidneys, ureters, and bladder (KUB); intravenous pyleogram; renal angiography; abdominal computerized tomography; and renal ultrasound. Advanced testing such as magnetic resonance imaging or guided renal biopsy may be indicated for complex disease states.

CONDITIONS/DISORDERS OF THE RENAL SYSTEM

Acute Kidney Injury (AKI)

Rather recently, the term acute renal failure has been replaced with the term acute kidney injury (AKI). AKI is a clinical condition which occurs in a rapid fashion and is commonly diagnosed by a decrease in glomerular filtration rate, and increase in BUN and Cr, and subsequent retention in metabolic waste products. Oliguria (less than 400 ml of urine output in a 24-hour period) is a clinical symptom which assists in the diagnosis. The mortality associated with AKI is significant, despite technological advances in critical care, particularly if not recognized early or if the patient is unresponsive to traditional treatment. The mortality rate can be as high at 85 percent. Even to the nephrologists, the pathophysiology of AKI is variable and not well understood. Dialysis remains the treatment of choice in AKI, provided that the patient meets criteria for dialysis.

Acute kidney injury can be classified into three major categories based on the clinical events which cause the condition: prerenal, intrarenal, and postrenal. However, in many cases, there may be multi-factorial causes of acute renal failure. Examples of these may be septic patients who also have a comorbidity of heart failure, patients who receive contrast media who are also on anti-inflammatory medications, and diabetic patients who suffer from obstructive renal calculi.

Prerenal conditions are those which cause reduced blood flow to the kidneys. The result of these conditions is *renal hypoperfusion and a decrease in the glomerular filtration rate.* There is a cascade of events which occur in prerenal conditions. This begins with vasoconstriction of the vasculature which supplies the critical filtering components (tubules) of the kidneys, followed by a reduced filtration of the blood, and reduced urine excretion. If treatment is initiated to counteract the hypoperfusion, such as vasopressors, increased fluid volume, or removal of nephrotoxins through dialysis, there is a strong likelihood that the condition can be reversed. Prerenal azotemia may affect as many as 70 percent of all critically ill patients. In traumatic injuries where significant muscle injury occurs, the acute elevation of the BUN and creatinine levels is due to the accumulation of fluid at the site of the muscle injury and loss of cellular membrane integrity, thus decreasing circulating fluid volume. In the septic patient, the cause of the hypoperfusion is due to the systemic inflammatory response. Examples of other causes of prerenal acute renal failure include hemorrhage, excessive diarrhea or vomiting, myocardial infarction, thrombosis of the renal artery, and anaphylactic shock.

Intrarenal conditions may be also described as intrinsic, primary, or parenchymal. Intrarenal damage is that which occurs in the nephron of the kidney either at the site of the glomeruli or in the tubules. Another name for this condition is acute tubular necrosis (ATN). This condition will be discussed at length in the following section. Approximately 25 percent of renal failure is due to an intrarenal cause. The mortality/morbidity of ATN is that 50 percent of patients die as a result of the condition, 25 percent require long term chronic dialysis due to a lack of kidney regeneration, and 25 percent recover with no long term effects. Some potential causes of intrarenal acute renal failure are malignant hypertension, acute glomerular nephritis, nephrotoxicity from heavy metals, and acute pylenephritis.

Finally, postrenal conditions are those which are due to obstruction in the urine flow in the key components beyond the kidney such as ureters or bladder. An example of this may be a renal calculi or tumor. A very small portion of patients actually show evidence of this type of renal failure. The treatment for this condition is to relieve the obstruction as quickly as possible.

In the critical care unit, it is important to manage the patient to reduce the likelihood of renal failure. It is the only truly effective remedy for AKI. In order to successfully achieve this, the patient must be constantly assessed for the risk of AKI. Care should be taken to avoid the use of nephrotoxic medications, particularly in the elderly population. Antibiotics should be evaluated for the risk/benefit to the patient, recognizing that aminoglycocides, as well as other antibiotics, pose a considerable risk of renal failure. Caution should be taken when using contrast mediums including evaluation of the creatinine clearance and pre-treatment with infusion of bicarbonate solutions to prevent kidney damage. Prevention of hypovolemia or vasoconstriction of critical renal vasculature should be undertaken early in the course of the symptoms.

Medical management of the patient in acute renal failure should focus on the following parameters: *fluid balance, electrolyte regulation, treatment of the causative factor, and promoting regeneration of functional kidney structures.* Secondarily, treatment of other symptoms such as decreased neurological function, skin conditions, and gastrointestinal disorders should also be considered important to the patient's recovery and should not be overlooked.

Fluid balance can be treated with a variety of interventions based on etiology of the AKI. Administration of fluids intravenously at a rate which will replace lost volume, as well as to maintain the perfusion to critical organs is necessary. In septic conditions, this may require large infusions of crystalloid solutions in a rapid fashion. Individual requirements may vary based on fever, blood loss, and other factors affecting perfusion. Colloids may be needed to expand intravascular volume in conditions where the mean arterial pressure, cardiac index, and/or pulmonary artery wedge pressure are low. These infusions may also be required to assist in the shift of fluid from the extracellular space to the intravascular space. Constant evaluation of hemodynamic parameters and serum electrolyte levels is necessary to judge the adequacy of the infusions. In cases where fluid administration does not significantly increase perfusion, vasopressor therapy may be required to elevate mean arterial pressure. Occasionally combination therapy of dopamine and furosemide therapy may reverse the oliguria.

In conditions where the patient is experiencing circulatory overload or interstitial edema, fluid restriction may be required. Monitoring of daily weights and accurate intake and output will provide information in regard to the fluid status.. In addition to fluid restriction, patients with intrarenal acute renal failure may require diuretic therapy (recognizing that in some cases diuretic therapy will worsen the AKI) and in advanced stages hemodialyis to acutely remove fluid, especially if there is cardiac or pulmonary compromise.

Management of electrolyte balance is also critical in the prevention of other complications which may occur as a result of AKI. **Hyperkalemia** occurs as a result of the inability of the kidney to reabsorb potassium from intravascular fluid. Clinical manifestations of hyperkalemia include EKG changes such as peaked T waves, lengthening of the QRS interval, and subsequently ventricular tachycardia. Levels may rise quickly to measurements of 6.0 mEq/L or higher. All potassium supplements are held, and if the patient is continuing to produce urine, diuretics may be ordered. If hyperkalemia requires immediate treatment, administer 100 ml of 50% glucose (D50) and 20 units of IV insulin with 1 mpule of calcium gluconate (for cardioprotection). The insulin forces the potassium out of the intravascular space and back into the intracellular space. Additionally, infusion of sodium bicarbonate (40–160 mEq) will promote excretion of potassium in the urine. Finally, oral or nasogastric tube administration of sodium polystyrene sulfonate (Kayexalate) will have an effect of binding with potassium in the bowel which would then be excreted in the stool, often administered in 15 or 30 gram doses.

Sodium imbalances may be categorized as hyponatremia or hypernatremia. Hypernatremia is essentially always the result of a free water deficit and requires adjustment in the amount of free water being administered to the patient. In contrast, hyponatremia is more complex. A full discussion of hyponatremia is beyond the discussion of the purpose of this review, but the critical care RN should understand that hyponatremia may be categorized as hypovolemic, euvolemic, or hypervolemic. Each of these categories has a different clinical treatment. Hypovolemic hyponatremia is treated with intravenous fluid administration. Euvolemic hyponatremia is treated with fluid restriction, where hypervolemic hyponatrema is treated with diuretic therapy. Hypertonic saline (three percent NS) is generally reserved for symptomatic patients with hyponatremia, but its use is decided by the treating physician.

Hypocalcemia and **hyperphosphatemia** occur in acute renal failure. Calcium and phosphorus have a converse relationship. Depletion of one causes elevation of the other in the serum, as reabsorption of calcium promotes excretion of phosphorus. The clinical manisfestations of this condition are nervous system excitement and irritability, and tetany. The treatment for hyperphosphatemia is administration of aluminum hydroxide orally or via nasogastric tube. This medication binds phosphorus in the bowel and excretion in the stool occurs. Calcium supplements such as Tums® or calcitonin can also be administered.

Diet restrictions may also be initiated with regard to protein, potassium, sodium and phosphorus. Patients need to be encouraged to take energy rich foods such as carbohydrates to promote necessary healing. Patients who are significantly malnourished may require total parenteral nutrition.

Chronic Renal Insufficiency (CRI)

Similar to acute renal failure, chronic renal failure is now referred to clinically as **chronic renal insufficiency (CRI)**. Patients may be admitted to the critical care unit with a history of CRI. This condition is the result of the progressive and primarily irreversible death of functional nephrons in the kidney. As mentioned earlier, the kidney may function normally even despite damage or loss of thousands of nephrons. One kidney may have up to a million nephrons. When there is approximately 75 percent loss of functional nephrons, the patient will have evidence of CRI and leads to end stage renal disease (ESRD). Currently, the treatment for CRI is dialysis. This can be in the form of either peritoneal dialysis or hemodialysis. Many years ago glomerularnephritis was the most common etiology behind CRI;

however, diabetes and hypertension have become the leading causes of CRI. Other causes of chronic renal insufficiency are renal vascular disorders, pyelonephritis, nephrotoxins, and congenital disorders.

Typically, the occurrence of chronic renal failure begins with an insult to the functional units of the kidneys, causing destruction of a significant number of nephrons. As a response, the remaining functional nephrons become hypertrophic and vasodilation occurs. Subsequently, the glomerular pressure and filtration increases. This is a temporary situation, as, over time, further injury to the surviving nephrons occurs. The exact cause of the additional injury, however, is hypothesized to be the constant stress of vasodilation and increased arterial blood pressure causing stenosis of the functional nephrons.

There are four stages of this progressive nephron loss: diminished renal reserve, renal insufficiency, end stage renal disease, and uremic syndrome. In the first stage the function of the kidneys is mildly reduced and the patient does not demonstrate significant symptoms of kidney failure. As the nephron loss increases, the patient develops renal insufficiency where there is evidence of impairment of the renal function and azotemia develops. The kidneys are unable to concentrate urine efficiently. At 90 percent nephron loss the patient has end stage renal disease and the patient must undergo dialysis to adequately filter water and solutes. Transplantation is considered if the patient is an appropriate candidate. The final stage is called uremic syndrome. The failure of the kidneys to function adequately causes a buildup of waste products and uremic waste.

Typically, the result of chronic renal failure is the inability of the kidney to adequately filter electrolytes and water, which causes a buildup in waste solutes and water retention. Over time without treatment the patient could show evidence of serious pulmonary consequences of increased fluid retention, such as pulmonary edema. Sodium and water is excreted in larger quantities into the intravascular space by the kidneys, causing water retention. The renin-angiotension secretion which is stimulated in response to the fluid overload causes hypertension. The BUN and Cr also rise dramatically as these products are not reabsorbed adequately by the viable nephrons. The effects are considered a viscous circle and continually worsen, causing a pattern of unrelenting symptoms.

Another condition that is commonly seen in patients with CRI is anemia. The cause of anemia of this type is the damaged kidney fails to excrete erythropoietin which stimulates the bone marrow to produce red blood cells. This is treated with the exogenous administration of erythropoietin.

Chronic renal failure can also lead to a condition where the bones are demineralized from the rise in phosphates in the serum caused by the decreased GFR. Phosphates bind with calcium, thus ionized calcium in the serum is decreased and the secretion of parathyroid hormone occurs. Subsequently, calcium is released from the bones. Similarly, chronic renal failure also causes a condition called osetomalacia, where the bones are literally partially absorbed and become weakened from the lack of calcium. The kidneys assist in the conversion of vitamin D along with the liver. This inability to produce active vitamin D prevents the reabsorption of calcium in the intestines and availability of calcium to the bone.

Acute Tubular Necrosis (ATN)

Acute tubular necrosis (ATN) is an acute renal disorder classified as *intrarenal* and is the most common form of this type. With as high as 75 percent of all cases being of this type, the majority of hospital acquired renal failure is ATN. Damage occurs to the renal tubular epithelium as a result of nephrotoxins or ischemic injury. If left untreated or is severe, the damage may spread to the basement membrane. Similar to those symptoms as described above in acute renal failure, the kidneys are unable to adequately concentrate urine, maintain acid-base balance, or regulate wastes.

There are many potential causes of ATN. The two types of ATN are described as **ischemic and toxic**. In situations where there is serious hypoperfusion to the kidneys, damage to the tubular cells membranes occurs, subsequently protein casts form and these, as well as, cellular debris obstruct the tubules. The *ischemia* and the obstructions further reduce flow to the kidneys and the ability of the afferent and efferent arterioles to autoregulate is seriously limited. Examples of ischemic ATN are hemorrhage, burns, sepsis, myocardial ischemia, pulmonary emboli, or obstetrical complications such as placenta previa or abruptio. The other type of ATN is *nephrotoxic*. There are drugs, bacterial endotoxins, and chemical agents which can cause damage to the renal tubular cells. In this type of ATN the basement membrane is not typically damaged and therefore can be reversed more frequently. Toxic agents which can cause this type of ATN are rhabdomyolysis, gram negative sepsis, aminoglycosides, contrast media, and street drugs.

ATN is classified into *four phases* based on the clinical course of the condition. **Initially**, the onset phase is difficult to detect as it occurs prior to cell injury. GFR is reduced due to hypoperfusion and decreased glomerular ultrafiltration pressure. This phase can last from a few hours to several days. If treatment is initiated during this phase, most likely there will be no permanent injury. The **second phase** is the oliguric/anuric phase. Oliguria most commonly occurs in ischemic ATN, whereas, nonoliguric ATN occurs in toxic exposure. This phase can last five to eight days in the patient with anuria and 10 to 16 days in the oliguric patient. Mortality can increase and be as high as 66 percent with oliguric ATN. **The third phase** is the diuretic phase where the patient has polyuria with urine outputs up to 4 L/day. In this stage, tubular function returns slowly and reabsorption by the kidney may not increase as quickly as the GFR. Fluid volume must be monitored closely to prevent hypovolemia. The **final stage** of ATN is the recovery phase. During this stage tubular function slowly returns to a normalized state. The period of recovery may be up to two years. In some instances, approximately 5 percent of cases of ATN, the patient may continue to require long term hemodialysis, while 33 percent will be left with renal insufficiency.

Renal Trauma

Traumatic renal injury is a result of the combination of force of both a penetrating or blunt injury and the pressure generated within the fluid-filled kidney as a result of that injury. The greatest majority (85 percent) of renal injury is blunt, while only about 10 to 20 percent is penetrating. The four main types of renal injury are contusions, lacerations, fractures of the parenchyma, and vascular injuries such as arterial tears. Contusions account for approximately 85 percent of non-penetrating renal injury. Motor vehicle accidents (MVA) are common causes of renal trauma, as are sports injuries and assaults. Penetrating trauma from gunshot, stabbing, or industrial accidents is associated with a high incidence of intra-peritoneal hemorrhage primarily from laceration of a vessel or the tearing of an artery. The physical exam is critical to the discovery and diagnosis of renal trauma. Some injuries are more evident than others, but due to the location of the kidneys, the diagnosis can be more difficult. The retroperitoneal space can hold a significant amount of undetected blood. Immediate diagnostic imaging is necessary such as CT scan, intravenous pyleogram, renal arteriogram, and general films of the ribs, kidneys, ureters, and bladder (KUB). The CT scan is the most commonly ordered diagnostic radiology exam. The patient may be admitted to the critical care unit for observation and monitoring, however, emergency surgical intervention is required in about 20 percent of the patients to stop hemorrhage and repair the injury. The other 80 to 85 perent of the patients will be treated with close monitoring and observation for complications which may rise as a result of the initial trauma.

Critical Electrolyte Imbalances

Hyperkalemia

Elevated potassium levels above 5.5 mEq/L is one of the most significant electrolyte imbalances, due to the effects on the myocardium. Acute and chronic renal failure is the primary cause of hyperkalemia due to the nephron's inability to excrete the potassium ion. Decreased renal perfusion can also reduce the excretion of potassium due to the limited availability of sodium for exchange. Other causes of hyperkalemia include acute cellular destruction and potassium release due to burns, trauma, acidosis, rhabdomyolysis, etc.; adrenal cortical insufficiency; and excessive intake or infusion of potassium chloride.

It is imperative that the critical care nurse monitor the potential cardiac effects of hyperkalemia, including continuous cardiac monitoring of QRS width, ST segment changes, and PR intervals. Asystole may be the result of a significantly elevated potassium level and the ability to resuscitate a patient with this condition is extremely difficult. Obtaining the patient's medical history relating to electrolyte imbalance including medical conditions and medication history is necessary to ascertain the potential cause of the hyperkalemia.

Treatment of this condition is the administration of IV glucose (one ampule of D50), insulin, and bicarbonate to force the movement of potassium back into the intracellular space for excretion by the kidneys. Kayexalate and sorbitol administration by oral or rectal routes should be done to more permanently remove the potassium via binding from the gastrointestinal tract. Administration of IV calcium chloride or gluconate to improve cardiac contractility is also indicated unless contraindicated in patients who take digoxin.

Hypokalemia

One of the most common causes of hypokalemia is the continued symptom of prolonged vomiting and/or diarrhea where the intake of potassium is considerably lower than the output. Other conditions which may cause hypokalemia include diuretic therapy without adequate potassium replacement, renal tubular acidosis, liver disease, and alkalosis.

Clinical manifestations of hypokalemia include weakness, muscular tenderness, respiratory changes, and EKG changes. In potassium levels below 3.5 mEq/L, the patient may experience depressed ST segments, flattened T waves, presence of a "U" wave, and ventricular dysrhythmias such as PVC's, PAC's, PAT, and AV blocks.

The treatment for hypokalemia is the administration of either IV or oral potassium supplements. For intravenous potassium in severe cases of hypokalemia, it is recommended that the patient have central venous access and administration be done over several hours. During this time it is important for the critical care nurse to monitor to assure that the patient does not develop hyperkalemia due to overcorrection.

Hypernatremia

Patients who show evidence of water retention and increased extracellular fluid volume will develop hypernatremia due to the inability to excrete sodium. In patients with normal renal function this condition is most likely due to a lack of ADH secretion or neurohypophyseal insufficiency such as in diabetes insipidus. For patients who do not have normal renal function, the cause is typically due to the inability of the renal tubules to respond to ADH secretion. The patient with hypernatremia will present with excessive weight gain, potential shortness of breath due to fluid overload, lethargy, muscle weakness, decreased urine output, and thirst.

METHODS OF DIALYSIS

There are three methods of dialysis, two of which have been used for many years, and one which has been recently developed.

Hemodialysis

Hemodialysis requires vascular access which can either been done as an acute intervention or through insertion of long term chronic intervention. In the critical care unit, most often the vascular access is inserted on an emergent basis by a physician who is trained in inserting central lines. Common sites for these line insertions are the internal jugular, subclavian, or femoral veins. The catheter used is a dual lumen catheter with a venous port (blue) for pulling blood flow and an arterial port (red) for returning the filtered blood.

More chronic or long term access can be obtained through a variety of *fistulas or grafts*. With these devices both the venous and arterial vasculature is accessed on a more permanent basis. The types are arteriovenous fistula, arteriovenous grafts, and arteriovenous shunts. An arteriovenous fistula grafts an artery with a vein such as the radial artery with the cephalic vein by creating an opening in both and anastomosing the two together. In an arteriovenous graft a tube is surgically implanted in the limb and tunneled in both the artery and the vein. Finally, the arteriovenous shunt requires a cutdown to be performed on both the artery and the vein, and a device is inserted in each and run through the skin externally between the two. Blood flows through the device via a T-connector where the dialysis connection occurs. This last device is not currently an access of choice due to frequency of complications such as thrombosis, infection, and skin erosion due the external device.

The treatment of hemodialysis works very similarly to the normal functional kidney. It takes the patient's blood and filters water, electrolytes, and toxins using the principles of osmosis, diffusion, and convection/ultrafiltration. A hollow fiber tube with seimpermeable membranes, called an extracorpeal dialyzer, is used to separate these components from the blood. A solution known as dialysate bathes the membranes and performs exchange of the blood and the bath through osmosis and diffusion to pull fluid, electrolytes, and toxins from the blood. Because the blood circulation does not have enough pressure to move the blood through the filtration device, a pump is used to provide a consistent flow of blood to the dialyzer.

Typically, this treatment takes three to four hours and in acute renal failure is performed daily, often at the bedside of the critical care patient. The dialysis patient must receive regional heparinization to prevent clotting of blood before it enters the dialyzer and while it is outside the body. The patient must be closely monitored for hemodynamic stability during the treatment. Inadvertent disconnect during the treatment can cause severe blood loss, so the patient must be maintained on a 1:1 observation by the dialysis nurse.

FIGURE 10.8 *Principles of Hemodialysis*

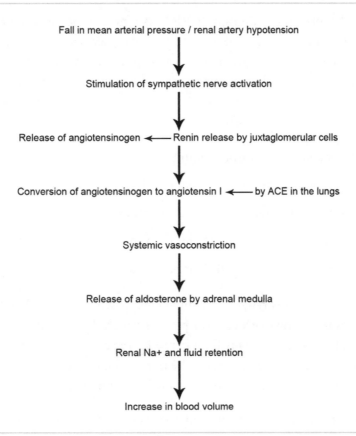

Fall in mean arterial pressure / renal artery hypotension

↓

Stimulation of sympathetic nerve activation

↓

Release of angiotensinogen ← Renin release by juxtaglomerular cells

↓

Conversion of angiotensinogen to angiotensin I ← by ACE in the lungs

↓

Systemic vasoconstriction

↓

Release of aldosterone by adrenal medulla

↓

Renal Na+ and fluid retention

↓

Increase in blood volume

Peritoneal dialysis

Peritoneal dialysis is done through an abdominal catheter that is placed surgically through the abdominal wall into the peritoneal space. The catheter has multiple holes at the end, which allow rapid infusion of dialysate into the abdominal wall. The peritoneal membrane, which covers the abdominal organs and overlies the capillary beds supporting the organs, serves as the filtering device. Under aseptic conditions, dialysate solution in infused into the abdominal cavity and left to dwell for a specific period of time. During this time, electrolytes and water are exchanged through the peritoneal membrane and filtered. After the dwelling time, the solution is drained from the abdomen. Recent abdominal surgery or past surgical interventions with history of adhesions or scarring are contraindications for peritoneal dialysis. Peritoneal dialysis is used for chronic renal failure and can be done in the patient's home after proper training. It can also be used for patients who are unable to tolerate hemodialysis due to hemodynamic instability.

Continuous Renal Replacement Therapy (CRRT)

Continuous renal replacement therapy (CRRT) is a new trend in acute care dialysis and requires specialized training, but can be done by the critical care nurse. CRRT mimics the functioning renal nephron in regulation of water, electrolytes and other solutes. The process is as the name implies a continuous treatment which occurs over the 24 hour period, and at a rate which is slower than the hemodialysis machine. Following are the five types of CRRT:

SCUF	Slow continuous ultrafiltration
CAVH	Continuous arteriovenous hemofiltration
CAVHD	Continuous arteriovenous hemodialysis
CVVH	Continuous venovenous hemofiltration
CVVHD	Continuous venovenous hemodialysis

The indications for using this type of system versus the conventional hemodialysis is multifold and includes the following: 1) slower process which the patient who is hemodynamically unstable can tolerate more easily than hemodialyis, 2) does not require the renal nurse to manage the system, and 3) cytokines can be removed more readily with high-permeability membranes. All of these therapies use a specialized hemofilter.

SCUF is used for the large amounts of fluid removal to achieve fluid balance. No dialysate or replacement fluids are used with this therapy if electrolytes or solutes are filtered. Patients who have been unresponsive to diuretic therapy may benefit from fluid removal using this treatment, particularly if there is pulmonary compromise due to the fluid overload.

CAVH uses an arterial access and an ultrafiltration pump to create a pressure where convection and ultrafiltration can be used to remove water and waste products. Physiological replacement fluids are used to replace the majority of ultrafiltrate extracted during this therapy since the focus on this therapy is removal of solutes. This is usually done pre-filter or post-dilution. The rate of exchange in either SCUF or CAVH is dependent on the membrane area, fiber diameter area, hematocrit, serum osmolality, pressure gradient, and blood flow.

Similarly, CAVHD requires an arterial access and adequate arterial hydrostatic pressure to move the blood through the filtering device. It is different than CAVH as dialysate solution is infused via a volumetric pump into the dialysis filter countercurrent to the blood flow to remove solutes and fluid. Blood is returned to the patient through a venous catheter after flowing through the hemofilter. The use of replacement fluid is optional as the purpose is to primarily remove waste or solutes.

In both CVVH and CVVHD, as the name implies, there does not need to be an arterial access. However, a roller pump is needed, as the venous circulation does not create the force necessary to create the flow through the system. In CVVHD dialysate solution is infused countercurrent into the hemofilter to increase filtration of both fluids and solutes. In CVVH the dialysate is infused into the blood. Prefilter replacement fluid may also be infused in either treatment.

SPECIAL CONSIDERATIONS FOR THE CRITICALLY ILL PATIENT WITH RENAL SYSTEM DISORDERS

The critical care nurse is responsible for the ongoing monitoring and intervention of all patients under her care. The patient with renal disorders poses some additional challenges with regard to fluid balance and electrolyte disturbances due to inefficient functioning of the filtering system of the kidneys. Nursing diagnosis which would apply to these conditions include fluid volume excess related to renal dysfunction, fluid volume deficit related to absolute loss, anxiety related to the fear of long term dialysis therapy and life-style changes, knowledge deficit due to new diagnoses, and potential for infection related to venous or arterial access devices.

During the initial admission history and physical assessment of the critically ill patient with a real or potential renal disorder, it is imperative to get a clear understanding of signs and symptoms which precipitated the condition. This includes history of cardiovascular diseases such as hypertension, congestive heart failure, or artherosclerosis. Diabetics are more prone to renal disorders due to vascular alterations as well. Changes in urine output either reduced or excess, appearance of urine, or patterns of urination should be noted.

The critical care nurse should provide ongoing monitoring of hemodynamic pressures, intake and outputs, daily weights, laboratory and radiological findings, and, in cases where the patient is on CRRT, will be required to provide ongoing management of the patient on a 1:1 basis to assure stable fluid balances. The challenge with renal patients is that they may experience both hypo- and hypertension, oliguria, anuria or polyuria, and cardiac dysrthymias which are either bradycardic or tachycardic based on the condition and diagnosis. Renal patients may also have electrolyte disturbances which are hypo- or hyper- as well. This diversity in findings requires the nurse's ongoing diligence and attention to detail.

Pharmacological management of renal patients includes the following classes of drugs: diuretics, methylxanthines, antiinfectives, cardiovascular drugs, anticonvulsants, electrolytes, and analgesics. Diuretics are commonly administered to address fluid excess in attempt to reduce the likelihood of dialysis treatments, balance outputs, and to assist the kidney in excretion of filtrate. Conditions such as hyperphosphetemia may require phosphate binding drugs such as "Renagel," while an erythrocyte stimulating drug such as "Epogen" may help the bone marrow increase production of red blood cells. Antiinfectives will be ordered to prevent or treat infections which may be a result of line, urine, or lung infections. Cardiac drug classifications also include beta blockers, ACE Inhibitors/ARB, calcium channel blockers, and antidysrhythmics. These medications may be required to treat the cardiac symptoms which may arise from electrolyte disturbances or uremic conditions. Intravenous or oral electrolytes will be used to supplement hypo- states. Patients in renal failure may need to have medication dosages altered based on metabolism and site of absorption and excretion in the kidneys, particularly antibiotics.

Another important aspect of pharmacological management is related to the patient on hemodialysis. Many drugs are dialyzed during treatments and therefore should not be administered until after completion of the treatment. Patients who are on hemodialysis or CRRT will require anticoagulation and therefore should be monitored for bleeding.

Multiorgan System

11

The multiorgan portion of the CCRN exam makes up 10 percent of the total number of questions.

This chapter covers a wide variety of conditions that affect multiple organ systems. This makes these patients very complex to care for, increases their length of stay in an Intensive Care Unit, increases the morbidity and mortality rates, and increases the cost of providing care. Topics covered include *injury, septic shock, systemic inflammatory response syndrome (SIRS), multiorgan dysfunction syndrome, toxic exposure,* and *toxic ingestions and inhalations.* Clinical manifestations and collaborative care will be discussed for each topic. The purpose of this chapter is to provide specific information necessary for the critical care RN to provide care for this vast group of conditions.

MULTISYSTEM TRAUMA: ADULT

Mechanism of Injury

The three most common mechanisms of injury are blunt trauma, penetrating trauma, and burns.

- **Blunt**—the *transmission of energy causes the injury.* This is the most common type of injury. Falls, crush injuries, motor vehicle crash, assault, motorcycle crash, bicycle crash, sports injuries are examples. The forces involved are acceleration, deceleration, shearing and crushing.

- **Penetrating**—an *object causes the injury as it passes through body tissues.* Gunshot wounds, shotgun wounds, stab wounds, impalements are examples. The forces involved are velocity and mass.

- **Burns**—*heat, chemical, electrical or thermal, causes tissue injury.* Other less common mechanisms of injury include bites, stings, inhaled and ingested poisons, and toxic exposure.

Clinical Manifestation

Clinical manifestation is specific to the mechanism of injury and is different in every patient. Examples of factors that affect clinical manifestation include age, gender, pre-existing illnesses, time between injury and treatment, and substance abuse.

Resuscitation and Collaborative Care

Injured patients need an organized and rapid approach to assessing their injuries, regardless of the mechanism of injury. The American College of Surgeons Committee on Trauma recommends performing a Primary and Secondary survey on all injured patients to identify and treat all life-threatening and non-life threatening injuries. The Primary Survey includes ABCDE. During this assessment all *life threatening injuries* are identified and treated. The survey does not proceed until an identified issue is addressed (i.e., patient not breathing—intubation and ventilation).

A = Airway: does the patient have a patent airway, is subcutaneous emphysema present

B = Breathing: is the patient able to breathe effectively, what color are the mucous membranes, is there thoracic penetration or flail chest

C = Circulation: what is the patient's volume status, are there obvious long bone or pelvic fractures, stop obvious bleeding, check peripheral pulses and capillary refill, draw labs including ABGs and type and cross

D = Disability: level of consciousness, pupils, motor and verbal response assess for spinal cord injury

E = Exposure: all clothing and jewelry must be removed, assess skin temperature, cover patient after primary survey is complete

Once the primary survey is complete, i.e., all life threatening injuries have been identified and treated, the secondary survey begins. This may be delayed by a trip to the operating room, angiography suite or interventional radiology. The secondary survey is a systematic head to toe assessment to identify all injuries the patient has sustained. During the secondary survey, a patient history, injury history, and further diagnostic studies are obtained. Information may be obtained from the patient, pre-hospital providers and/or friends and family when available. During this time a definitive plan for care of the patient is formulated.

Fluid Resuscitation

Most injured patients need some degree of fluid resuscitation. The goal of fluid resuscitation is to restore adequate circulating fluid volume and oxygen delivery to the tissues. Remember that vital signs are just one piece of the puzzle. In the setting of an injured patient, urine output, capillary refill, and level of consciousness are often more sensitive indicators of the adequacy of resuscitation. Crystalloids and blood products are the resuscitation fluids of choice for injured patients. Colloids such as dextran and hetastarch do not have hemoglobin carrying capacity and research has not shown that colloids are more effective than crystalloids in resuscitating injured patients. Potential adverse effects of the above mentioned colloids include large fluid shifts, anaphylaxis, and coagulopathy.

Crystalloids

Crystalloid solutions are clear fluids made up of water glucose, and electrolytes, i.e., normal saline, lactated ringers, etc. The formula to determine the volume of crystalloid to be administered initially is three millilitres of crystalloid should be given for each millilitre of blood lost (3 ml crystalloid: 1 ml blood loss). In the setting of resuscitation, crystalloids are categorized as shown in table 11.2.

Blood and Blood Products

Transfusion of blood and blood products during resuscitation is limited to hemodynamically unstable patients who have lost blood and need volume expansion and oxygen carrying capability. In an emergency situation, when there is no time to obtain a type and cross match for blood products, type specific or O-negative blood may be administered. Replacement of coagulation factors, such as platelets or fresh frozen plasma (FFP) or

TABLE 11.1 *Parameters That Reflect Adequacy of Resuscitation*

Parameter	Normal	What it indicates
Lactate	.3 to 2.2 mmo/L	A rising lactate indicates inadequate tissue perfusion and oxygenation
Base Deficit	–2 to +3 mEq/L	An increasing base deficit (> –2), indicates decreased perfusion and oxygenation
Urine Output	30 cc/hr in an adult	Less than 30 cc/hr indicates inadequate circulating volume or kidney perfusion
Capillary Refill	< 2 seconds	Prolonged capillary refill indicates decreased perfusion to the extremities

TABLE 11.2

	Solutions	Contents	Uses	Effect	Miscellaneous
HYPOTONIC	D5W (5% Dextrose in Water)	Dextrose and free water, no electrolytes	Not used to resuscitate injured patients who are volume depleted.	Cause leakage of fluid into interstitial and intracellular spaces.	Monitor patient for fluid overload, total body edema, and hyperglycemia.
	D5 ½ NS (5% Dextrose and 0.45% Normal Saline)	Dextrose, sodium, and chloride	Commonly used as a maintenance fluid, not a resuscitation fluid.	No significant effect on intravascular volume, increases total body edema.	Monitor patient for hyperglycemia and total body edema.
	D5 ¼ NS (5% Dextrose and 0.225% Normal Saline)	Dextrose, sodium, and chloride	Commonly used as a maintenance fluid, not a resuscitation fluid.	No significant effect on intravascular volume, increases total body edema.	Monitor patient for hyperglycemia and total body edema.
ISOTONIC	NS (0.9% Normal Saline)	Sodium and chloride	Used for volume replacement in hypovolemic patients, used with blood transfusions, and used to replete low serum sodium.	No significant fluid shifts across cellular membranes or vessels.	Monitor patient's serum sodium during infusion to prevent hypernatremia. Monitor patient for fluid overload.
	LR (Lactated Ringer's)	Sodium, chloride, potassium, calcium, and lactate, similar to concentration in human plasma	Used to resuscitate volume depleted trauma and burn patients. Can also be used to replete volume lost from vomiting, dehydration or diarrhea.		Lacking the magnesium and phosphate in human plasma.
HYPERTONIC	3% Normal Saline	Saline	Used cautiously in patients due to sodium load.	Draws fluid from cells and interstitial spaces into vessels.	Monitor serum sodium, monitor for fluid overload.

cryoprecipitate should occur only in the presence of active bleeding or if interventional procedures are to be undertaken emergently. Autotransfusion is commonly used in patients with chest injuries. It is not useful in patients with abdominal injuries due to potential contamination of blood from spilled gastric contents.

- Platelets: Given if platelet count falls below 50,000

- Fresh frozen plasma: Administered if PT/INR or PTT is higher than 1.5 times control

- Cryoprecipitate: Given for Fibrinogen levels < 0.8g/l

Additional aspects of collaborative care for injured patients involve continued monitoring and treatment of deficits in oxygenation, ventilation, circulation, perfusion, mobility, skin integrity, nutrition, and pain. It is also essential to maintain patient safety at all times, assess and treat the patient and family's psychosocial status, and initiate discharge planning and teaching when it is appropriate.

Sequelae of Multisystem Trauma

The following is a list of potential complications of multisystem trauma and their causes. The nurse plays an integral part in the prevention of and early recognition of the signs and symptoms of these potentially fatal conditions.

Pressure Ulcers
Inadequate tissue perfusion, direct trauma to tissue, edema, that results from prolonged bed rest

Atelectasis/Pneumonia
Chest trauma, pain, head injury, inhalation injury, aspiration, prolonged immobility or bed rest, intubation, multiple transfusions, massive fluid resuscitation

Deep Vein Thrombosis (DVT)
Endothelial injury (traumatic or iatrogenic), venous stasis (due to hypovolemia, immobility, etc.), prolonged immobilization

Pulmonary Embolism/Fat Embolism
Fractures, head and/or spinal cord injury, hypotension, hypovolemia, shock, prolonged immobilization

Hypovolemic Shock
Massive blood loss or continued bleeding, significant dehydration for cutaneous loss in severe large surface area burns

Infection/Sepsis
"Dirty wounds," open wounds, indwelling lines and catheters, depressed immune system, advanced age, history of immunosuppression or diabetes, malnutrition, massive blood transfusion

Adult Respiratory Distress Syndrome (ARDS)

Head injuries, multiple major fractures, pulmonary contusion, massive transfusion, immunosuppression, ongoing shock, aspiration

Acute Kidney Injury (AKI, previously referred to as Acute Renal Failure)

Long periods of hypoperfusion or hypovolemia, renal trauma, vasopressors, antibiotics, contrast medium, rhabdomyalysis, transfusion reactions, pre-existing renal disease, obstruction of the renal tubular system (e.g., nephrolithiasis)

Disseminated Intravascular Coagulation (DIC)

Shock, massive transfusion or mismatched blood, sepsis, near drowning, hypothermia, venomous bites, crush injuries

Systemic Inflammatory Response Syndrome (SIRS)

Widespread inflammation including organs and systems not involved in the initial injury, increased temperature, increased WBC, increased metabolic rate

Multiple Organ Dysfunction Syndrome

Hemorrhage, massive blood transfusion, shock, sepsis, prolonged tissue hypoxia, toxic exposure

Sepsis and Septic Shock

Septic shock is one type of distributive shock that involves all organ systems. Critically ill patients are at increased risk for developing sepsis and septic shock. Technology has enabled us to prolong the life of patients who would have previously died from their initial insult. Blood urine, and sputum cultures will be positive for bacterial growth. The most commonly implicated organisms are either gram negative bacilli, such as E-coli or gram-positive cocci like methicillin-resistant Staphylococcus aureus (MRSA). The list of potential infectious agents is significantly broadened in immunocompromised and transplant patients. The emergence of antibiotic resistant bacteria has also contributed to the rising rates of sepsis and septic shock. Septic shock due to viral pathogens is uncommon in adults. Many cases of septic shock are from hospital acquired or nosocomial infections. These pathogens commonly enter the body through the pulmonary, urinary, or gastrointestinal tract. Line sepsis involves infection of an indwelling IV catheter. Generally, if "line sepsis" is being considered, the medical team will provide antibacterial coverage for gram-positive organisms with vancomycin until speciation and antibiotic sensitivities are known from the cultures sent. Central venous lines and pulmonary artery catheters necessary for care of critically ill patients are commonly implicated. To decrease a patient's risk of developing line sepsis, it is imperative to use sterile techniques during insertion of all indwelling lines. The use of antibiotic coated and impregnated catheters has been found to have little effect on reducing the rate of line sepsis. As soon as line sepsis is suspected, the line must be removed.

Clinical Manifestations

There is a continuum of infection which involves sepsis, severe sepsis, and septic shock. The clinical manifestations of the "sepsis continuum" are listed below.

Sepsis

Systemic response to infection that includes *two or more of the following:* T > 38° C or < 36° C (100.4° F or 96.8° F), HR > 90 beats per minute, RR > 20 breaths per minute, or $PaCO_2$ < 32mmHg, WBC > 12,000 cells/mm^3, or >10% bands (immature WBCs)

Severe Sepsis

All of the above with the addition of organ dysfunction and hypoperfusion. The earliest signs are change in mental status (up to 72 hours before the onset of severe sepsis) and decreasing urine output. Increasing lactic acid levels and base deficit are also present.

Septic Shock

Sepsis with *hypotension and inadequate perfusion* unaffected by adequate fluid resuscitation. These patients often are on inotropic and vasoactive agents in an attempt to augment cardiac function, making hypotension difficult to assess. Increases in lactic acid levels or base deficit and continued decreases in mental status and urine output are common. If not successfully treated, multiple organ systems will begin showing signs of dysfunction.

Collaborative Care

The priorities of care for the patient with sepsis and septic shock are *identification and treatment of the infecting pathogen.* Treatment goals are directed toward maintaining oxygenation, ventilation, circulation, perfusion, skin integrity, nutrition, and pain control. It is also important to ensure patient safety, prevent hazards of immobility, and address any psychosocial issues the patient and family might have. Clinically, the patient will be intubated and mechanically ventilated, may have a pulmonary artery catheter to monitor fluid/volume status and cardiac output, and potentially need vasoactive and/or inotropic support. Antibiotics are administered according to culture results. Broad spectrum antibiotic coverage may be initiated prior to obtaining culture results, then streamlined when the pathogens are positively identified.

Systemic Inflammatory Response Syndrome (SIRS)

A syndrome characterized by a widespread inflammatory response to an insult.

Clinical Manifestation

Two or more of the following are present; T > 38° C or < 36° C, HR > 90 beats per minute, RR greater than 20 per minute, WBC > 12,000 cells/mm^3, less than 4,000 cells/mm^3 or > 10% bands on differential. There is often no infectious pathogen identified. When SIRS is caused by documented infection, it is called sepsis.

Collaborative Care

Treatment goals are similar to that of septic shock and center around restoring adequate oxygenation and tissue perfusion. Being that no infectious source is usually identified, administration of antibiotics has no effect on SIRS, although some may consider starting empiric antibiotics if the suspicion for infection is high.

Multiorgan Dysfunction Syndrome (MODS)

At the end of the shock continuum, organs begin to fail due to continued lack of adequate oxygenation and perfusion.

- The failure of one organ causes the failure of subsequent organs. The lungs often fail first and are followed by the liver, GI tract, kidneys, hematologic system and finally the heart. Early identification and meticulous monitoring of patients at risk for developing MODS is the best way to decrease morbidity and mortality.

- The treatment of MODS is largely supportive, treatment specific to one system has been found to be ineffective, the mortality rate of MODS approaches 75 percent.

TOXIC EXPOSURE

Chemical Exposure: Nerve Agents

Nerve agents are organic chemicals (organophosphates) that disrupt the mechanism by which nerves transfer messages to organs. The disruption is caused by blocking acetylcholinesterase, an enzyme that normally relaxes the activity of acetylcholine, a neurotransmitter. Nerve agents are classified as **G Agents** (Sarin, Somon, and Tabun) or **V Agents** (VX). These agents can be absorbed either through the respiratory tract or through the skin. They are easily vaporized or aerosolized, enabling them to spread over large areas.

Clinical Manifestations

Sarin has no odor, therefore patients may not initially be aware of exposure. Soman has a fruity or camphor-like odor and Tabun has a very faint fruity odor. Being that these odors are not unusual, patients exposed to either Soman or Tabun may not initially be aware of exposure. Signs and symptoms of exposure to **G Agents** develop within seconds to hours of exposure. Patients with *minimal to moderate exposure* present with non-life threatening symptoms that include runny nose, watery eyes, small pinpoint pupils, eye pain, blurred vision, drooling, excessive sweating, cough, chest tightness, tachypnea, diarrhea, increased urine output, confusion, drowsiness, weakness, headache, nausea, vomiting, abdominal pain, tachycardia or bradycardia, and hypotension or hypertension. With *significant exposure,* signs and symptoms are life-threatening and include change in level of consciousness ending in unconsciousness and seizure, paralysis, respiratory failure and death. Patients exposed to **V Agents** display the same signs and symptoms as those exposed to G agents.

Collaborative Care

Initial care for patients exposed to both G and V agents includes *removal of all clothing and thorough decontamination.* Health care professionals involved in decontamination procedures must wear full body protection to avoid exposure to both G and V agents. Early administration of *Atropine and pralidoxime (Protopam)* within minutes of exposure has been shown to be effective and is also indicated to block acetylcholine receptors.

Blood Agents

This is a group of toxins that are carried by the blood and travel throughout the body, ultimately affecting every body system. These agents exert their effect at the cellular level, e.g., cyanide.

Clinical Manifestations

Even minimum exposure to cyanide, either by breathing, absorption via the skin, or ingestion cause *immediate signs and symptoms* including tachypnea, restlessness, dizziness, weakness, headache, nausea, vomiting, and tachycardia. After exposure to large amounts of cyanide via any of the above mentioned portals, the patient immediately develops seizures, hypotension, bradycardia and unresponsiveness. Patients who are exposed to large amounts of cyanide immediately develop acute lung injury which leads to respiratory failure and death. Patients exposed to small or moderate amounts of cyanide can survive, but may have long term cardiac and brain damage.

Collaborative Treatment

Decontamination is the initial step in treatment of patients exposed to cyanide. Health care workers involved in the decontamination must wear full body protection to avoid exposure to cyanide. All of the patient's clothing must be removed and the body thoroughly cleansed with soap and water. Pharmacologic treatment of cyanide poisoning includes the administration of amyl nitrate, IV sodium nitrate, and sodium thiosulfate.

Vesicant or Blister Agents

Exposure to vesicant or blister agents such as HD (sulfur mustard), HN (nitrogen mustard), L (Lewisite), or CX (Phosgene) may not immediately be apparent to the patient, as neither agent has an identifying odor.

Clinical Manifestations

Patients exposed to mustard gas may not develop signs and symptoms 2 to 24 hours after exposure, depending on the amount of agent the person is exposed to. Initially, the patient's skin becomes red and itchy, then it turns yellow and blisters. Within an hour of exposure, the patient may experience non-specific symptoms of skin irritation, pain, swelling and tearing. Severe exposure may produce blindness lasting up to 10 days. Respiratory signs and symptoms mimic those of a cold and include runny nose, sneezing, hoarseness, bloody nose, sinus pain, shortness of breath, and cough. Exposure to Phosgene causes immediate cutaneous pain with accompanying blanching surrounded by red rings (within 30 seconds of exposure) Hives appear within 30 minutes and after 24 hours the blanched areas turn brown, the skin dies and a scab is formed. Pain and itching continue until the wound is healed. Phosgene in the eyes causes severe eye pain and temporary blindness along with tearing. Respiratory symptoms of phosgene exposure include immediate signs of upper respiratory tract irritation, runny nose, hoarseness and sinus pain along with shortness of breath, cough, and with large exposure, pulmonary edema. Data on Lewisite exposure has been largely obtained from animal models.

Collaborative Care

Initial treatment of patients exposed to vesicant or blistering agents involves *decontamination*, including the removal of all clothing. Health care professionals involved in the decontamination effort must wear protective body suits to avoid exposure to the agents. There are *currently no antidotes* for exposure to vesicant or blistering agents and the care is largely supportive.

Pulmonary or Inhaled Agents

Chemicals that cause rapid and severe irritation to the respiratory tract include ammonia, chlorine, phosgene, ricin, and carbon monoxide.

Clinical Manifestations

The severity of signs and symptoms is directly related to the amount and duration of exposure. Immediate symptoms are manifested in three categories: muscarinic, nicotinic, and central nervous system. **Muscarinic** manifestations include bradycardia, hypotension, rhinorrhea, bronchorrhea, bronchospasm, cough, respiratory distress, increased salivation, nausea, vomiting, diarrhea, abdominal pain, urinary and fecal incontinence, blurred vision, miosis, diaphoresis, and increased lacrimation. **Nicotinic** effects include muscle fasciculations, cramping and weakness, diaphragmatic failure, hypertension, and tachycardia, mydriasis and pallor. **Central nervous system** manifestations include altered mental status, anxiety, emotional lability, restlessness, confusion, ataxia, tremors, seizures, and coma. Symptoms of **carbon monoxide poisoning** vary widely depending on the level of exposure and can include headache, dizziness, nausea, flu-like symptoms, fatigue, shortness of breath on exertion, impaired judgment, chest pain, confusion, depression, hallucinations, seizures, impaired memory, and cherry red skin.

Collaborative Care

Decontamination is the first priority of care in patients exposed to ammonia, chlorine and phosgene. All clothing must be removed and the body washed thoroughly with soap and water to limit further exposure. There is *no antidote* for ammonia, chlorine or phosgene exposure; hence treatment is symptomatic. Patients with high levels of exposure to inhaled agents may be intubated, mechanically ventilated, and admitted to an intensive care unit. The patient's condition may warrant use of hemodynamic monitoring and support of circulation with the use of vasoactive and/or inotropic agents.

Biologic Exposure

Biologic agents are categorized into two categories, A and B. **Category A** includes anthrax, botulism, plague, smallpox, tularemia, and viral hemorrhagic fevers. These agents are easily spread person to person and have a high mortality rate. **Category B** includes brucellosis and ricin. Category B agents are moderately easy to transmit person to person and cause increased morbidity, but low mortality after exposure.

Clinical Manifestations

Anthrax is a spore-forming bacteria that is not easily spread from person to person. There are three routes of exposure to anthrax, all with different manifestations. **Cutaneous exposure** is the most common (95 percent of all exposures). The spore enters the body via a cut in the skin. Within two days of exposure, a small raised itchy bump resembling an insect bit is noted; this bump evolves into a vesicle eventually becoming a painless ulcer with a black necrotic center. **Inhalation** of the spore initially presents with signs and symptoms of the common cold including malaise, sore throat, low-grade fever, and muscle aches. The symptoms quickly progress to acute respiratory failure and shock. **Gastrointestinal exposure** is generally due to eating meat contaminated with the anthrax spore. Signs and symptoms resemble acute inflammation of the gastrointestinal tract including anorexia, nausea and vomiting, blood stools and uncontrolled diarrhea.

Botulism (Clostridium botulinum) is not spread from one person to another. Exposure can be either *foodborne,* from eating meat, canned fruit jam, honey, or from a wound infected with the toxin-producing bacteria. Signs and symptoms may not be apparent for up to two weeks after exposure but most commonly appear within 12–36 hours of exposure. The botulism toxin is a *muscle-paralyzing agent.* Symptoms include double or blurred vision, drooping eyelids, slurred speech, dysphagia, dry mouth, and muscle weakness that always involves the shoulders first and progresses downward.

Plague (Yersinia pestis) is a bacteria common to rodents and their fleas. Plague can be bubonic, pneumonic, or septicemic. **Bubonic plague**, the most common, is contracted via a flea bite or thru a cut in the skin. Exposure is manifested by swollen and very tender lymph nodes accompanied by a painful swollen glands, called a *bubo,* approximately two to six days after exposure. It is not spread person to person. **Pneumonic plague** is contracted by inhaling aerosolized particles or droplets from very close contact with an infected person or animal. Signs and symptoms include headache, fever, weakness, aggressive pneumonia with shortness of breath, chest pain, and cough with watery and/or bloody sputum. Within two to four days of exposure, respiratory failure and shock develop. **Septicemic plague** is not spread person to person and is commonly a complication of the other two forms of plague but can occur on its own. The signs and symptoms are similar to bubonic and pneumonic plague without the development of buboes. Abdominal pain and internal bleeding may occur with septicemic plague.

Smallpox is caused by two viruses, variola major/minor, that has been eradicated in the United States except for laboratory stockpiles. **Variola minor** produces very mild signs and symptoms, is rare, and is much less serious. **Variola major** has four sub categories: *ordinary,* the most frequent type (90 percent of all exposures); *modified,* a mild form in previously vaccinated individuals; *flat* and *hemorrhagic,* both of which are severe and fatal. Clinical manifestations include fever (greater than or equal to 101° F), followed by a rash with firm deep seated vesicles or pustules that are all at the same stage of development. The incubation period is approximately 1 to 17 days and is not contagious during this time. Smallpox is highly contagious once the rash appears. The rash starts as small red spots in the mouth and on the tongue that spreads to the face, arms, legs, hands and feet. Within 24 hours of appearance, the mouth and tongue rash becomes pustules.

Exposure to **tularemia** or rabbit fever is most common from an infected tick bite; the bacteria is found in rodents and rabbits. Tularemia can also be transmitted from touching the dead animal or eating or drinking from infected sources. The bacteria can also be inhaled. Exposure to a small amount of bacteria can cause symptoms in approximately three to five days. Clinical manifestations include chills, enlarged groin or underarm lymph nodes, fever, headache, joint stiffness, muscle pain, red spots on the skin that enlarge over time and progress to an ulcer, shortness of breath, sweating, and weight loss and pneumonia.

Collaborative Treatment

Diagnosis of exposure to anthrax is by history. Early treatment (within seven days) to cutaneous exposure with tetracyclines, fluoroquinolones, or penicillins is usually curative. Lack of treatment carries a 20 percent mortality rate. Exposure by inhalation carries a 75 percent mortality rate, even with aggressive treatment with antibiotics, intubation, mechanical ventilation, and circulatory support. Gastrointestinal exposure has up to a 60 percent mortality rate with aggressive treatment, as mentioned above. There is currently a vaccine available for anthrax, but it is only recommended for active duty military personnel, persons working directly with anthrax spores in the laboratory, or persons who work with animals or animal hides that can potentially be infected. Vaccination of the general public is not currently recommended.

Diagnosis of exposure to **botulism** is presumptive and based on the patient's history. Treatment for presumed exposure must be initiated long before the confirmatory laboratory tests are available. These tests include culture of feces, gastric secretion, vomitus, serum, and/or wounds. Treatment includes an anti-toxin stored at the Centers for Disease Control that reduces the severity of the symptoms if given early in the post-exposure period. Persons exposed to the botulism toxin usually survive after weeks to months of supportive treatment including aggressive intensive care unit treatment with intubation, mechanical ventilation, and circulatory support.

The diagnosis of exposure to **plague** relies on the patient's history. Laboratory tests include bronchial washings and blood and tissue from the patient. *Immediate treatment with antibiotics* for patients with pneumonic plague is essential for survival. Streptomycin, gentamycin, the tetracyclines, or chloramphenicol are recommended for treatment. Intensive care unit treatment with intubation, mechanical ventilation and circulatory support are essential, as death occurs within four days without appropriate treatment. Plague has not been reported east of the Rocky Mountains in the United States.

Exposure to **smallpox** is fatal if left untreated; those who survive exposure are left with deep scars, possible blindness and arthritis. Treatment is supportive with intravenous fluid, pain medication and antipyretics. Antibiotics are given only to treat secondary infections. A vaccine is currently available but is not recommended for the general public.

Collaborative treatment for **tularemia** includes blood and sputum cultures, a thorough history of potential for exposure and treatment with antibiotics. The tetracyclines and fluoroquinolones are given orally and streptomycin or gentamycin can be given intramuscularly or intravenously. Inhaled tularemia can evolve into a life-threatening pneumonia if not treated.

Nuclear/Radiation Exposure

There are two types of radiation, *ionizing and non-ionizing.* Non-ionizing does not cause tissue damage and will not be discussed here. Ionizing radiation causes an immediate effect on human tissues. In the event of a radiation or nuclear event, everything including soil and water, at the site of the blast would be vaporized. The vapors mix with radioactive material, eventually cool and fall back to earth as dust; this is referred to as the "fallout" and can be carried over a large area. Anything the fallout lands on becomes contaminated with radiation. Injury to humans and animals can be from the blast itself or from exposure to radioactive fallout and its contaminants.

Acute Radiation Syndrome (ARS)

Acute Radiation Syndrome occurs when the *entire body is exposed to a high dose of radiation* over a short period of time. Persons at the site of nuclear blasts or accidents are most likely to develop ARS. There are four stages of ARS: the Prodromal stage, the Latent stage, the Manifest Illness stage, and the Recovery/Death stage.

Clinical Manifestations

In the **Prodromal stage** of ARS, symptoms can appear almost immediately, including nausea, vomiting and diarrhea, lasting minutes to days. In the **Latent stage,** the exposed person looks and feels healthy for the next few hours to weeks. After this brief respite from symptoms, the **Manifest Illness stage** begins and lasts hours to months. Symptoms of this stage include anorexia, fatigue, fever, nausea, vomiting, diarrhea, temporary blindness, and possibly seizures and coma. Skin manifestations range from red, itchy skin to severe burns depending on the level of exposure. The skin may also take months to heal. The final stage of ARS is the **Recovery/Death stage** which may take years to complete.

Collaborative Care

Treatment is based on the severity of exposure and the signs and symptoms the patient exhibits. Survival depends on the severity of exposure and the syndrome with which the patient presents. Survival of patients with **Bone Marrow Syndrome** decreases as the dose of radiation increases; the cause of death in this group is bone marrow destruction and hemorrhage. Patients presenting with **GI Syndrome** are not likely to survive. Death is within two weeks of exposure from irreparable changes and destruction of the GI tract and bone marrow. Patients develop infection, dehydration, and electrolyte imbalance. Patients presenting with **CV/CNS Syndrome** usually die within three days of exposure from circulatory collapse, increased intracranial pressure secondary to cerebral edema, vasculitis and meningitis. Initial care of patients with ARS includes stabilization of the ABC's, physiologic monitoring, treatment of major injuries (burns, fractures, etc.), and blood work for CBC with total lymphocyte count and HLA prior to any transfusion. Continued treatment is based on symptoms.

Toxic Ingestion

- **Lye (sodium hydroxide)** is found in cements, clinitest tablets, drain and oven cleaners and many household cleaners. Injury from ingestion is caused by the alkaline nature of the substance.

- **Anitfreeze (Ethylene glycol)** is found in antifreeze, engine coolants, and brake fluids. Ingestion is considered a medical emergency. The lethal dose is approximately 100 cc or 1.4–1.6 ml/kg but as little as 30 cc has been know to be fatal in an adult. Inhalation of ethylene glycol is unlikely. It is only mildly irritation to the mucous membranes and skin and is not absorbed thru the skin.

Clinical Manifestations

Clinical manifestations of exposure to **lye** include shortness of breath, pneumonitis, edema, burning eyes nose and mouth and lips, esophageal burns, blood vomitus and diarrhea, and necrotic skin. Symptoms may progress to severe abdominal pain, cardiovascular collapse, severe metabolic acidosis, and skin necrosis within 12 hours of ingestion.

Ethylene glycol is rapidly absorbed by the gastrointestinal tract (within one to four hours of ingestion), the main route of exposure. Ingestion leads to systemic toxicity that begins with central nervous system dysfunction. Cardiac and pulmonary failure develops within 24–72 hours. Metabolic acidosis, dehydration and renal failure requiring hemodialysis develop within this time period also.

Collaborative Care

Initial treatment is administration of activated charcoal and gastric lavage. Vomiting is not induced as the ingested chemical will burn the GI tract a second time when the patient vomits. An initial chest x-ray is obtained; the patient is kept NPO and may undergo endoscopy or esophagoscopy. Intravenous fluid is administered to enhance renal clearance. Sodium bicarbonate is given intravenously to correct acidosis with a pH of < 7.2. With ethylene glycol ingestion, intramuscular pyridoxine and thiamine are given to control symptoms of bleeding. Fomepizole (Antizol) is given intravenously with an initial loading dose, followed by twice daily doses. Intubation, mechanical ventilation, cardiovascular support and fluid resuscitation are necessary with large ingestions. Early hemodialysis may be instituted to augment treatment of acidosis and prevent renal insufficiency. Diagnosis and treatment must be prompt to achieve the best outcome.

Toxic Inhalation

- **Carbon Monoxide**, also known as the silent killer, has a slower onset of the signs and symptoms of toxicity. Risk for exposure to carbon monoxide is high in the following: industrial workers, persons unable to escape a fire in an enclosed space, personnel at fire scenes, persons using gas powered generators during power outages, and persons in running vehicles that are poorly ventilated.

Clinical Manifestations

Assessment of oxygen saturation is not reliable in patients with carbon monoxide poisoning because carbon monoxide binds to hemoglobin at a higher affinity than oxygen which causes the patient's O_2 saturation to be erroneously elevated. Signs and symptoms of carbon monoxide poisoning include headache, dizziness, nausea, flu-like symptoms, fatigue, shortness of breath on exertion, impaired judgment, chest pain, confusion, depression, hallucinations, agitation, vomiting, abdominal pain, drowsiness, visual changes, fainting, seizures, impaired memory, and cherry red skin (seen in 2–3 percent of severely poisoned patients). Chronic smokers normally have carboxyhemoglobin levels as high as 10 percent. Patients with carboxyhemoglobin levels of 10–20 percent begin to show signs of toxicity and those with levels of > 25 percent show signs of severe exposure.

Collaborative Care

The priority of care for patients exposed to carbon monoxide is to administer 100 percent oxygen. The half-life of carbon monoxide is reduced from approximately five hours to an hour with this treatment. Collaborative care of patients with high levels of exposure to inhaled agents may include the patient being intubated, mechanically ventilated and admitted to an intensive care unit. The patient's condition may warrant use of hemodynamic monitoring and support of circulation with the use of vasoactive and/or inotropic agents.

PEDIATRIC MULTIORGAN

Age-Specific Patterns of Injury

The number one cause of unintentional injury related deaths in children varies according to age. Airway obstruction (including suffocation and choking) is the leading cause of unintentional injury related death in infants less than one year of age. In children one to four years of age, drowning is the number one cause of death followed by motor vehicle crash, pedestrian injury, burns and airway obstruction. Children five to nine years of age die most often from injuries suffered in motor vehicle crashes, followed by pedestrian injury, drowning, burns, and bicycle crashes. Ten to 14-year-olds' leading cause of death from unintentional injury is motor vehicle crash, followed by pedestrian injury, drowning, fire, and bicycle crashes. Deaths occur more often around the child's home between May and August and in the late afternoon and evening hours when children of this age are often unsupervised. Pancreatic injuries are commonly sustained during contact with the handlebars of a bicycle during a bicycle crash.

Clinical Manifestations

Clinical presentation is specific to the type of injury sustained but airway management is age-specific. In young children the trachea is very compliant, the gums are more vascular, and the teeth are poorly anchored. A large tongue and gastric dilatation may compromise respiratory status. Cuffed endotracheal tubes are rarely used in children less than 8 years of age. Cervical spine injuries are uncommon in children less than 12 years of age due to the greater mobility and elasticity of the cervical spine but should always be suspected in a child with an altered level of consciousness or one who is unable to cooperate with a clinical examination. Appropriate cervical spine stabilization should be maintained. Closed head injuries are common in young children due to the increased head to body ratio, the lack of myelination of the brain, and the thinner, more pliable cranial bones. Serum amylase is not a reliable indicator of the extent of pancreatic injury in children. Health care providers must always consider abuse when assessing an injured child whose injury pattern does not match the history provided by the child's parents or guardians. Abuse is more common in children presenting with blunt trauma. Shaken baby syndrome (in infants < 2 years of age), is manifested by retinal hemorrhages, subdural and/or subarachnoid bleeds in the absence of other external trauma.

Collaborative Care

Heart rate, respiratory rate, and blood pressure are age-dependent in children and are noted below:

TABLE 11.3

	Infant < 2 years old	Preschool (2–4 years old)	School Age (5–16 years old)
Heart Rate	< 140 beats per minute	< 120 beats per minute	< 100 beats per minute
Respiratory Rate	20–40 per minute	16–30 per minute	14–20 per minute
Systolic Blood Pressure	80 + 2x age in years	80 + 2x age in years	80 + 2x age in years
Diastolic Blood Pressure	2/3 systolic blood pressure	2/3 systolic blood pressure	2/3 systolic blood pressure

Infants and small children have poor thermoregulatory control so warning lights/blankets and warmed resuscitation fluids are recommended. Intravenous access is often difficult in injured children, especially infants. The intraosseous route may be used in this setting. Due to the smaller blood volume in children and infants there is little room for error. Infants in shock present with either hyper- or hypoventilation, mottled skin, erratic heart rate and blood pressure, glucose intolerance and metabolic swings. In these patients, urine output is the best indication of cardiovascular status. In infants a urine output of > 2 mg/kg/hr is optimal and in young children > 1 mg/kg/hr is desired. Non-operative management is the standard of care in the stable child with solid organ injury (liver, spleen). Failure of this method will manifest early. Within the first 12 hours after injury, decreasing hematocrit, urine output, and blood pressure, and rising respiratory and heart rates indicate failure of non-operative management. Changes in the child's abdominal exam and level of consciousness may also be noted. Exploratory laporotomy may be necessary in children with suspected pancreatic injury as non-operative management is often not reliable.

Injury prevention is of extreme importance with this age group. Parents of newborns should be taught the importance of proper car set use and how to babyproof their home. Car seat and booster seat use according to the American Association of Pediatrics guidelines should be stressed. Children should never ride in the bed of a pickup truck. Helmet use for bicycles, skateboards, and certain team sports must be emphasized. Water safety for all age groups including infants and toddlers should be included in injury prevention programs. This education needs to continue throughout childhood and adolescence, and include the child as soon as he or she is able to understand simple safety concepts.

TABLE 11.4

Age	Recommendation
Infants	Infants should always ride in the backseat in a rear-facing car seat until they are 1 year of age and weigh at least 20 pounds. Infant car seats should never be installed in the front seat of a vehicle.
Toddlers, preschoolers	Children 1 year of age and at least 20 pounds can ride forward-facing in the backseat of a vehicle. It is best for children to ride rear-facing as long as possible.
School-aged children	Booster seats are for older children who have outgrown their forward-facing car seats. Children should ride in a booster seat until the adult seat belts fit correctly (usually when a child reaches about 4' 9" in height and is between 8 and 12 years of age). School age children should always ride in the backseat of a vehicle.
Older children	Children who have outgrown their booster seats should ride in a lap and shoulder belt; they should ride in the backseat of a vehicle until they are at least 13 years of age.

Traumatic Asphyxia

In young children, traumatic asphyxia is often caused by being crushed under furniture or a motor vehicle's tires. As the child approaches adulthood, strangulation, suicide, and being pinned under a motor vehicle are the leading causes of traumatic asphyxia.

Clinical Manifestations

In young children, the chest wall is very compliant, making compression of the heart and lungs more likely. Clinical manifestations of asphyxia include cervical and facial petechial hemorrhage, cyanosis, vascular engorgement, and subconjunctival hemorrhage. Cyanosis above the third or fourth rib may also be present.

Collaborative Care

Treatment is directed toward the symptoms the child exhibits. In severe traumatic asphyxia, CPR is the initial treatment. Supportive treatment may continue for several days in the intensive care unit if intubation, mechanical ventilation, and cardiovascular stabilization are necessary.

Burns

Mechanism of Injury

Burn injury in children can be caused by flames, scalding hot liquids, electricity, or the inhalation of toxic substances. In infants, bathing related scalds and child abuse are the most common mechanism of injury. In toddlers, hot liquid spills—either accidental or abusive— and low voltage burns from electrical outlets are the most common mechanism of injury. The most common mechanism of injury in the school age child is a flame burn from playing with matches. Teenagers most commonly sustain burns from volatile agents, electricity, and flames due to cigarette smoking.

Clinical Manifestations

The most common cause of scald burns in young children is pulling hot liquids off the stove or counter onto themselves; therefore, the burn commonly involves the head, face, neck and shoulders. Their hypermetabolic response to injury often approaches 200 percent of their basal metabolic rate. In school age children, flame burns are more common and are often more serious, a hypermetabolic response of >200 percent of their basal metabolic rate is common as is anemia, thrombocytopenia, increased fibrinogen, systemic immunosuppression and increased capillary leak. There is an initial decreased cardiac output which normalizes with fluid resuscitation. Hyperthermia increases insensible fluid loss. The stress response decreases glycogen stores and causes hypoglycemia. The severity of the burn is determined by the depth of burn, the total body surface area (TBSA) involved, the anatomical location of the burn, the age and pre-burn health of the patient, and the presence or absence of an inhalation injury. Hypertension is common in 7–10 year old boys, with seven percent of those at risk for developing hypertensive encephalopathy. If the pattern of burn injury is not consistent with the reported mechanism of injury, abuse must be suspected.

Classification of Burns

- **Depth of Burn:** First degree or superficial partial thickness burns involve the epithelial layer of the skin. Patient complaints of pain and erythema are evident. Sunburn is an example. Second degree or deep partial thickness burns involve damage into the dermis. Patient complaints of extreme pain due to exposure of nerve endings, blistering and edema are evident. Third degree or full thickness burns involve all layers of the skin into the subcutaneous fat. The nerve endings are destroyed so patients do not complain of pain. Difficulty breathing and the development of compartment syndrome with circumferential burns is a concern with these burns. Fourth degree burns include all layers of the skin, subcutaneous fat, bone, muscle, and/or joints. No pain is experienced with this type of burn. The degree or depth of a burn may not be evident for up to 72 hours post injury.

- **Percent Body Surface Area Burned (BSAB):** The two most commonly used methods for estimating burn size are the **Rule of 9's** and the **Lund Browder Chart.** Both are illustrated below:

TABLE 11.5 *Rule of 9's*

	Infants	**Toddlers**	**Adults**
Head and neck	21%	18%	9%
Each arm	10%	9%	9%
Chest		18%	18%
Back and abdomen each	13%	18%	18%
Buttocks	5%		
Each leg	13.5%	13.5%	18%
Genitals	1%	1%	1%

TABLE 11.6 *Lund-Browder Chart*

Age in years	0–1	1–4	5–9	10–18	Adult
Head	19%	17%	13%	10%	7%
Neck	2%	2%	2%	2%	2%
Anterior trunk	13%	13%	13%	13%	13%
Posterior trunk	13%	13%	13%	13%	13%
Right buttock	2.5%	2.5%	2.5%	2.5%	2.5%
Left buttock	2.5%	2.5%	2.5%	2.5%	2.5%
Genitalia	1%	1%	1%	1%	1%
Right upper arm	4%	4%	4%	4%	4%
Left upper arm	4%	4%	4%	4%	4%
Right lower arm	3%	3%	3%	3%	3%
Left lower arm	3%	3%	3%	3%	3%
Right hand	2.5%	2.5%	2.5%	2.5%	2.5%
Left hand	2.5%	2.5%	2.5%	2.5%	2.5%
Right thigh	5.5%	6.5%	8.5%	8.5%	9.5%
Left thigh	5.5%	6.5%	8.5%	8.5%	9.5%
Right lower leg	5%	5%	5.5%	6%	7%
Left lower leg	5%	5%	5.5%	6%	7%
Right foot	3.5%	3.5%	3.5%	3.5%	3.5%
Left foot	3.5%	3.5%	3.5%	3.5%	3.5%

Collaborative Care

If neither of these charts is available, the patient's palm, including the fingers, is approximately one percent of their body surface area. This can be used to roughly estimate the percent of body surface area that is burned. Daily weights are essential in burned children; a weight loss of greater than one percent of their baseline per day for more than five consecutive days is indicative of a need to change the nutritional plan. Pain management with intravenous morphine sulfate is the gold standard. Anxiolytics may be added as needed. Intramuscular or subcutaneous routes are not used for medicine administration in burn patients as absorption is unreliable. Wound management is determined by the specific injury, and includes cleaning, debridement, antimicrobial ointments, and bandaging. Wounds are evaluated at specified time intervals depending on the severity of the wound. Superficial and partial thickness burns often heal on their own without surgery in 7 to 14 days. Deep partial thickness and full thickness burns need surgical eschar debridement and split thickness skin grafting to heal. Early excision and grafting is the recommended treatment if the patient is otherwise stable.

Initial evaluation and stabilization of the patient's ABC's must be undertaken along with evaluation of potential associated injuries. Signs and symptoms of inhalation injury include hoarse voice; soot on the face, in the nose or mouth; singed eyebrows, eyelashes, or nasal hairs; cutaneous burns on the face; and mucosal edema. A patient with a compromised airway or the potential for a compromised airway should be intubated and mechanically ventilated before airway edema develops. Circulatory support with intravenous fluid resuscitation is necessary in patients with a total surface area burn of > 15 percent. With smaller burns, oral and enteral fluid resuscitation often is adequate. Once the burn size has been estimated, fluid resuscitation can be calculated and begun. The Baxter/ Parkland or Consensus formula are two of the most frequently used formulas to estimate fluid resuscitation. Lactated Ringers is the fluid of choice for the first 24 hours of resuscitation in both of these formulas. Using the Baxter/Parkland formula you estimate 4 cc of Ringers multiplied by the patient's weight in kilograms times the percent total body surface area burn (4 cc/kg/%TBSA). Half of the total is infused in the first eight hours post burn, the remaining half is infused equally over the next 16 hours. If you use the Consensus formula, the only difference is to use 2–4 cc of Ringers in adults and 3–4 cc in children, with the rest of the formula remaining the same. Both of these formulas arrive at a suggested amount of crystalloid to be infused; this amount may need to be increased or decreased. Patients who sustained electrical or inhalation injury may require additional fluid during the first 24 hours post burn to achieve adequate resuscitation. Urine output is the best indicator of adequate fluid resuscitation with 1 cc/kg of urine each hour the goal for children.

Hemolytic Uremic Syndrome

A common cause of acute renal failure in children aged six months to four years who have been exposed to e-coli. Exposure is via undercooked meat, unwashed produce, unpasteurized dairy products or juice and potentially from petting farm animals. The child may also be exposed to e-coli in a pool or lake contaminated with feces.

Clinical Manifestations

Up to one week after exposure, the child looks pale, is irritable, bruises easily, and possible bleeds from the nose or mouth. Signs of gastroenteritis are vomiting, cramps and bloody diarrhea. Toxins from the e-coli enter the child's bloodstream and destroy red blood cells, causing renal failure. Urine output may be decreased, urine may be dark red, and peripheral edema may be present due to fluid retention.

Collaborative Care

Children may need short term hemodialysis to restore renal function. Intravenous fluid replacement, maintaining normal serum sodium levels, transfusion of red blood cells, and limiting dietary protein are all potential treatments depending on the severity of the illness. Children may become hypertensive due to the renal failure and need to be treated with angiotension converting enzyme (ACE) inhibitors. Most children recover completely with no long term sequelae.

Septic Shock

Children less than 36 months of age are at increased risk of developing sepsis due to the immaturity of their immune systems. A rectal temperature of equal to or greater than 100.4° F is presumed to have a serious bacterial infection (SBI). A urinary tract infection is the most common cause in children 2 to 36 months old. After 3 months of age, children are still at risk for community-acquired pathogens but the risk of serious bacterial infection and/or bacteremia decreases.

Clinical Manifestations

Systemic signs of infection, including fever, hypotension, tachycardia, tachypnea, lethargy or difficulty consoling the child, are common presenting symptoms. A child may be septic and not run a fever, making history and physical a very important part of the evaluation. Meningococcal sepsis affects healthy school age children with males being most likely to develop this type of sepsis and die; this finding parallels the adult literature. Group A Streptococcus and Haemophilus influenzae are other common causes of sepsis in school age children. During the winter, respiratory syncytial virus (RSV) is a common cause of sepsis in children. Nosocomial infection is frequently from Klebsiella or Enterobacter and commonly affects children with prior health problems who are chronically debilitated and/or immunosuppressed.

Collaborative Care

Lab work including CBC with diff, urinalysis and urine C+S should be sent on all children presenting with the above signs and symptoms. Blood cultures may be sent if indicated. Treatment is with third generation cephalosporins intravenously for children between 31 and 60 days of age, ampicillin is added if the infant is severely ill. Children between 2 and 36 months of age are treated symptomatically with antipyretics and antibiotics appropriate for the culture results. Hospital admission, intubation, mechanical ventilation and cardiovascular support in an intensive care unit may be necessary especially if the child's sepsis progresses to septic shock.

Systemic Inflammatory Response Syndrome (SIRS)

A syndrome characterized by systemic inflammation that, if left untreated, progresses to organ failure and death.

Clinical Manifestation

The patient presents with increases in non-culture positive markers of inflammation such as C-reactive protein (CRP) and, in children, 2 or more of the following:

- Temperature > 38.5° C or < 36° C

- Tachycardia > 2 standard deviations above normal for age

- Respiratory Rate > 2 standard deviations above normal for age, or need for mechanical ventilation for an acute process that is unrelated to a neuromuscular disease or the administration of general anesthesia.

- Leukocyte count either high or low for age or > 10 percent immature neutrophils.

Collaborative Care

Treatment goals are similar to that of septic shock and center around restoring adequate oxygenation and tissue perfusion. Being that no infectious source is usually identified, administration of antibiotics has no effect on SIRS.

Multiple Organ Dysfunction Syndrome (MODS)

In children, MODS is broken down into two categories: primary and secondary. Primary is defined as an immediate response to injury. Secondary MODS is a component of SIRS and has a higher associated mortality rate and entails a longer hospital stay.

Clinical Manifestation

Children develop MODS earlier in the course of an illness than do adults. Organs fail simultaneously not sequentially, with the GI tract and liver rarely being involved. Mortality is less frequent and is estimated to occur in between 25 and 50 percent of children who develop MODS.

Collaborative Care

Treatment is supportive in an intensive care unit and depends on the symptoms the child exhibits. Those with secondary MODS may require intubation, mechanical ventilation, enteral nutrition, cardiovascular, and renal support.

TOXIC EXPOSURE

Chemical Exposure: Nerve Agents

Nerve agents are organic chemicals (organophosphates) that disrupt the mechanism by which nerves transfer messages to organs. The disruption is caused by blocking acetylcholinesterase, an enzyme that normally relaxes the activity of acetylcholine, a neurotransmitter. Nerve agents are classified as G Agents and V Agents. G Agents include Sarin, Soman, and Tabun. The V agent is VX. These agents can either be absorbed through the respiratory tract or through the skin. They are easily vaporized or aerosolized, enabling them to spread over large areas.

Clinical Manifestations

Sarin has no odor so patients may not initially be aware of exposure. Soman has a fruity or camphor-like odor and Tabun has a very faint fruity odor. Being that these odors are not unusual, patients exposed to either Soman or Tabun may not initially be aware of exposure either. Signs and symptoms of exposure to G Agents develop within seconds to hours or exposure. Patients with minimal to moderate exposure present with non-life threatening symptoms that include runny nose, watery eyes, small pinpoint pupils, eye pain, blurred vision, drooling, excessive sweating, cough, chest tightness, tachypnea, diarrhea, increased urine output, confusion, drowsiness, weakness, headache, nausea, vomiting, abdominal pain, tachycardia or bradycardia, and hypotension or hypertension. With prolonged exposure, signs and symptoms are life-threatening and include change in level of consciousness ending in unconsciousness and seizure, paralysis, respiratory failure and death. Patients exposed to V Agents like VX display the same signs and symptoms as those exposed to G agents.

Collaborative Care

Initial care for patients exposed to both G and V gents includes removal of all clothing and thorough decontamination. Health care professionals involved in decontamination procedures must wear full body protection to avoid exposure to both G and V agents. Early administration of Atropine and pralidoxime (given within minutes of exposure to be effective) are also indicated to block acetylcholine receptors.

Blood Agents

Blood agents are a group of toxins that are carried by the blood and travel throughout the body, ultimately affecting every body system. These agents exert their effect at the cellular level. Cyanide is an example of a blood agent.

Clinical Manifestations

Even minimal exposure to cyanide, either by breathing, absorption via the skin or ingestion, causes immediate signs and symptoms including tachypnea, restlessness, dizziness, weakness, headache, nausea, vomiting, and tachycardia. After exposure to large amounts of cyanide via any of the above mentioned portals of entry, the patient immediately develops seizures, hypotension, bradycardia and unresponsiveness. Patients who are exposed to large amounts of cyanide immediately develop acute lung injury which leads to respiratory failure and death. Patients exposed to small or moderate amounts of cyanide can survive but may have long term cardiac and brain damage.

Collaborative Treatment

Decontamination is the initial step in treatment of patients exposed to cyanide. Health care workers involved in the decontamination must wear full body protection to avoid exposure to cyanide. All of the patient's clothing must be removed and the body thoroughly cleansed with soap and water. Pharmacologic treatment of cyanide poisoning includes the administration of amyl nitrate, IV sodium nitrate, and sodium thiosulfate.

Vesicant or Blister Agents

Exposure to vesicant or blister agents such as HD (sulfur mustard), HN (nitrogen mustard), L (Lewisite), or CX (Phosgene) may not be immediately apparent to the patient, as none of these agents has an identifying odor.

Clinical Manifestations

Patients exposed to mustard gas may not develop signs and symptoms for 2 to 24 hours after exposure depending on the amount of mustard gas the person is exposed to. Initially, the patient's skin becomes red and itchy then turns yellow and blisters. Within an hour of exposure, the patient may experience non-specific symptoms of skin irritation, pain, swelling and tearing. Severe exposure may produce blindness lasting up to 10 days. Respiratory signs and symptoms mimic those of a cold and include runny nose, sneezing, hoarseness, bloody nose, sinus pain, shortness of breath, and cough.

Exposure to phosgene causes immediate cutaneous pain with accompanying blanching surrounded by red rings within 30 seconds of exposure. Hives appear within 30 minutes and after 24 hours the blanched areas turn brown, the skin dies and a scab is formed. Pain and itching continue until the wound is healed. Phosgene in the eyes caused severe eye pain and temporary blindness along with tearing. Respiratory symptoms of phosgene exposure include immediate signs of upper respiratory tract irritation, runny nose, hoarseness and sinus pain along with shortness of breath, cough, and, with large exposure, pulmonary edema. Data on Lewisite exposure have been obtained largely from animal models.

Collaborative Care

Initial treatment of patients exposed to vesicant or blistering agents involves decontamination, including the removal of all clothing. Health care professionals involved in the decontamination effort must wear protective body suits to avoid exposure to the agents. There are currently no antidotes for exposure to vesicant or blistering agents and the care is largely supportive.

Pulmonary or Inhaled Agents

Chemicals that cause rapid and severe irritation to the respiratory tract include ammonia, chlorine, phosgene, and ricin.

Clinical Manifestations

The severity of signs and symptoms of exposure to ammonia, chlorine and phosgene are directly related to the amount and duration of exposure. Immediate symptoms are manifested in three categories. **Muscarinic** manifestations include bradycardia, hypotension, rhinorrhea, bronchorrhea, bronchospasm, cough, respiratory distress, increased salivation, nausea, vomiting, diarrhea, abdominal pain, urinary and fecal incontinence, blurred vision, miosis, diaphoresis, and increased lacrimation. **Nicotinic** effects include muscle fasciculations, cramping and weakness, diaphragmatic failure, hypertension and tachycardia, mydriasis and pallor. **Central nervous system** manifestations include anxiety, emotional lability, restlessness, confusion, ataxia, tremors, seizures and coma.

Signs and symptoms of ricin exposure manifest within a few hours and include respiratory distress, fever, cough, nausea, chest tightness, sweating, pulmonary edema, respiratory failure and death. If the patient survives the first three to five days after exposure, he is likely to survive.

Collaborative Care

Decontamination is the first priority of care for patients exposed to ammonia, chlorine and phosgene. All clothing must be removed and the body washed thoroughly with soap and water to limit further exposure. There is no antidote for ammonia, chlorine, phosgene, or ricin exposure, making symptomatic care the treatment of choice. Care of patients with high levels of exposure to pulmonary or inhalation agents may include the patient being intubated, mechanically ventilated and admitted to an intensive care unit. The patient's condition may warrant use of hemodynamic monitoring and support of circulation with vasoactive and/or inotropic agents.

Biologic Exposure

Biologic agents are categorized into two categories, A and B. Category A includes anthrax, botulism, plague, smallpox, tularemia, and viral hemorrhagic fevers. These agents are easily spread person to person and have a high mortality rate. Category B includes brucellosis and ricin. Category B agents are moderately easy to transmit person-to-person and cause increased morbidity but low mortality after exposure.

Clinical Manifestations

Anthrax is a spore-forming bacterium that is not easily spread from person-to-person. There are three routes of exposure to anthrax, each with different manifestations. Cutaneous exposure is the most common (95 percent of all exposures). The spore enters the body via a cut in the skin. Within two days of exposure, a small raised itchy bump resembling an insect bit is noted. This bump evolves into a vesicle, eventually becoming a painless ulcer with a black necrotic center. Inhalation of the spore initially presents with signs and symptoms of the common cold, including malaise, sore throat, low-grade fever, and muscle aches. The symptoms quickly progress to acute respiratory failure and shock. Gastrointestinal exposure is generally due to eating meat contaminated with the anthrax spore. Signs and symptoms resemble acute inflammation of the gastrointestinal tract: anorexia, nausea and vomiting, blood stools and uncontrolled diarrhea.

Botulism (Clostridium botulinum) is not spread from one person to another. Exposure can be from food (eating meat infected with the toxin-producing bacteria) or from a wound infected with the bacteria. Signs and symptoms may not be apparent for up to two weeks after exposure but most commonly appear within 12–36 hours. The botulism toxin is a muscle-paralyzing agent. Symptoms include double or blurred vision, drooping eyelids, slurred speech, dysphagia, dry mouth, muscle weakness that always involves the shoulders first, then progresses downward.

Plague (Yersinia pestis) is a bacteria common to rodents and their fleas. Plague can be bubonic, pneumonic, or septicemic. Bubonic plague, the most common, is contracted via a flea bite or thru a cut in the skin. Exposure is manifested by swollen and very tender lymph nodes accompanied by a painful swollen gland called a bubo approximately two to six days after exposure. It is not spread person-to-person. Pneumonic plague is contracted by inhaling aerosolized particles or by inhaling droplets from very close contact to an infected person or animal. Signs and symptoms include headache, fever, weakness, aggressive pneumonia with shortness of breath, chest pain, and cough with watery and/or bloody sputum. Within two to four days of exposure, respiratory failure and shock develop. Septicemic plague is not spread person-to-person and is commonly a complication of the other two forms of plague but can occur on its own. The signs and symptoms are similar to bubonic and pneumonic plague without the development of buboes. Abdominal pain and internal bleeding may occur with septicemic plague.

Smallpox (variola major) has been eradicated in the United States except for laboratory stockpiles. There are two types of smallpox: variola major and minor. Variola minor produces very mild signs and symptoms, is rare, and is much less serious. Major has four sub categories: ordinary, the most frequent type (90 percent of all exposures); modified, a mild form in previously vaccinated individuals; flat, and hemorrhagic, both of which are severe and fatal. Clinical manifestations include fever greater or equal than 101 degrees followed by a rash of firm, deep seated vesicles or pustules with no known other cause that are all at the same stage of development. The incubation period is approximately 1 to 17 days and is not contagious. However, smallpox is highly contagious once the rash appears. The rash starts as small red spots in the mouth and on the tongue that spread to the face, arms, legs, hands and feet, and within 24 hours the mouth and tongue rash become pustules. Exposure to tularemia or rabbit fever is most commonly acquired from an infected tick bite; the bacteria are found in rodents and rabbits. Tularemia can also be transmitted from touching the dead animal or eating or drinking from infected sources. The bacteria can also be inhaled. Exposure to a small amount of bacteria can cause symptoms in approximately three to five days. Clinical manifestations include chills, enlarged groin or underarm lymph nodes, fever, headache, joint stiffness, muscle pain, red spots on the skin that enlarge over time and progress to an ulcer, shortness of breath, sweating, weight loss, and pneumonia.

Collaborative Treatment

Diagnosis of exposure to anthrax is by history. Early treatment (within seven days) to cutaneous exposure with tetracyclines, fluoroquinolones, or penicillins is usually curative. Lack of treatment carries a 20 percent mortality rate. Exposure by inhalation carries a 75 percent mortality rate even with aggressive treatment with antibiotics, intubation, mechanical ventilation and circulatory support in the intensive care unit setting. Gastrointestinal exposure has up to a 60 percent mortality rate with aggressive treatment as mentioned above. There is currently a vaccine available for anthrax but it is recommended only for active duty military personnel, persons working directly with anthrax spores in the laboratory, or persons who work with animals or animal hides that are potentially infected. Vaccination of the general public is not currently recommended.

Diagnosis of exposure to botulism is presumptive and based on the patient's history. Treatment for presumed exposure must be initiated long before the confirmatory laboratory tests are available. These tests include culture or feces, gastric secretion, vomitus, serum, and/or wound cultures. Treatment includes an anti-toxin stored at the Centers for Disease Control that reduces the severity of the symptoms if given early in the post-exposure period. Persons exposed to the botulism toxin usually survive after weeks to months of supportive treatment including aggressive intensive care unit treatment with intubation, mechanical ventilation, and circulatory support.

The diagnosis of exposure to plague relies on the patient's history. Laboratory tests including bronchial washing, blood and tissue from the infected individual are obtained but results are not available for several days. Immediate treatment of antibiotics for patients with pneumonic plague is essential for survival. Streptomycin, gentamycin, the tetracyclines and/or chloramphenicol are recommended for treatment. Intensive care unit treatment with intubation, mechanical ventilation and circulatory support are essential as death within 4 days occurs without appropriate treatment. Plague has not been reported east of the Rocky Mountains in the United States.

Exposure to smallpox is fatal if left untreated; those who survive are left with deep scars, possible blindness, and arthritis. Treatment is supportive with intravenous fluid, pain medication and antipyretics. Antibiotics are given only to treat secondary infections. A vaccine is currently available but is not recommended for the general public.

Diagnosis and treatment of tularemia includes blood and sputum cultures, a thorough history of potential for exposure, and treatment with antibiotics. The tetracyclines and streptomycin are not given to children until all permanent teeth have erupted. The fluoroquinolones are given orally or gentamycin can be given intramuscularly or intravenously. Inhaled tularemia can evolve into lifethreatening pneumonia if not treated.

Nuclear/Radiation Exposure

There are two types of radiation, **ionizing** and **non-ionizing**. Non-ionizing does not cause tissue damage and will not be discussed here. Ionizing radiation causes immediate effect on human tissues. In the event of a radiation or nuclear event, everything including soil and water, at the site of the blast would be vaporized. The vapors mix with radioactive material, eventually cool and fall back to earth as dust or fallout which can be carried over large areas. Anything the fallout lands on becomes contaminated with radiation. Injury to humans and animals can be from the blast itself or from exposure to radioactive fallout and its contaminants.

- **Acute Radiation Syndrome (ARS):** Acute radiation syndrome occurs when the entire body is exposed to a high dose of radiation over a short period of time. Persons at the site of nuclear blasts or accidents are most likely to develop ARS. The risk of developing ARS is elevated in children due to their higher minute ventilation which allows a greater exposure to radioactive gas. Fetuses in utero have an increased risk of developing cancer when exposed to radiation. Also, children are more likely to develop psychological issues after a radiation disaster.

Clinical Manifestations

Clinical manifestations that appear within minutes to days include nausea, vomiting, and diarrhea, and last only minutes to days with the exposed person looking and feeling healthy for the next few days. After this brief respite from symptoms, anorexia, fatigue, fever, nausea, vomiting, diarrhea, temporary blindness, and possibly seizures and coma develop and last from hours to months. Skin manifestations range from red, itchy skin to severe burns depending on the level of exposure. The skin may take months to heal.

Collaborative Care

Treatment of children is based on the severity of exposure and the signs and symptoms patients exhibit, as well as their blood cell counts. Survival depends on the dose of radiation the patient was exposed to. Most fatalities are due to bone marrow destruction and its sequelae, and they occur within a few months of exposure. Ultimate recovery may take years.

Toxic Ingestion: Poisoning

Sixty percent of all accidental poisonings occur in children less than 6 years old. Children are curious and often swallow harmful things as they are unaware of their danger. Children less than six years of age most commonly swallow drugs, cosmetics, personal care agents, cleaning products, and foreign bodies.

Clinical Manifestations

Clinical manifestations depend on what was ingested. Non-steroidal anti-inflammatory drugs cause headaches, gastrointestinal upset, dizziness, ringing in the ears, vision disturbances, hypotension, tachycardia, hypothermia, and bleeding. Analgesics and opioids cause nausea, vomiting, diarrhea, seizures, CNS depression, respiratory distress and potential liver dysfunction if the drug contained Tylenol. Antihistamines cause CNS depression anticholinergic effects, hypotension, muscle weakness, seizures, and dysrhythmias. Rat and mouse poison cause anticoagulant effects for up to seven weeks and may cause gastrointestinal and/or genitourinary bleeding, intracranial bleeding, or bleeding from mucous membranes. Household plants cause burning and irritation of the mucous membranes, nausea , vomiting, shortness of breath, jitteriness, gastric irritation, and decreased level of consciousness. Household cleaning products cause mucous membrane irritation and burning, abdominal pain, bloody diarrhea, and esophageal and gastric destruction. Personal care products like perfumes, mouthwashes and cosmetics cause central nervous system depression and respiratory depression secondary to the alcohol in the products. Hypoglycemia may also be present.

Collaborative Care

Initial treatment for pill ingestion is gastric lavage with activated charcoal. With opioid ingestion, naloxone (Narcan) may be administered along with N-acetylcysteine. For ingestion of antihistamines, IV fluid may be necessary, EEG monitoring for central nervous system depression and sodium bicarbonate for the treatment of dysrhythmias. Vomiting is not induced with ingested material that is alkaline in nature, as further damage from burning would occur. Luckily, children usually ingest a small amount of poison and the effects are short lived and minimal. All medicines given to children are dosed according to body weight.

Toxic Inhalation

Mercury released by heating systems and vacuum cleaners can produce toxic levels of exposure in children. Exposure to the amount of mercury in a thermometer that has been aerosolized is enough to produce developmental acrodynia in children. Other signs and symptoms may manifest within three hours of high levels of mercury exposure. There is no toxic reaction to ingesting this amount of mercury in children. Carbon monoxide, also known as the silent killer, has a slower onset of the signs and symptoms of toxicity. Children at risk of developing carbon monoxide poisoning are those who ride in the back of an enclosed pick-up truck, are unable to escape from an burning enclosed space, are in a home that uses a portable heater or gas powered generator, or are in the bow of an improperly ventilated boat.

Clinical Manifestations

Signs and symptoms of low level mercury exposure are pneumonitis, cough, dyspnea, nausea, vomiting, tremors, weight loss and rash. Prolonged exposure to high levels of mercury can produce pulmonary edema, pneumothorax, respiratory failure and death. Assessment of oxygen saturation is not reliable in patients with carbon monoxide poisoning because carbon monoxide binds to hemoglobin at a higher affinity than oxygen which causes the patients O_2 saturation to be erroneously elevated. Signs and symptoms of carbon monoxide poisoning include headache, dizziness, nausea, flu-like symptoms, fatigue, shortness of breath on exertion, impaired judgment, chest pain, confusion , depression, hallucinations, agitation, vomiting, abdominal pain, drowsiness, visual changes, fainting, seizures, impaired memory, and cherry red skin (seen only in two to three percent of severely poisoned patients). Patients with carboxyhemoglobin levels of 10 to 20 percent begin to show signs of toxicity and patients with carboxyhemoglobin levels of > 25 percent show signs of severe exposure.

Collaborative Care

Treatment for exposure to mercury includes thoroughly washing the area with soap and water. Chelation with antibiotics has not been proven effective in controlled studies. Supportive therapy for presenting signs and symptoms is commonly indicated. The priority of care for patients exposed to carbon monoxide is to administer 100 percent oxygen. The half-life of carbon monoxide is reduced from approximately five hours to one hour with this treatment. Patients with high levels of exposure to pulmonary and inhalation agents may include the patient being intubated, mechanically ventilated and admitted to an intensive care unit. The patient's condition may warrant use of hemodynamic monitoring and support of circulation with the use of vasoactive, or inotropic agents may be necessary also.

NEONATAL MULTIORGAN

Asphyxia

- **Pathophysiology:** Perinatal or neonatal asphyxia is due to compression of the umbilical cord in the mother's body, placental abruption, severe meconium aspiration, congenital cardiac or pulmonary abnormalities, birth trauma, or airway obstruction.

Clinical Manifestation

An Apgar score of 0–3 for longer than five minutes, a pH of < 7, or a Base Excess greater than 12 on umbilical cord arterial blood gasses are indicative of hypoxia and metabolic acidosis, which confirm asphyxia. The neonate may exhibit seizures, coma, hypotonia and/or multisystem organ failure. Hypoxic ischemic injury in utero may cause severe central respiratory depression called "secondary apnea." A neonate with this form of asphyxia is unresponsive to tactile stimulation; intubation and mechanical ventilation must be instituted immediately after birth. If meconium aspiration is suspected, the neonate may have atelectasis, airway obstruction, or a pneumothorax. Neonates born with narcotic-induced asphyxia exhibit signs of apnea and hypotonia.

Collaborative Care

Treatment of perinatal or neonatal asphyxia is aimed at minimizing the sequelae. Immediate recognition and resuscitation is imperative to restore blood flow and oxygenation to the brain thereby limiting secondary damage. Continued lack of perfusion and oxygenation will cause hypoxic ischemic encephalopathy to worsen. Intubation and mechanical ventilation with high concentration oxygenation is initiated. Hemodynamic support is instituted as indicated.

Initial treatment of meconium aspiration includes clearing the airway of meconium as soon as the head has been delivered. If the meconium is thick or has particulate matter in it, intubation and mechanical ventilation is recommended. Treatment of an infant born with narcotic-induced depression includes the administration of nalaoxone, 0.02 mg/kg either IM or IV, to reverse the effects of narcotics.

Sequelae

The prognosis depends on the degree of asphyxia, but the long-term outlook includes the development of cerebral palsy, developmental delays, visual and hearing impairment, learning disabilities and behavioral issues.

Life-threatening Maternal–Fetal Complications

- **Birth Trauma:** Causes of birth trauma include a prima gravida mother, cephalo-pelvic disproportion, extremes of labor, oligohydramnios, breech presentation, forceps or vacuum extraction, very low birth weight, prematurity, fetal macrosomia, large fetal head, and fetal anomalies.

- **Birth-related injuries:** Soft tissue birth related injuries include abrasions, petechia, ecchymosis, lacerations, intra-abdominal injury and subconjunctival or retinal hemorrhage. Musculoskeletal injuries include skull fractures, clavicle fractures, long bone fractures, sternocleidomastoid injury, facial nerve palsy, radial nerve palsy, and brachial or lumbosacral plexus injury. Cephalohematomas are caused by subperiosteal hemorrhage in the parieto-occipital area. Facial nerve palsy may be due to compression by forceps or from spontaneous compression against the sacrum during delivery. Fracture of clavicle may occur during a difficult breech delivery. Midshaft long bone fractures most commonly occur during manipulation of the arms or legs in a breech delivery. Brachial plexus injury is due to traction on or avulsion of cranial nerve roots following prolonged labor and/or difficult delivery.

Clinical Manifestations

Cephalohematomas present as fluctuant swelling on the second day of life, and if large enough, they may cause anemia and jaundice. In an infant with facial nerve palsy the paralyzed side of the face appears smooth and full with obliteration of the nasolabial fold. The eye may remain persistently open and the corner of the mouth droops. With crying, the mouth is drawn to the side that is not paralyzed. Spontaneous improvement usually occurs. Infants with a fractured clavicle or long bone fracture exhibit swelling, pain deformity and limb shortening on the affected limb. The infant holds the arm limply along the body with the forearm pronated. Symptoms of brachial plexus injury include loss of movement and reflexes in the affected limb including the Moro response, but the grasp remains.

Collaborative Care

In infants with facial nerve paralysis, if the eye on the affected side remains open, cover the eye with a moist patch to prevent corneal abrasion. Treatment of a fractured clavicle in an infant includes arm and shoulder immobilized for 7 to 10 days. Treatment of long bone fracture in the neonate is immobilization with casting. Newborns have a great capacity for bone remodeling and complete union is usually complete in three to four weeks. Treatment of brachial plexus injury is expectant, but with braces and physical therapy most recover in four months to two years.

- **Genetic disorders:** The following potentially life-threatening fetal genetic disorders can be detected before birth: cystic fibrosis, congenital adrenal hyperplasia, Duchenne's muscular dystrophy, hemophilia A, alpha and beta thalassemia, Huntington's chorea, polycystic kidney disease, sickle cell disease, Tay-Sach's disease, neural tube defects like spina bifida and Down Syndrome.

Clinical Manifestation

Clinical manifestation is based on the genetic disorder.

Collaborative Care

Initial care of the neonate born with a genetic disorder depends on the disorder itself. As with any neonate, appropriate care includes evaluation and stabilization of the ABCs and should be followed by a complete physical exam.

- **Maternal Fetal transfusion:** Rh factor incompatibility occurs when the mother is Rh negative and is carrying an Rh positive fetus. Complications are uncommon with the first pregnancy but without proper immunization, mild to severe fetal complications may develop during subsequent pregnancies.

Clinical Manifestation

No maternal signs and symptoms are evident with Rh factor incompatibility. The fetus may exhibit anemia, jaundice, hydrops fetalis, cardiac failure, cerebral alterations and even death.

Collaborative Care

Diagnosis can be made by a variety of methods. Serum sampling for blood type of the mother and father, amniocentesis, fetal biophysical profile, fetal blood sampling via the umbilical cord, and ultrasound are some of the methods. Single or multiple intrauterine transfusions of the fetus via cannulization of the umbilical cord may be necessary. Long term, indwelling arterial and venous catheterization into placental vessels is currently being researched.

- **Abruption placenta:** Abruption placenta is the separation of a normally implanted placenta prior to the birth of the fetus. Diagnosis is usually made during the third trimester of pregnancy. Trauma accounts for a small number of cases. Maternal hypertension, (both chronic and pregnancy induced) is a major risk factor. Cocaine related abruption is being seen more frequently. Risk of abruption increases with the premature rupture of membranes.

Clinical Manifestation

Vaginal bleeding, abdominal pain, contractions and uterine tenderness are the most common presenting symptoms.

Collaborative Care

Diagnosis is made by history and ultrasound. The patient is often hypovolemic but may have misleadingly normal vital signs. Constant monitoring of maternal vital signs, fetal monitoring (external), insertion of a large bore IV, crystalloid infusion and foley catheter insertion are the standards of care. Baseline lab work including hematocrit, electrolytes, renal function, coagulation studies, and type and crossmatch are sent. If the fetus is immature and abruption is mild, expectant treatment is indicated. If the abruption is severe, immediate delivery is indicated; vaginal versus cesarean birth is decided according to the fetal and maternal condition.

- **Placenta Previa:** Placenta previa is an uncommon pregnancy complication that can cause excessive bleeding before or during delivery. The placenta will detach from the lower part of the uterus as the cervix begins to open in preparation for labor. This can cause severe vaginal bleeding. There are three specific types of placenta previa. In total placenta previa, the placenta completely covers the cervix. In partial placenta previa, the placenta partly covers the cervix. In marginal placenta previa, the placenta approaches the edge of the cervix. The development of placenta previa is more common in women who have already delivered a baby, had a previous cesarean section, had placenta previa with a previous pregnancy, are 35 years of age or older, smoke, are carrying multiples, or have had previous uterine surgery.

Clinical Manifestations

Painless, bright red vaginal bleeding in the second half of pregnancy is the main sign of placenta previa.

Collaborative Care

Placenta previa is diagnosed through ultrasound, either during a routine prenatal appointment or after an episode of vaginal bleeding. The treatment of marginal placenta previa is bed rest at home with limited to no sitting and standing. A vaginal delivery may be attempted with marginal placenta previa. Severe bleeding from placenta previa may necessitate bed rest in the hospital, transfusion and drugs (tocolytics), to prevent pre-term labor (before 37 weeks gestation). A planned cesarean section at 36 weeks is the optimal outcome of treatment for placenta previa requiring hospital bed rest. Steroids may be given pre-delivery to achieve maximal maturity of the fetal lungs. Monitoring the patient for severe vaginal hemorrhage before delivery, during labor and delivery, and for the first few hours after delivery is imperative as hemorrhage can lead to hypovolemic shock and death.

Lab work for hematocrit, acid base balance, renal function and clotting time along with type and cross match is sent. Severe maternal hemorrhage may prompt an emergency C-section regardless of fetal age.

Low Birth Weight/Prematurity

Premature or preterm birth is before 37 weeks gestation but not all premature babies have very low or low birth weight and thus have a decreased risk of chronic health problems.

Causes

Women of extremes in age or those who receive no prenatal care are at increased risk for delivering a low birth weight infant. Premature birth and intrauterine growth retardation are other causes of low birth weight.

Criteria

Babies born weighing less than 5 pounds, 8 ounces (2,500 grams) are considered low birth weight and are at increased risk for chronic health problems. Very low-birth weight babies are those who weigh less than 3.5 pounds or 1,500 grams at birth. They have the highest risk of chronic health problems due to the immaturity of their organ systems.

Clinical Manifestations

Preterm labor frequently results in the birth of a premature, low-birth weight baby. Mothers at risk for developing preterm labor are those who had preterm labor resulting in a premature birth in a previous pregnancy, are pregnant with multiples, or have cervical or uterine abnormalities. Mothers with pre-pregnancy chronic health conditions such as hypertension, diabetes, cardiac, pulmonary or renal disease, or those who develop acute pyelonephritis during pregnancy have a significant risk of developing preterm labor and delivering a preterm infant. Smoking not only slows fetal growth but mothers who continue to smoke throughout pregnancy are at a two times higher risk of developing preterm labor and delivering a small, premature infant. Abuse of illegal drugs such as cocaine has been associated with preterm delivery. Low-birth weight babies are at an increased risk of developing life threatening complications during the newborn period. Many of these babies are admitted to a neonatal intensive care unit. Respiratory distress syndrome (RDS) is seen in babies born before the 34th week of gestation. Due to the immaturity of their lungs, they lack sufficient amounts of surfactant to keep the end alveoli open. Intraventricular hemorrhage (IVH) occurs in some very low birth weight babies most commonly during the first three days of life and range from mild to severe. Many of these hemorrhages resolve spontaneously and leave the infant with no long term effect; the most severe hemorrhages cause increased intracranial pressure secondary to cerebral edema. Another problem seen in babies born before 34 weeks gestation is patent ductus arteriosus or PDA.

Premature infants often do not have the murmur characteristic of PDA in full term infants; they display signs and symptoms of fluid overload such as tachypnea, increased work of breathing, poor feeding and sweating while feeding. Yet another complication of premature birth is necrotizing enterocolitis or NEC. The intestines of premature infants are fragile and immature and are very sensitive to changes in blood flow and the development of infection. Infants who develop NEC are typically already in the neonatal intensive care unit due to prematurity and have other complications of premature birth. Manifestations of NEC usually appear after a feeding and include lethargy, periods of apnea, difficulty with thermoregulation, increased respiratory distress, decreasing platelet count, and feeding intolerance evidenced by yellow/green vomitus, increased abdominal distention and bloody stool. Retinopathy of prematurity (ROP), also called retrolental fibroplasias, is an abnormal growth of blood vessels in the eye that leads to minor to severe vision loss in babies born before 32 weeks gestation or those weighing less than 1250 grams. The smaller the neonate, the higher the risk of developing ROP.

There are 5 stages of ROP:

STAGE	Vessel Growth	Treatment	Vision
I	Mildly abnormal	Resolves spontaneously	Eventually normal
II	Moderately abnormal	Resolves spontaneously	Eventually normal
III	Severely abnormal, vessels may become enlarged and twisted	Resolves spontaneously unless vessels enlarge and become twisted—then laser or cryotherapy is indicated	Eventually normal unless laser or cryotherapy is performed, which causes loss of peripheral vision but preservation of central vision
IV	Partially detached retina	Scleral buckle	Potentially normal with scleral buckle therapy, if left untreated child will have mild to severe visual disturbances
V	Completely detached retina	Scleral buckle or vitrectomy	Same as stage IV

Collaborative Care

Aerosolized exogenous surfactant has been shown to improve alveolar function and oxygenation in babies with RDS. Some babies with RDS will need supplemental oxygen and may need endotracheal intubation and mechanical ventilation.

Treatment of PDA in premature infants may include administering indomethacin or ibuprofen both of which have been shown to help close PDAs. Depending on the size of the infant, transcatheter closure devices may be used; surgical closure is undertaken if the infant is in distress. If the infant shows no signs of distress, it will be given time to grow and a transcatheter closure device will be attempted when it reaches an appropriate size.

Care of the infant with NEC is insertion of an NG tube, making the infant NPO, IV fluids, blood cultures, hemoccult of stool, and antibiotics. Surgical intervention is needed only if there are continuing signs of systemic infection, radiological evidence of intestinal perforation, worsening physical exam, or declining cardiovascular and/or pulmonary function. The goal of surgical treatment is to remove all of the necrotic tissue. Occasionally infants will develop short gut syndrome due to the amount of dead intestine and need total parenteral nutrition for life. Death from NEC is directly related to overwhelming infection or extreme prematurity.

Care of infants with ROP is summarized in the table above.

Septic Shock

Infants between 1 and 28 days of age are presumed to have a serious bacterial infection (SBI) if they have fever. Fever of unknown origin (FUO) is a febrile illness with no known source; viral infections are the most common cause of FUO. Occult bacteremia is a febrile illness with positive blood cultures but no systemic signs of infection. Low or very low birth weight neonates and/or those with underlying conditions are at increased risk for developing sepsis.

Clinical Manifestations

Early onset sepsis is seen less than 72 hours after birth and is often related to low birth weight, prolonged rupture of membranes, infected amniotic fluid, maternal fever, difficult or prolonged labor or meconium aspiration. Hypothermia, respiratory distress, delayed capillary refill and cyanosis are signs of early onset sepsis. S.agalactiae (group B strep) is the most commonly implicated organism in early onset sepsis. Late onset sepsis occurs after 72 hours and is usually nosocomial in nature. Clinical manifestations include feeding difficulties, lethargy and hypothermia. Frequently implicated pathogens are Klebsiella, Pseudomonas, Candida and Enterococcus.

Collaborative Care

CBC with differential, urinalysis, urine C&S and lumbar puncture are indicated in neonates suspected of being septic. All neonates under 30 days of age are admitted to the hospital. Treatment is with a third-generation cephalosporin or gentamycin. Acyclovir is used if respiratory syncytial virus (RSV) is suspected. Antibiotics are continued until cultures show no bacterial growth at 48 hours. Sepsis in neonates can quickly progress to include shock, bleeding, renal failure and death. Early endotracheal intubation, mechanical ventilation, physiologic monitoring and circulatory support may be necessary in neonates with septic shock.

TOXIC EXPOSURE

Fetal Exposure to Drugs and Alcohol

Exposure of the fetus to drugs and/or alcohol can cause congenital deformities, chronic health problems and learning and developmental delays. Alcohol, illegal and prescription drugs have been implicated. All women planning to become pregnant or who find themselves pregnant should talk with their physician about the drugs—either illegal or prescribed that they are taking and should not drink alcohol.

Clinical Manifestations

Infants born with fetal alcohol syndrome are at an increased risk for premature birth, low birth weight and small gestational age. They exhibit facial abnormalities including small head circumference, narrow small eyes with large epicanthal folds, small upper jaw and short upturned nose. They exhibit increased muscle tone, hyperactivity, sleeping and sucking difficulties, tremors, agitation and crying. Signs of withdrawal will develop 24–48 hours after birth but may be delayed as neonatal metabolism of alcohol is slower than adults. Physical exam may reveal a murmur from either an ASD or a VSD, abnormal joints of the hand, feet, finger, and toes and skin hemangiomas. The neonate may have failure to thrive. As the child matures he or she may be at increased risk for learning and/or developmental delays, mental retardation and low IQ. Infants born to mothers who abuse drugs are usually premature, have low birth weight and are also addicted to drugs. Within 72 hours of birth, they will exhibit signs of withdrawal including tremors, irritability, red, dry skin, fever, sweating, diarrhea, excessive vomiting and seizures that include periods of apnea and back arching. Infants whose mothers routinely took stimulants exhibit lethargy for the first few days then are easily overstimulated and go from sleeping to loud crying within seconds. This pattern can last well into the preschool years.

Collaborative Care

Care of the neonate with either fetal alcohol syndrome or exposure to drugs is largely supportive. Treatment of withdrawal is according to symptoms, the judicial use of opioids and phenobarbital is recommended. Treatment of associated birth defects is also instituted. Admission to a neonatal intensive care unit for intravenous fluid administration, medicine administration, and physiologic monitoring is advocated.

Professional Caring and Ethical Practice Using the Synergy Model

12

HISTORY

The American Association of Critical-Care Nurses (AACN) established the Certification Corporation in 1975 with a mandate to develop the critical care registered nurse (CCRN) certification examination program. The purpose of this program was to have a method for developing, maintaining, and promoting high standards for the critical care nursing practice. The end outcome of the certification process is the best possible care of critically ill patients and their families in a respectful, healing, and humane health care environment. Initially, requirements for certification included hours worked in a critical care setting, the number and type of tasks performed, and an examination based on body systems.

Starting in the late 1980s, health care in the United States implemented multiple system changes. They included:

- Diagnostic related groups (DRGs) for payment of hospital care

- Legally mandated nurse-to-patient ratios

- Shorter lengths of hospitalization

- Increased use of unlicensed assistive personnel

All of this change impacted the bedside nurses' ability to advocate and provide optimal patient care. Much discussion in the media sought to identify problem areas such as critical care nurse burnout, erosion of the bedside nurse's autonomy, and how to measure quality of care.

In 1992, AACN developed a vision of health care systems driven by the needs of patients and families, where critical care nurses were able to maximize their contribution to patient care. At the same time, the Certification Corporation commissioned a think tank to develop a conceptual model of certified nursing practice. Over the next several years, the group developed the Synergy Model for Patient Care. In 1995, the Synergy Model was adopted for use in certifying critical care nursing practice. The first testing for certification with the new model was in 1999.

SYNERGY MODEL FOR PATIENT CARE

The basic premise of the model is based on the writings of Virginia Henderson (1960). She described the nurse-patient-family relationship as nurses "doing what patients and their families need for them to do." All patients have similar needs and therefore, experience these needs across a wide range, from health to illness. Logically, the more compromised a patient is, the more severe or complex his needs. Nursing practice is driven by the needs of patients and their family, and it requires nurses to be proficient in multiple dimensions of care. When nurse competencies relate to patient needs and the characteristics of the nurse and patient synergize, optimal patient outcomes can result.

There are four components of the Synergy Model for Patient Care: **core concepts**, **patient and family characteristics**, **nurse competencies (characteristics)**, and **outcomes**. The core concepts include the following ideas:

- The needs and characteristics of patients and families influence and drive the competencies of the nurse.

- Synergy occurs when individuals work together in ways that move them toward a common goal (Curey 1998).

- Active partnership between the patient and nurse will result in optimal outcomes.

Patient and family characteristics include resiliency, vulnerability, stability, complexity, resource availability, participation in care, participation in decision-making, and predictability. **Nurse competencies** (characteristics) include clinical judgment, advocacy/moral agency, caring practices, collaboration, systems thinking, response to diversity, clinical inquiry, and facilitation of learning. **Outcomes** can be patient-derived, nurse-derived, or system-derived.

PATIENT CHARACTERISTICS

Resiliency is the capacity to return to a restorative level of functioning using compensatory and/or coping mechanisms. The ability to bounce back from an insult is influenced by multiple factors such as age, comorbidities, and intact compensatory mechanisms. The levels of resiliency are:

Minimal	Moderate	High
Unable to respond	Moderate response	Respond and maintain
Coping failure	Begin coping	Intact coping response
Minimal reserves	Moderate reserves	Strong reserves
Brittle		High endurance

Vulnerability is the susceptibility to actual or potential stressors which can adversely affect patient outcomes. It can be impacted by the patient's health behaviors or physiological make-up. The levels of vulnerability are:

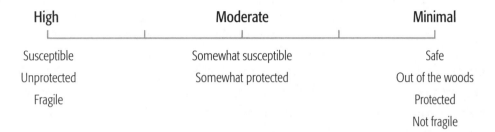

High	Moderate	Minimal
Susceptible	Somewhat susceptible	Safe
Unprotected	Somewhat protected	Out of the woods
Fragile		Protected
		Not fragile

Stability is the ability to maintain a steady-state of equilibrium. The patient and family response to therapies and nursing interventions can have an impact on the patient's stability. The levels of stability are:

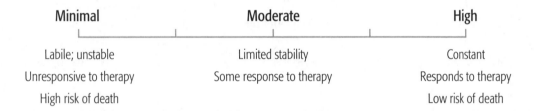

Minimal	Moderate	High
Labile; unstable	Limited stability	Constant
Unresponsive to therapy	Some response to therapy	Responds to therapy
High risk of death		Low risk of death

Complexity is the intricate entanglement of two or more systems. Systems refer to either emotional or physiological states of the body, family dynamics, therapies, or the environmental interactions with the patient. When multiple systems are involved, the patient displays more complex patterns. The levels of complexity are:

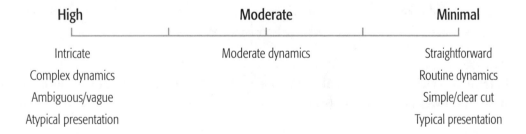

High	Moderate	Minimal
Intricate	Moderate dynamics	Straightforward
Complex dynamics		Routine dynamics
Ambiguous/vague		Simple/clear cut
Atypical presentation		Typical presentation

Resource availability is the level of resources (technical, fiscal, personal, psychological, social) that the patient/family/community brings to the situation. When a patient or her family brings more resources to the health care situation, there is greater potential for a positive outcome. The levels of resource availability are:

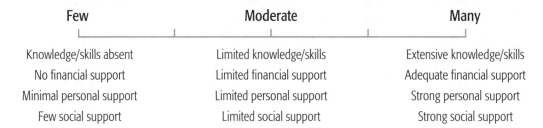

Few	Moderate	Many
Knowledge/skills absent	Limited knowledge/skills	Extensive knowledge/skills
No financial support	Limited financial support	Adequate financial support
Minimal personal support	Limited personal support	Strong personal support
Few social support	Limited social support	Strong social support

Participation in care is the extent to which patient/family engages in all aspects of care. Patient and family participation can be influenced by cultural background, educational background, and resource availability. The levels of participation are:

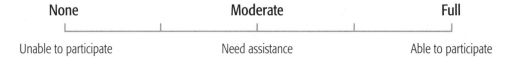

None	Moderate	Full
Unable to participate	Need assistance	Able to participate

Participation in decision-making refers to the extent to which patient/family engages in decision-making. Patient and family involvement in clinical decision-making can be influenced by their knowledge level, capacity to make decisions, cultural background, and the level of inner strength during a crisis. The levels of participation are:

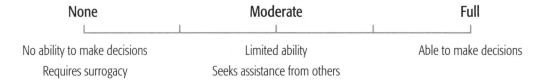

None	Moderate	Full
No ability to make decisions	Limited ability	Able to make decisions
Requires surrogacy	Seeks assistance from others	

Predictability is a characteristic that allows one to expect a certain course of events or course of illness. The levels of predictability are:

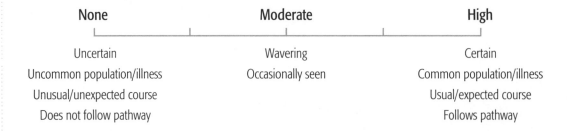

None	Moderate	High
Uncertain	Wavering	Certain
Uncommon population/illness	Occasionally seen	Common population/illness
Unusual/unexpected course		Usual/expected course
Does not follow pathway		Follows pathway

NURSE CHARACTERISTICS

Critical care nursing is an integration of knowledge, skills, experience, and individual attitudes. The nurse characteristics are bedside competencies that are essential for the provision of care to critically ill patients and their families. The development of clinical knowledge was first described by Patricia Benner (1984), in her landmark book *From Novice to Expert*.

Clinical judgment includes clinical reasoning, decision-making, critical thinking, and a global grasp of the situation. This is coupled with nursing skills acquired through a process of integrating formal and informal experiential knowledge and evidence-based guidelines. This integration of knowledge assists the critical care nurse to make the appropriate clinical decisions during the course of care given to the patient and her family. The levels of clinical judgment are:

Novice	Competent	Expert
Collects basic level data	Collects/interprets complex data	Synthesizes multiple data
Follows written directions	Makes routine decisions	Sees the 'big picture'
Questions own decisions	Seeks help appropriately	Collaborates as needed
Delegates decisions	Recognizes patterns/trends	Responds dynamically
Includes extraneous data	Focuses on key elements	Recognizes limits

Advocacy/moral agency is working on another's behalf and representing the concerns of the patient/family and nursing staff. This includes serving as a moral agent in identifying and helping to resolve ethical and clinical concerns within and outside the clinical setting. Since nursing has a unique relationship with patients and their families, they are often the voice for those who cannot speak for themselves. The levels of advocacy and moral agency are:

Novice	Competent	Expert
Advocates for patient/self	Advocates for patient/family	Works for patient/family
Self assesses own values	Incorporates patient values	Advocates for patient/family
Aware of ethical conflicts	Supports ethical decisions	Uses all resources
Functions in own values	Moral decisions inconsistent	Patient rights drive decisions
Aware of patient rights	Acknowledges patient/family rights	Empowers patient/family
Accepts death as outcome	Assists with dying process	Achieve professional relationships

Caring practices are nursing interventions that create a compassionate, supportive, and therapeutic environment for patients and staff, with the aim of promoting comfort, healing and prevention of unnecessary suffering. These activities include vigilance, engagement, and responsiveness of caregivers, including family and health care personnel. These caring practices create a safe environment for sick patients. An overwhelming fear of many patients and their families is that they will experience unrelenting pain or suffering. Pain assessment and management are fundamental caring practices. The levels of caring practices are:

Novice	Competent	Expert
Focuses on basic needs	Responds to subtle changes	Anticipates changes/needs
Uses standards/protocols	Provides individualized care	Engages patient/family
Maintains save environment	Uses caring practices	Needs determine care
	Optimizes environment	Promotes safety/comfort
		Facilitates safe passage

Collaboration is working with patients, families, and health care providers, in a way that promotes and encourages each person's contribution toward achieving optimal and realistic patient and family goals. This involves multidisciplinary work with colleagues and community. The bedside nurse knows the care environment best and is able to assemble a team together and focus on the best interest of the patient and family. The levels of collaboration are:

Novice	Competent	Expert
Willing to be taught	Willing to teach/mentor others	Serves as role model/teacher/mentor
Attends team meetings	Preceptors and teachers	Facilitates team meetings
Open to assistance	Involved in multidisciplinary care	Involved in pat outcomes community leader

Systems thinking includes the body of knowledge and tools that allow the nurse to manage whatever environmental and system resources exist for the patient, family, and staff, within or across all systems. Integral to systems thinking is the ability to understand how one decision can impact the whole system. Nurses, using a global perspective in clinical decision-making, have the ability to negotiate the needs of the patient and family through the health care system. The levels of systems thinking are:

Novice	Competent	Expert
Uses strategies/standards	Care based on patient need	Care driven by patient/family needs
Poor problem resolution	Finds system solutions	Global view of system problem
Patient/family isolated environment	Negotiates care decisions	Navigates problems for patient/family
Self as key resource	Reacts to patient/family needs	Optimizes patient/family outcomes

Response to diversity is the sensitivity to recognize, appreciate and incorporate differences into the provision of care. Differences may include cultural beliefs, spiritual beliefs, gender, race, ethnicity, lifestyle, socioeconomic status, age, values, and the use of alternative and complementary therapies. Nurses need to recognize the individuality of each patient while observing for patterns that respond to nursing interventions. The competent nurse asks about differences and considers the impact on patient care, but the expert nurse tailors the care environment to meet the diversity needs of the patient and family. The levels of response to diversity are:

Novice	Competent	Expert
Assesses; uses standards	Asks; considers impact on care	Anticipates patient/family needs
Care is based on own beliefs	Accommodates differences	Incorporates differences
Recognizes barriers to care	Assists incorporation of system culture	Adapts culture to needs
	Seeks to meet patient/family needs	Reduces/eliminates barriers; uses EBP for outcomes

Clinical inquiry is the ongoing process of questioning and evaluating practice and providing informed practice. Creating practice changes through research utilization and experiential learning. Clinical inquiry evolves as the nurse moves from novice to expert. At the expert level the nurse individualizes standards and guidelines to meet the patient needs. Clinical inquiry is all about observing, asking questions, finding the evidence, and making practice changes. The levels of clinical inquiry are:

Novice	Competent	Expert
Does not question practice	Adapts standards to pt needs	Improves based on research
Uses EBP when directed	Applies EBP (if no conflict)	Questions practice
Needs more learning	Accepts direction for change	Seek answers to EBP questions
Seeks assistance	Seeks alternative care practices	Lifelong learner
Data collector	Research team member	Evaluates EBP and implements

Facilitation of learning means that the nurse is able to facilitate learning for patients and families, nursing staff, other members of the health care team, and the community using both formal and informal learning. Education is based on the individual strengths and weaknesses of the patient and family. Creative methods need to be used to ensure patient and family comprehension.

Novice	Competent	Expert
Uses standard educational materials	Adapts educational material to needs	Modifies/develops content
Keeps teaching separate from care	Educates as part of patient care	Pt/fam involved in teaching
Provides information	Teaches based on needs	Individualizes teaching
Basic knowledge of needs	Uses various teach methods	Collaborates teaching needs
Pt/fam are passive learners	Pt/fam has input in teaching	Negotiates teaching needs

OUTCOMES

Optimal outcomes happen when the patient characteristics and nursing characteristics are matched. Since the Synergy Model views the patient and family as active participants, the outcomes measured must be patient and family driven. The *three levels of outcomes* discussed are **patient-driven**, **nursing-driven**, and **system-driven**.

Patient-driven outcomes include functional changes, behavioral changes, comfort, trust, quality of life, and satisfaction. *Nurse-driven outcomes* include: physiological changes, the presence or absence of complications, and the extent treatment objectives were obtained. *System-driven outcomes* include readmission rates, length of stay, and resource utilization for each case (Curley, 1998).

Patient-Driven Outcomes

Patients and their families require competence, caring, and trust from nurses when they are vulnerable and powerless. Trust is the result of the patient and family developing a caring relationship with the nurse. The nurse demonstrates her competence to the patient and family by being attentive to their concerns, empowering, and teaching them. Without trust between the nurse, patient, and family relevant information can be lost or ignored. To patients and their family, nursing care that comforts them is the most basic service that caregivers can provide. Caring practices that create a therapeutic and compassionate environment are a large component of the patient's quality of care outcomes. Patient satisfaction measures related to nursing care usually include technical and professional factors, trusting relationships, and educational experiences.

Nurse-Driven Outcomes

The critical care nurse monitors and manages therapies, based on trends physiological changes, in a timely and competent manner. By knowing the trajectory of specific illnesses, the nurse can respond with the appropriate changes needed to assist the patient to a positive outcome. Using vigilance and clinical judgment, the nurse creates a healing environment that provides safe passage for the vulnerable patient. Safe passage mandates the absence of complications (iatrogenic injury, infection, and hazards of immobility).The extent that treatment objectives are attained within a predictable timeframe is a nursing derived outcome variable. A high degree of collaboration and positive communication between critical care nurses and other health care professionals is associated with lower mortality rates, lower rates of nosocomial infections, shorter lengths of stay, and high patient satisfaction rates regarding care.

System-Driven Outcomes

The overriding goal of health care systems is to give the high quality care at reasonable cost for the greatest number of patients. Elevated readmission rates add to the personal and financial burden of providing health care. Third-party payers (insurance companies, Medicare, Medicaid) are no longer paying for multiple admissions to the same hospital for the same diagnosis or complications from that diagnosis. The critical care nursing competencies are instrumental in decreasing complications, length of stay, and readmissions. Nurses play a critical role in coordination of the patient's care, which maximizes resource utilization and minimizes cost to the health care system.

ETHICAL ISSUES

Ethics is defined as the system or code of morals of a particular person, religion, group, or profession. The American Nurses Association (ANA) is the major source of ethical guidance for the nursing profession. The ANA code of ethics is based on the underlying assumption that nursing is concerned with the protection, promotion, and restoration of health; prevention of illness; and the alleviation of patient suffering. The critical care nurse encounters ethical issues on a daily basis. Some of these ethical issues include do not resuscitate (DNR) orders, withdrawal of support, new technologies, and new protocols. Since the critical care nurse may have developed a therapeutic relationship with the patient and family, it is important that she be involved with any discussion of the ethical dilemma.

ANA Code of Ethics for Nurses

1. The nurse, in all professional relationships, practices with compassion and respect for the inherent dignity, worth, and uniqueness of every individual, unrestricted by considerations of social or economic status, personal attributes, or the nature of health problems.

2. The nurse's primary commitment is to the patient, whether an individual, family, group, or community.

3. The nurse promotes, advocates for, and strives to protect the health, safety, and rights of the patient.

4. The nurse is responsible and accountable for individual nursing practice and determines the appropriate delegation of tasks consistent with the nurse's obligation to provide optimum care.

5. The nurse owes the same duties to self as to others, including the responsibility to preserve integrity and safety, to maintain competence, and to continue personal and professional growth.

6. The nurse participates in establishing, maintaining, and improving health care environments and conditions of employment conducive to the provision of quality health care and consistent with the values of the profession through individual and collective action.

7. The nurse participates in the advancement of the profession through contributions to practice, education, administration, and knowledge development.

8. The nurse collaborates with other health professionals and the public in promoting community, national, and international efforts to meet health needs.

9. The profession of nursing, as represented by associations and their members, is responsible for articulating nursing values, for maintaining the integrity of the profession and its practice, and for shaping social policy.

From the American Nurses Association (2001). Code of ethics for nurses with interpretive statements. Washington, DC: American Nurses Association.

The American Association of Critical-Care Nurses (AACN) has included the ethics of care and ethical principles within its mission, vision, and values statements. An ethic of care is a moral orientation. Essential to an ethic of care are trust, compassion, collaboration, and accountability. Traditional nursing ethical principles provide a basis for assessment and decision-making. These principles include autonomy, beneficence, nonmaleficence, futility, justice, veracity, fidelity, and confidentiality.

Autonomy

The principle of autonomy recognizes the rights of individuals to self determination. This is rooted in society's respect for individuals' ability to make informed decisions about personal matters. Autonomy has become more important as social values have shifted to define medical quality in terms of outcomes that are important to the patient rather than medical professionals. The increasing importance of autonomy can be seen as a social reaction to a "paternalistic" tradition within health care. Respect for autonomy is the basis for informed consent and advance directives. Autonomy can often come into conflict with beneficence when patients disagree with recommendations that health care professionals believe are in the patient's best interest. Individuals' capacity for informed decision-making may come into question during resolution of conflicts between autonomy and beneficence. The role of surrogate medical decision makers is an extension of the principle of autonomy. Paternalism is the term used when health care providers make decisions for the patient based on the rationale that it is in the patient's best interest. This practice denies the patient the autonomy to make his own decisions.

Beneficence

Beneficence is the concept of doing good and preventing harm to humanity in general. This requires that one promote the well-being of patients and infers that harms and benefits are balanced, leading to positive or beneficial outcomes.

Nonmaleficence

The concept of non-maleficence is embodied by the phrase, "first, do no harm." The critical care nurse has a duty to remove the patient from or prevent harmful situations.

Beneficence and nonmaleficence are on opposite ends of a continuum and are often carried out differently.

Futility

This principle states that care should not be given if it is futile in terms of improving patient comfort or the medical outcome. In recent years there has been increased use of advanced directives including living wills and durable powers of attorney for health care. In many cases, the "expressed wishes" of the patient are documented in these directives, and this provides a framework to guide family members and health care professionals in decision-making when the patient is incapacitated. Undocumented expressed wishes can also help guide decision-making in the absence of advanced directives. "Substituted judgment" is the concept that a family member can give consent for treatment if the patient is unable (or unwilling) to give consent himself. The key question for the decision-making surrogate is not "What would you like to do," but instead, "What do you think the patient would want in this situation?" Courts have supported family's arbitrary definitions of futility to include simple biological survival.

Justice

The principle of justice requires that health care resources be distributed fairly and equitably among groups of people. This is especially important to critical care since a majority of health care resources are used in this practice setting.

Veracity

The principle of veracity requires that persons are obligated to tell the truth when communicating with others. Some cultures do not place a great emphasis on informing the patient of the diagnosis, especially when cancer is the diagnosis. Even American culture did not emphasize truth-telling in a cancer case, up until the 1970s. In American medicine, the principle of informed consent takes precedence over other ethical values, and patients are usually at least asked whether they want to know the diagnosis.

Fidelity

Involves the notions of loyalty, faithfulness, and honoring commitments. Patients and families must be able to trust the nurse and have faith in the therapeutic relationship if growth is to occur. Therefore, the nurse must take care not to threaten the therapeutic relationship or to leave obligations unfulfilled.

Confidentiality

Confidentiality is commonly applied to conversations between health care professionals and patients. Legal protections prevent health care professionals from revealing their discussions with patients, even under oath in court. Confidentiality is mandated by HIPAA laws, specifically the Privacy Rule, and various state laws, some more rigorous than HIPAA. Confidentiality is challenged in cases such as the diagnosis of a sexually transmitted disease in a patient who refuses to reveal the diagnosis to a spouse, or in the termination of a pregnancy in an underage patient, without the knowledge of the patient's parents.

Ethical Decision-Making

Ethical cases are not always straightforward or 'black and white' and often involve circumstances with multiple side-issues and distractions. The most common ethical issues seen in critical care units are allocation of scarce critical care resources, informed consent, organ donation, confidentiality, and foregoing treatment. It is often difficult to know that a true ethical dilemma exists. Thompson & Thompson (1985) identified three criteria to be used for defining moral and ethical dilemmas in clinical practice: an issue with different options, an awareness of the different options, and the choice of one option compromises the option not chosen. Rushton & Scanlon (1998) listed warning signs that can assist the critical care nurse with recognizing ethical dilemmas.

- Is the situation emotionally charged?

- Has the patient's condition changed significantly?

- Is there confusion or conflict about the facts?

- Is there increased hesitancy about the right course of action?

- Is the proposed action a deviation from customary practice?

- Is there a perceived need for secrecy around the proposed action?

When these warning signs occur, the critical care nurse needs to reassess the situation and then determine if an ethical dilemma exists. Finding a morally justifiable resolution to ethical dilemmas can be difficult for patients, families, and health care professionals. Using a systematic, structured process is a helpful way of approaching ethical decision-making.

TABLE 12.1 *Ethical Decision-Making Models*

M.O.R.A.L. Model (Crisham, 1992)	Ethical Decision-Making Process (Aiken, 1994)	ERC Plus Model (Ethics Resource Center, 2008)
1. Massage the dilemma	1. Collect, analyze, interpret the data or information	1. Define the problem
2. Outline the options/ possibilities	2. State the dilemma clearly	2. Identify available alternative solutions to the problem
3. Review criteria and resolve	3. Consider choices of action based on ethical principles	3. Evaluate the identified alternatives
4. Affirm the position	4. Analyze the advantages and disadvantages of each action	4. Make the decision
5. Look back	5. Make a decision that resolves the dilemma	5. Implement the decision
		6. Evaluate the decision

Ethical Decision-Making Process

1. Identify the dilemma. Gather as much information as you can that will illuminate the situation. In doing so, it is important to be as specific and objective as possible. Writing ideas on paper may help you gain clarity. Outline the facts, separating out innuendos, assumptions, hypotheses, or suspicions.

2. Determine the nature and dimensions of the dilemma. There are several avenues to follow in order to ensure that you have examined the problem in all its various dimensions. Consider the ethical principles of autonomy, nonmaleficence, beneficence, justice, and fidelity. Decide which principles apply to the specific situation, and determine which principle takes priority for you in this case. In theory, each principle is of equal value, which means that it is your challenge to determine the priorities when two or more of them are in conflict. Review the relevant professional literature to ensure that you are using the most current professional thinking in reaching a decision. Consult with experienced professional colleagues and/or supervisors. As they review with you the information you have gathered, they may see other issues that are relevant or provide a perspective you have not considered. They may also be able to identify aspects of the dilemma that you are not viewing objectively. Consult your state or national professional associations to see if they can provide help with the dilemma.

3. Generate potential courses of action. Brainstorm as many possible courses of action as possible. Be creative and consider all options. If possible, enlist the assistance of at least one colleague to help you generate options.

4. Consider the potential consequences of all options and determine a course of action. Considering the information you have gathered and the priorities you set, evaluate each option and assess the potential consequences for all the parties involved. Ponder the implications of each course of action for the client, for others who will be affected, and for yourself as a counselor. Eliminate the options that clearly do not give the desired results or cause even more problematic consequences. Review the remaining options to determine which option or combination of options best fits the situation and addresses the priorities you have identified.

5. Evaluate the selected course of action. Review the selected course of action to see if it presents any new ethical considerations. Apply three simple tests to the selected course of action to ensure that it is appropriate. The three tests are justice, publicity, and universality. In applying the test of justice, assess your own sense of fairness by determining whether you would treat others the same in this situation. For the test of publicity, ask yourself whether you would want your behavior reported in the press. The test of universality asks you to assess whether you could recommend the

same course of action to another nurse in the same situation. If the course of action you have selected seems to present new ethical issues, then you'll need to go back to the beginning and reevaluate each step of the process. Perhaps you have chosen the wrong option or you might have identified the problem incorrectly. If you can answer in the affirmative to each of the questions, thus passing the tests of justice, publicity, and universality, and you are satisfied that you have selected an appropriate course of action, then you are ready to move on to implementation.

6. Implement the course of action. Taking the appropriate action in an ethical dilemma is often difficult. Once a decision has been reached, it often comes after much thought and consideration and rarely is there complete agreement among all of the interested parties.

7. After implementing your course of action, it is good practice to follow up on the situation to assess whether your actions had the anticipated effect and consequences. The evaluation of the outcome can be used as a basis for future decision-making. If the outcome is not as planned, it may be possible to modify the plan or to use an alternative that was not originally chosen.

Legal Accountability

Each state has a Nurse Practice Act that defines the scope of practice that provides guidance for acceptable nursing roles. Standards of care are any established measure of extent, quality, quantity, or value. There are many established standards including usual and customary practice, institutional guidelines, association guidelines, and legal precedent. The ANA and AACN have established standards of practice. Many hospitals have developed standards for practice within the institution. Critical care units have standards of care, policies, and protocols for specific groups/types of patients or specific procedures (ACLS; intensive insulin therapy; blood transfusion policies).

Professional Liability

Professional liability includes *professional negligence, malpractice, and delegation.* **Negligence** is the failure to do what any reasonable, prudent nurse would do under similar circumstances or an act or failure to act that leads to injury of another person. There are six specific elements that must be established to determine negligence. These elements are:

- **Duty** to protect the patient from an unreasonable risk of harm
- **Breach of duty:** Failure to do what a reasonable, prudent nurse would do under the same or similar circumstances
- **Proximate cause:** Proof that the harm to the patient was preventable

- **Injury:** Proof of harm done to the patient

- **Direct cause of injury:** Proof that the nurse's conduct was the cause or contributed to the patient's injury

- **Damages:** Proof of actual loss, damage, pain, or suffering caused by the nurse's behavior

Malpractice

Malpractice is a specific type of negligence that takes into account the status of the care-giver and the standard of care. There are two types of malpractice: professional misconduct and malpractice. Professional misconduct is the improper discharge of professional duties or the failure to meet the standard of care, resulting in harm to the patient. Malpractice is the failure to utilize the prevailing professional standard or failure to anticipate conse-quences of the nurse's actions. The majority of malpractice and negligence that occurs in the critical care environment include failure to prevent falls, medication errors, failure to assess changes in clinical status, and failure to notify the primary health care professional of changes in patient status.

Delegation and Supervision

When delegating, the nurse must ensure appropriate assessment, planning, implemen-tation and evaluation. The delegation decision-making process, which is continuous, is described below.

I. **Delegation criteria.**

   A. Nursing Practice Act.

      1. Permits delegation.

      2. Authorizes task(s) to be delegated or authorizes the nurse to decide delegation.

   B. Delegator qualifications.

      1. Within scope of authority to delegate.

      2. Appropriate education, skills and experience.

      3. Documented/demonstrated evidence of current competency.

   C. Delegatee qualifications.

      1. Appropriate education, training, skills and experience

      2. Documented/demonstrated evidence of current competency.

   Provided that this foundation is in place, the licensed nurse may enter the continuous process of delegation decision-making.

II. Assess the situation.

A. Identify the needs of the patient, consulting the plan of care.

B. Consider the circumstances/setting.

C. Assure the availability of adequate resources, including supervision.

If patient needs, circumstances, and available resources (including supervisor and delegatee) indicate patient safety will be maintained with delegated care, proceed to step III.

III. Plan for the specific task(s) to be delegated.

A. Specify the nature of each task and the knowledge and skills required to perform.

B. Require documentation or demonstration of current competence by the delegatee for each task.

C. Determine the implications for the patient, other patients, and significant others.

If the nature of the task, competence of the delegatee, and patient implications indicate patient safety will be maintained with delegated care, proceed to IV.

IV. Assure appropriate accountability.

A. As delegator, accept accountability for performance of the task(s).

B. Verify that delegatee accepts the delegation and the accountability for carrying out the task correctly.

If delegator and delegatee accept the accountability for their respective roles in the delegated patient care, proceed to V–VII.

V. Supervise performance of the task.

A. Provide directions and clear expectations of how the task(s) is to be performed.

B. Monitor performance of the task(s) to assure compliance to established standards of practice, policies and procedures.

C. Intervene if necessary.

D. Ensure appropriate documentation of the task(s).

VI. Evaluate the entire delegation process.

A. Evaluate the patient.

B. Evaluate the performance of the task(s).

C. Obtain and provide feedback.

VII. Reassess and adjust the overall plan of care as needed.

From National Council of State Boards of Nursing. Delegation: Concepts and decision-making process. National Council position paper, retrieved June 6, 2008, from http://www.ncsbn.org/regulation/ uap_ delegation _documents_delegation.asp.

The act of delegation must ensure that the critical care nurse coordinates safe and effective patient care. Delegation allows the nurse to perform functions that only a registered nurse can perform and it utilizes the full potential of the health care team to maximize positive patient outcomes. The Five Rights of Delegation provide an additional resource to facilitate decisions about delegation. They are:

- **Right Task**
  One that is delegable for a specific patient

- **Right Circumstances**
  Appropriate patient setting, available resources, and other relevant factors considered

- **Right Person**
  Right person is delegating the right task to the right person to be performed on the right person

- **Right Direction/Communication**
  Clear, concise description of the task, including its objective, limits and expectations

- **Right Supervision**
  Appropriate monitoring, evaluation, intervention, as needed, and feedback

PART III

Practice Test

CCRN Practice Test

Try to answer the following 150 questions in three hours to mirror the conditions you will find on test day. Good luck!

1. A patient with heart failure should be taught which factor most useful in monitoring this condition clinically?

   A. Ejection fraction

   B. Cholesterol panel

   C. Cardiac output

   D. Coronary atherosclerosis

2. A 73-year-old male is admitted to the ICU. He appears to be in respiratory distress with worsening tachypnea (rate of 41) and use of accessory muscles. He is also anxious. Oxygenation with supplemental oxygen has been unsuccessful due to compliance. What is the most appropriate next step?

   A. Prompt initiation of BiPap with FiO_2 of 100%

   B. Prompt initiation of CPAP with FiO_2 of 100%

   C. Prompt administration of sedation to increase compliance

   D. Prompt intubation and initiation of mechanical ventialtion

3. Your 12-year-old patient has a 45 percent, deep partial thickness, total body surface area (TBSA) burn and a hematocrit of 55 percent 12 hours after being admitted to the Burn Unit. Your next best action would be:

   A. increase the IV fluid rate per protocol.

   B. decrease the IV fluid rate per protocol.

   C. give 2 units of packed red blood cells (PRBCs) per protocol.

   D. give 1mg/kg of lasix (furosemide) IV per protocol.

4. The nephron is the smallest functional unit of the kidney. It is composed of a tubular system, where the processes of reabsorption, secretion, and excretion occur. Choose the appropriate components of the tubular system in the proper order in which the filtrate passes.

   A. Glomerulus, Bowman's capsule, loop of Henle, collecting tubule

   B. Collecting tubule, distal tubule, loop of Henle, proximal tubule

   C. Proximal tubule, loop of Henle, distal tubule, collecting tubule

   D. Afferent arteriole, juxtaglomerular apparatus, efferent arteriole

5. An increase in the concentration of the final hormone product of the hypothalamic-hypophysis axis (e.g., testosterone) will cause which of the following?

  A. Inhibition of the hormone-releasing hormone from the hypothalamus (Gonadotropin Releasing Hormone)

  B. Increase of the hormone-releasing factors from the hypothalamus (Gonadotropin Releasing Hormone)

  C. Increased hormone production of luteinizng hormone by the anterior pituitary

  D. Increased testosterone production by the testes

6. Ruptured plaque occluding a cerebral artery is a common cause of:

  A. transient ischemic attack (TIA).

  B. hemorrhagic stroke.

  C. myocardial infarction.

  D. ischemic stroke.

7. The use of sequential compression devices (SCDs), Ted hose, and/or low molecular weight heparin are important measures to directly prevent which of the following?

  A. Myocardial infarction

  B. Pulmonary embolus

  C. Deep vein thrombosis (DVT)

  D. COPD exacerbation

8. Evaluating whether there is an elevation in leukocytes as a sign of infection can be difficult in a patient who is taking:

  A. herbal remedies.

  B. corticosteroids.

  C. acetominophen.

  D. NSAIDs.

9. The most likely cause of elevation of direct bilirubin is:

  A. intestinal (small bowel) obstruction.

  B. obstructive jaundice.

  C. gastroesophageal reflux disease.

  D. hepatitis A.

10. Which of the following nursing interventions will help the patient feel safe in the critical care setting?

  A. Not allowing family members to remain at the bedside.

  B. Asking the charge nurse's help before making any decisions.

  C. Conversing with him by telling him your plans for after work.

  D. Responding quickly to a his call bell or need for assistance

11. The hormones of the adrenal medulla are under the control of which structure?

  A. Hypothalamus

  B. Posterior pituitary

  C. Anterior pituitary

  D. Autonomic nervous system

12. A patient who is four days post-operative coronary bypass grafting (CABG) has an ON-Q device to control incisional pain. The physician orders removal of the ON-Q catheter. You encounter resistance as you attempt to remove the catheter. What is the priority nursing action?

    A. Remove catheter, since some resistance is common after four days; ensure black tip is intact.

    B. Stop removing catheter and obtain an x-ray immediately.

    C. Stop removing catheter and notify the physician of your findings.

    D. Stop removal process, change the patient's position, and retry removal of catheter in 30–60 minutes.

13. Leukopenia in a patient with viral infection, overwhelming bacterial infection, or bone marrow disorder may demonstrate:

    A. the patient has used all the available leukocytes to fight the infection and is unable to reproduce them at the necessary rate to successfully post an immune response.

    B. the patient has no need for the body to stimulate an immune response with these types of infections, and therefore there is no need to produce additional leukocytes.

    C. the bone marrow is selective in the production of cells for the body and may inhibit production in these situations.

    D. the CBC is unable to accurately count WBC when antibiotics are being used.

14. Which of the following is a warning sign that can alert the critical care nurse that an ethical dilemma may exist?

    A. There is no need for secrecy about a proposed intervention.

    B. Family members are confused about what is happening to the patient.

    C. The proposed course of action follows customary practices.

    D. The situation is emotionally stable.

15. A nurse should recognize that a patient who is taking Lopressor (Metoprolol) is at most risk for developing which of the following clinical manifestations?

    A. Hypertension

    B. Drug-induced cardiogenic syndrome

    C. Bradycardia

    D. Tachycardia

16. Which of the following factors is the primary consideration when applying a model for ethical decision-making?

    A. Court's wishes

    B. Family's wishes

    C. Patient's wishes

    D. Staff's wishes

17. What percentage of the resting cardiac output do the kidneys receive?

    A. 40 percent

    B. 20–25 percent

    C. 10–15 percent

    D. 5 percent

18. Bilirubin is the result of a breakdown of

    A. hemoglobin.

    B. white blood cells.

    C. amylase.

    D. bile.

19. A patient with 4 hours of chest pain has acute ST elevation in leads V_1–V_2. You understand that the location of the infarction is to be:

    A. lateral

    B. septal

    C. inferior

    D. anterior

20. The lateral aspect of the skull beneath the temporal bone just above the ear is the most common site of injury for:

    A. epidural hematoma.

    B. intracerebral hemorrhage.

    C. subarachnoid hemorrhage.

    D. subdural hematoma.

21. A patient presents with tachypnea, tachycardia and hypotension. A pulmonary embolus is suspected. Which of the following is the quickest/easiet imaging to order to make the diagnosis, assuming normal renal function and no known allergies?

    A. Pulmonary angiography

    B. CT chest with IV contrast

    C. CT chest without IV contrast

    D. V/Q perfusion scan

22. Your patient is receiving D5 ½ NS as a maintenance IV fluid. The physician has ordered a transfusion of packed red blood cells (PRBCs) for a low hematocrit. Prior to hanging the blood, you know to prime the blood administration tubing with which of the following fluids?

    A. 5% dextrose in water

    B. Lactated ringers solution

    C. .9% normal saline

    D. 3% normal saline

23. The anterior pituitary receives stimulation from the hypothalamus through the:

    A. vascular system.

    B. sympathetic nervous system.

    C. parasympathetic system.

    D. central nervous system.

24. A 52-year-old male is intubated and on a ventilator following cardiac bypass surgery. Which of the following assessment tools would be the most appropriate to determine the patient's pain level?

    A. The FACES scale

    B. The pain intensity scale

    C. The PQRST method

    D. The Jacox scale

25. When giving a nurse a health history, a patient reports all of these conditions. Which one would indicate a risk for the development of gastrointestinal bleeding?

    A. Arthritis relieved by nonsteroidal anti-inflammatory medication

    B. Diabetes mellitus controlled with oral medications

    C. Hypertension with slight pedal edema

    D. Bronchitis with persistent cough

26. A patient diagnoses with acute pericarditis, as evidenced by global ST elevation. How many of the 12 leads will show reciprocal ST segment depression?

    A. One

    B. Two

    C. Three

    D. None of the leads

27. Which of the following compounds is found in an antiseptic cream frequently used to treat burn wounds?

    A. Silver

    B. Copper

    C. Gold

    D. Tin

28. A 67-year-old female with hypertensive urgency is being monitored for response to a new antihypertensive medication. The elderly husband asks if he can sit next to her and hold the patient's hand. Which of the following responses would be best for you to say?

    A. "No, further stimulation may make her blood pressure worse."

    B. "No, your presence may make her anxious."

    C. "No, it interferes with my taking her blood pressure."

    D. "Yes, and I will continue to monitor her."

29. The following drugs may produce leucopenia except:

    A. Analgesics/anti-inflammatory drugs.

    B. Antibiotics.

    C. Antineoplastics.

    D. Diuretics.

30. Calculate cerebral perfusion pressure by:

    A. adding the ICP to the MAP.

    B. multiplying the MAP by the ICP.

    C. subtracting the ICP from the MAP.

    D. subtracting the MAP from the ICP.

31. A patient with advanced Parkinson's disease is just admitted to the ICU with hypoxia. A tracheal aspirate showed the presence of multiple organisms. The CCRN may expect antibiotic coverage for:

    A. aspiration pneumonia.

    B. community-acquired pneumonia.

    C. nosocomial pneumonia.

    D. COPD exacerbation.

32. Electrocardiographic changes which result from hyperkalemia are:

    A. widened QRS, elevated ST segment, lengthening PR interval.

    B. prolonged QT segment, bradycardia.

    C. U waves, ST depression, ventricular irritability; i.e., PVC's.

    D. tachycardia, ventricular irritability.

33. An ethical dilemma is a situation requiring a choice between which of the following?

    A. Morally acceptable, but opposing alternatives

    B. Morally unreasonable, but legal alternatives

    C. Legal but immoral alternatives

    D. Illegal but morally acceptable alternatives

34. A common clinical finding of SIADH (syndrome of inappropriate antidiuretic hormone) may include which symptoms?

    A. Mental status changes

    B. Tachycardia

    C. Polyuria

    D. Polydipsia

35. A healthy 40-year-old female is admitted to the ICU post-operatively from an elective surgical procedure, where she received a general anesthetic. She is somnolent. The physician requests an ABG, which returns as pH of 7.2, $PaCO_2$ 62, PaO_2 75, and HCO_3- 25. This patient has a:

    A. respiratory alkalosis.

    B. metabolic acidosis.

    C. metabolic alkalosis.

    D. respiratory acidosis.

36. The medication fenoldopam (Trade name: Corlopam) is ordered for a patient with hypertensive crisis. You will need to monitor for which of the following side effects?

    A. Hypokalemia, headache, and reflex tachycardia

    B. Hypokalemia, headache, and bradycardia

    C. Hyperkalemia, headache, and reflex tachycardia

    D. Hyperkalemia, headache, and reflex tachycardia

37. Treatment of hyperkalemia includes which of the following?

    A. Fluid bolus of 500 cc NS

    B. Administration of $NaHCO_3$, CaCl, insulin and glucose, and/or kayexalate and sorbitol

    C. Administration of an antiarrythmic

    D. Dietary restrictions for fluid and sodium

38. Which of these clinical manifestations should a nurse recognize as most significant when assessing a patient with intestinal obstruction?

    A. Vomiting

    B. Fever

    C. Constipation

    D. Sweating

39. Which of the following is an **unacceptable** way to administer a central painful stimulus?

    A. Pinching and twisting the trapezius muscle

    B. Pressing on the superior orbital rim

    C. Pushing up and inward at the angle of the jaw

    D. Twisting a nipple

40. A 68-year-old female, recovering in the ICU from complications following an emergency colostomy expresses concern about who will take care of her at home. The nurse learns that she and her 75-year-old husband live on the second floor of an apartment building that has no elevator. In addition, the husband is having difficulty understanding how to care for the patient's wounds. Which of the following nursing interventions would be most appropriate?

    A. Ask the patient's grown daughter to move in for a short time to provide care.

    B. Consult with the patient's insurance carrier for nursing home placement.

    C. Contact case management or social work for a home nursing consult.

    D. Reinforce information about wound care and provide reassurance to the spouse.

41. Erythropoietin is manufactured approximately 90 percent of the time in:

    A. bone marrow.

    B. kidneys.

    C. liver.

    D. lungs.

42. You are caring for a patient diagnosed with Systemic Inflammatory Response Syndrome (SIRS). You know that one difference between SIRS and sepsis is:

    A. blood cultures are positive with SIRS and not with sepsis.

    B. blood cultures are negative with SIRS but are positive with sepsis.

    C. temperature elevation is found only in SIRS.

    D. tachycardia is found only in sepsis.

43. A post-cardiac catheterization patient reports severe back pain and dizziness. The patient has no history of back pain. Which of these actions should a nurse take?

    A. Give the patient an analgesic.

    B. Obtain the patient's blood pressure.

    C. Instruct the patient to turn to his side.

    D. Lower the patient's head-of-bed.

44. A patient is brought into the ICU after being involved in a motor vehicle accident. He is in respiratory distress. On physical exam you notice that the left side of his chest is moving inwards as he inhales and the remaining chest wall expands. Based on this observation, you suspect that the patient is suffering from:

    A. pneumothorax.

    B. pulmonary hemorrhage.

    C. flail chest.

    D. atrial fibrillation.

45. Which of the following modalities would **NOT** be used to treat SIADH?

    A. Fluid restriction

    B. Diuretic administration

    C. Administration of 3% saline

    D. Kayexalyate enemas

46. A Native American from a nearby reservation is admitted from the ED with a diagnosis of hepatic encephalopathy. He has a 25-year history of alcoholism and was found unresponsive at home. On admission he is unresponsive, BP 148/74, HR 110, jaundiced, and has abdominal ascites. A peritoneal tap is performed and the patient's blood pressure drops to 86/64 and breathing becomes labored with RR 32 and SpO_2 of 84%. The patient is intubated and ventilated. The family, after consulting with the tribal elders, chooses to withdraw support. They request that a tribal drummer be allowed to drum and sing as their parent dies. Another nurse expresses concern about the noise and disruption that this will cause. Which of the following would be the most appropriate response to the coworker?

   A. "We will have the ceremony outside in the garden."

   B. "The physician has approved the ceremony in the room."

   C. "Don't you understand what this ceremony means to them?"

   D. "What concerns do you have about the ceremony?"

47. Using the Parkland Formula, calculate the first eight hour fluid resuscitation needs of a 40 kg patient with a 65 percent total body surface area (TBSA) burn.

   A. 502 cc

   B. 10400 cc

   C. 5200 cc

   D. 1040 cc

48. A goal of therapy for a patient with congestive heart failure is to:

   A. decrease preload, increase afterload, and increase cardiac output.

   B. increase preload, increase afterload, and increase cardiac output.

   C. increase preload, decrease afterload, and increase cardiac output.

   D. decrease preload, decrease afterload, and increase cardiac output.

49. Ischemic injury to the kidney will usually commence when:

   A. mean arterial pressure is < 60 mm/Hg for > than 40".

   B. mean arterial pressure is > 60 mm/Hg, however, urine output is < 30 ml/hr.

   C. mean arterial pressure is intermittently < 60 mm/Hg over a 60" period.

   D. systolic BP < 100 mm/Hg.

50. A 35-year-old female is admitted to the critical care unit for possible organ rejection. The patient's history includes a liver transplant approximately 1 year ago after she had an acute episode of hepatitis which significantly damaged her liver. Her symptoms might include:

   A. elevated liver enzymes.

   B. hematuria.

   C. bradycardia.

   D. normal temperature.

51. A 14-year-old male is admitted to the PIUC, with a diagnosis of meningococcemia, requiring intubation, ventilation, and vasoactive drips to maintain blood pressure. He is treated with antibiotics and sedation. The patient recovers quickly and the physician wants to extubate the patient as soon possible. The patient is awake, responsive, and cooperative. Which of the following is the most appropriate action?

   A. Describe the extubation process to the patient.

   B. Immediately extubate the patient.

   C. Administer a sedative to calm the patient.

   D. Contact the parents to obtain consent.

52. On interview, you are reviewing the medication records of a 35-year-old female admitted to the ICU. Which one of the following would suggest an increased risk of deep vein thrombosis?

   A. Use of oral contraceptive pills

   B. Use of daily ASA

   C. Use of a daily multivitamin

   D. Use of a proton pump inhibitor for acid reflux

53. Meningeal irritation is indicated by:

   A. nuchal rigidity.

   B. Homan's sign.

   C. Babinski's reflex.

   D. flaccid paralysis.

54. Four days after sustaining a partial thickness or second-degree burn of the hand, what would be the highest priority of care during your shift?

   A. Pain management

   B. Body image

   C. Airway maintenance

   D. Fluid volume management

55. As the physician is working up a septic patient in the critical care unit for DIC, the nurse may note the following laboratory findings:

   A. Normal or increased platelet count.

   B. Normal or increased fibrinogen level.

   C. Normal d-dimer.

   D. Elevated PT and PTT.

56. A nurse understands that the presence of hepatojugular reflux (HJR) is an indication of right-sided heart failure. To determine if a patient has hepatojugular reflux, the nurse should:

   A. place patient's head-of-bed at 45-degrees, compress the upper right abdomen for 30 to 45 seconds, assess for pronounced jugular vein distension.

   B. place patient's head-of-bed at 45-degrees, compress the upper left abdomen for 30 to 45 seconds, assess for pronounced jugular vein distension.

   C. place patient in trendelenburg, compress the lower left abdomen for 30 to 45 seconds, assess for pronounced jugular vein distension.

   D. place patient in trendelenburg, compress the upper left abdomen for 30 to 45 seconds, assess for pronounced jugular vein distension.

57. The critical care nurse should recognize that major complications of diabetes insipidus could include:

   A. dehydration.

   B. hyponatremia.

   C. hyperkalemia.

   D. bradycardia and hypertension.

58. A 65-year-old male with a history of COPD, diagnosed by pulmonary function tests, is admitted to the ICU in respiratory distress after his wife called 911 because he was gasping for air. He is hypoxic with oxygen saturation of 83 percent and has a mildly elevated WBC count. What are the appropriate measures to treat this patient?

   A. Beta agonist and steroids

   B. Beta agonist, steroids only, and chest x-ray

   C. Beta agonist, steroids, and broad spectrum antibiotics

   D. Beta agonist, steroids, broad spectrum antibiotics, chest x-ray, blood/urine cultures

59. The clinical manifestations of hyperphosphatemia and hypocalcemia are similar due to the reciprocal relationship in the reabsorption and secretion of these electrolytes in the kidneys. These symptoms include:

   A. muscle weakness and apathy.

   B. muscular irritability, twitching, seizure activity.

   C. obtundation.

   D. thirst, dehydration.

60. A patient with pancreatitis receiving lactulose asks the nurse how the medication will help. Which response is appropriate? Lactulose

   A. helps the body decrease ammonia.

   B. increases the pH of the intestine.

   C. causes increased urine output.

   D. deceases the bilirubin level.

61. Which of the following behaviors is an example of families trying to obtain some control over the situation?

   A. Going to work and visiting once a day.

   B. Sleeping at the patient's bedside.

   C. Refusing to help feed the patient.

   D. Closing their eyes when entering the room.

62. A patient suffers a myocardial contusion after CPR. The patient's heart rate is 142 bpm, cardiac output is 2.8 L/min, and heart tones are significantly distant. The nurse should prepare for which of the following procedures or surgeries?

   A. Cardiac surgery

   B. Cardiac catheterization

   C. Echocardiogram

   D. Pericardiocentesis

63. Which cerebral component is responsible for reabsorbing cerebrospinal fluid?

   A. Lateral ventricle

   B. Dura mater

   C. Arachnoid villi

   D. Subarachnoid cisterns

64. Which lab test should always be run simultaneously with ionized calcium levels?

    A. Sodium

    B. Potassium

    C. Albumin

    D. Hematocrit

65. All of the following are categories of clinical conditions which may result in acute renal failure, **except**:

    A. prerenal.

    B. intrarenal.

    C. postrenal.

    D. uremic.

66. While suctioning an intubated and ventilated patient, the nurse notes that the ventilator alarm is malfunctioning. Which of the following would be the most appropriate action for the nurse to take?

    A. Reset the ventilator alarm and monitor it closely for the next few hours.

    B. Notify the physician of the problem.

    C. Report the occurrence to the FDA.

    D. Contact respiratory therapist monitoring to ensure the patient is safe and prepare to replace the ventilator, and report the occurrence to the appropriate department.

67. Which of the following illustrate collaborative management for the critically ill patient with septic shock?

    A. Ambulate three times a day, withhold nutrition, and consult speech therapy

    B. Consult physical therapy, reposition patient as tolerated, withhold nutrition

    C. Administer enoxaparin sodium (Trade name: Lovenox) for deep vein thrombosis prophylaxis, reposition patient as tolerated, administer nasoenteral feedings

    D. Monitor vital signs once a shift, out of bed to the chair, and regular diet

68. A nurse is doing initial assessments on four patients. Which of these manifestations, if present, should cause a patient to be given priority?

    A. Cirrhosis without ascites

    B. Pancreatitis with ascites

    C. A palpable right kidney

    D. Hepatitis and peripheral edema

69. Which of the following is an indication for an immediate needle thoracostomy and/or chest tube placement?

    A. Chest radiograph with 5 cm of air between the chest wall and the lateral margin of lung parenchyma

    B. Dyspnea with exposure to a methacholine challenge

    C. Irregularly irregular cardiac rhythm

    D. Tachypnea, dyspnea, and fever

70. A patient on the unit has suffered frontal head injuries from an auto accident. Which type of impairment may result from injury to the frontal lobe?

    A. Loss of sensation

    B. Loss of vision

    C. Alterations in hearing

    D. Alterations in personality

71. A client with a recent bowel obstruction is prescribed all of the following medications. Which medication should the nurse question?

    A. Celebrex®

    B. Lortab®

    C. Lipitor®

    D. Caduet®

72. When assessing a patient who has undergone coronary artery bypass grafting, which of these findings would indicate hypovolemic shock secondary to post-operative hemorrhage?

    A. Low CO, low CVP, low BP, and increased heart rate

    B. Low CO, normal CVP, low BP, and normal heart rate

    C. High CO, normal CVP, low BP, and increased heart rate

    D. High CO, low CVP, low BP, and normal heart rate

73. Calcitonin is released by which gland?

    A. Pituitary

    B. Adrenal

    C. Parathyroid

    D. Thyroid

74. All of the following are effects of leukemia on the body **except**:

    A. uncontrolled proliferation of white blood cells which invade various areas of the body.

    B. excessive use of metabolic substrates by the growing cancerous cells.

    C. rapid deterioration in the normal protein tissues of the body.

    D. patient is less likely to be at risk for infection.

75. Priority nursing care for a patient with an acute dissecting descending aortic aneurysm includes:

    A. maintain above normal blood pressure.

    B. monitor BUN and creatinine laboratory values.

    C. pain relief and blood pressure control.

    D. maintain below normal blood pressure.

76. A patient was in respiratory distress and found to have a pneumothorax. She fully recovered after a needle thoracostomy and chest tube placement. Repeat routine chest radiograph shows air in the mediastinum. Chest tube is functioning properly. Which of the following is the correct course of action?

    A. Do nothing and simply observe.

    B. Remove the chest tube.

    C. Insert the chest tube further.

    D. Prepare to place the patient on BiPAP.

77. A patient with a balloon-pump is admitted to the CVIC unit. The charge nurse utilizes the Synergy model by assigning which of the following to care for him?

    A. The nurse with the most seniority on the unit.

    B. The nurse with the most experience with balloon-pumps.

    C. The new graduate who will gain experience from this assignment.

    D. The nurse who has the room next to this patient.

78. A 23-year-old male was riding his bike in a triathlon race when he hit a large stone in the road, causing his bike to veer off the road and crash into a tree. He hit the tree at his back just below the rib cage on the right side. Able to rise, upon standing he found himself with severe pain in the lower right retroperitoneal area. The first aid personnel at the scene noted a significant contusion to the right retroperitoneal region upon examination and informed the young man to go to the nearest ED to be evaluated. Upon evaluation, the patient's vital signs are stable; however, he has severe tenderness in the right retroperitoneal region. The most likely initial radiology procedure the physician would order is:

    A. abdominal CT scan.

    B. intravenous pyelogram (IVP).

    C. renal arteriogram.

    D. chest x-ray.

79. Your patient's lactic acid level has risen from 2 mmol/L to 6 mmol/L 8 hours after a motor vehicle crash. You know that this likely indicates:

    A. appropriate fluid resuscitation.

    B. the need to start total parenteral nutrition (TPN) immediately.

    C. inadequate tissue perfusion.

    D. the need to transfuse 20 units of cryoprecipitate immediately.

80. The three precipitating factors of deep venous thrombosis include all **but**:

    A. Venous stasis or impaired blood flow.

    B. Malignancy.

    C. Alteration or injury to the vascular endothelium.

    D. Hemophilia A.

81. A patient is admitted to the ICU and is mechanically ventilated on volume control. The family is at the bedside and is curious as to what this means. Which of the following correctly explains the nature of volume control ventilation?

    A. The ventilator prevents the patient from taking in too much volume.

    B. The ventilator controls the amount of tidal volume delivered to the patient in each breath.

    C. The ventilator has a set volume to deliver in a day and will stop after this volume has been administered, to allow the patient to breath on his own.

    D. The patient controls the amount of tidal volume in each breath, but the ventilator controls the IPAP and EPAP.

82. The primary purpose of the CSF is to:

    A. transport oxygen to the brain.

    B. manufacture neurotransmitters.

    C. cushion the brain and spinal cord.

    D. maintain cerebral perfusion pressures.

QUESTIONS 83 AND 84 REFER TO THE FOLLOWING SCENARIO.

A 48-YEAR-OLD FEMALE IS ADMITTED TO THE UNIT WITH POSSIBLE SYNCOPAL EPISODE. She currently is awake although she is nervous and anxious. Her vital signs are:

BP 178/108; P 160; RR 28; T 39° C. During your initial exam, you note she has exophthalmos and her skin is warm and wet.

83. Given the above information, what condition could be present?

    A. Myxedema

    B. Parathyroid crisis

    C. Thyroid storm

    D. Aldosterone crisis

84. Which of the following treatments would be given in this situation?

    A. Calcitonin

    B. Propranolol (Brand name: Inderal)

    C. Normal saline

    D. Parathyroid hormone

85. Select the statement which best describes an arterial occlusive problem.

    A. Affected limb is pink, warm, painful, and has a pulse.

    B. Affected limb is white, cold, painful, and pulseless.

    C. Affected limb is cyanotic, cool, edema, and pulseless.

    D. Affected limb is white, cool, edema, and has a pulse.

86. A neonate, diagnosed with anencephaly, is admitted to the NICU immediately after delivery. Compassionate care is implemented. The father of the baby expresses his wish that he does not want the mother to ever see the baby, stating that it would be "too devastating" for her. Which of the following actions should the nurse do?

    A. Agree with the father regarding maternal visitation.

    B. Contact the hospital clergy for parental support.

    C. Tell the father that his request cannot be honored.

    D. Give the father his own picture of the baby.

87. A patient is scheduled for a surgical procedure involving the gastrointestinal tract. The patient asks what a Billroth II procedure involves. The best answer by the nurse is there will be a(n)

    A. partial removal of part of the large intestine.

    B. complete excision of the stomach.

    C. anastomosis of the gastric remnant to the jejunum.

    D. creation of rectangular stomach flap.

88. The parietal lobe is responsible for which function?

    A. Hearing

    B. Sensory integration

    C. Motor function

    D. Vision

89. Which of the following laboratory results would be most important for the nurse to assess in a premature infant born to a mother with type O negative blood prior to discharge from the hospital?

    A. Hemoglobin

    B. Hematocrit

    C. Bilirubin

    D. Urinalysis

90. You are caring for a toddler who sustained burns to his entire head, neck and right arm circumferentially, including his hand. Using the Rule of 9s you estimate that his total body surface area (TBSA) burn is approximately:

    A. 35 percent.

    B. 7 percent.

    C. 15 percent.

    D. 27 percent.

91. For a patient who has an intraaortic balloon pump, which of the following findings requires immediate nursing intervention?

    A. 150 mmHg pressurized Heparin (1,000U/500 ml NS) bag connected to arterial pressure line

    B. Low Helium alarm warning

    C. Similar aortic and arterial blood pressure readings

    D. Loss of left arm distal pulses, chest discomfort, or low urine output

92. The pathway which is called the common pathway in the coagulation cascade and is activated when the initial insult is a result of damaged tissues or trauma is:

    A. Intrinsic pathway.

    B. Extrinsic pathway.

    C. Hypercoagulability.

    D. Erythropoietin mechanism.

93. In the polyuric stage of ATN, what are the most important nursing considerations?

    A. Restricting fluid intake, monitoring electrolyte levels

    B. Monitoring for fluid depletion and electrolyte levels

    C. Administering hypertonic solution

    D. Administering diuretic therapy

94. An infant is born at 32 weeks and admitted to the NICU. The infant is noted to have spells of apnea on the monitor. After a thorough physical exam, the infant is diagnosed with apnea of prematurity (AOP). Knowing this it would be important to:

    A. consider assessing and monitoring the infant for gastroesophageal reflux.

    B. place the infant on a ventilator.

    C. initiate BiPAP.

    D. initiate CPAP.

95. A 62-year-old male who has recently had valve replacement and been discharged on Coumadin® presents to the emergency department with hematuria. His INR is 2.1, Hgb is 9.5 and Hct 37%. What would be the initial course of treatment?

    A. FFP infusion

    B. Cryoprecipitate infusion

    C. Platelet infusion

    D. Administration of Vitamin K

96. The child you are caring for has sustained an isolated inhalation injury diagnosed by signed nasal hairs, oral burns, and respiratory distress. She is intubated. You know that a common complication for this group of patients is:

    A. Anaphylactic shock.

    B. Chronic renal failure.

    C. Gram-negative sepsis.

    D. Bronchopneumonia.

97. A patient with pancreatitis calls the nurse to report trouble breathing and his pulse oximetry shows a saturation of 89 percent. What action should receive priority?

    A. Assess blood pressure.

    B. Check oxygen saturation levels.

    C. Administer oxygen.

    D. Give the prescribed medication for pain.

98. Parathyroid hormone (PTH) release is stimulated by which humoral event?

    A. Decreased calcium

    B. Decreased magnesium

    C. Decreased cortisol

    D. All of the above.

99. The most common cause today of chronic renal failure is:

    A. poorly controlled diabetes.

    B. sepsis.

    C. glomerulonephritis.

    D. renal vein thrombosis.

100. A stroke in which area of the brain would cause aphasia?

    A. Left hemisphere

    B. Right hemisphere

    C. Pons

    D. Cerebellum

101. A 36-year-old female is seen to the Emergency Department. The patient and her family do not speak English and are unable to communicate with the health care team. Which of the following methods would be most effective, when coordinating care with the family of this patient?

    A. Use a translation service.

    B. Have a bilingual family member translate.

    C. Use ancillary staff for explanations.

    D. Use a communication board.

102. If the patient demonstrates a decorticate posture, which of the following should the nurse expect to find?

    A. Flexion of both upper and lower extremities.

    B. Flexion of elbows, extension of the knees, and plantar flexion of the feet.

    C. Extension of upper extremities and flexion of lower extremities.

    D. Extension of elbows and knees, plantar flexion of feet, and flexion of the wrists.

103. Which of these manifestations, if identified in a patient who has suffered a myocardial infarction, should a nurse associate with the development of a papillary muscle rupture?

    A. Abrupt onset of shortness of breath and no neck vein distension

    B. Abrupt onset of chest pain and holosystolic murmur

    C. Abrupt onset of shortness of breath and acute neck vein distention

    D. Abrupt onset of chest pain and no murmur or neck vein distension

104. A premature infant is diagnosed with apnea of prematurity (AOP). The **best** course of treatment initially would be:

    A. initiation of BiPAP.

    B. administration of supplemental oxygen.

    C. initiation of BiPAP and acid reflux prophylaxis.

    D. initiation of supplemental oxygen and acid reflux prophylaxis.

105. A patient with gastroesophageal reflux is complaining of chest discomfort and shortness of breath following a meal. Which of the following interventions should the nurse carry out first?

    A. Position the patient in high Fowler's position.

    B. Assist the patient to cough and take deep breaths.

    C. Reassure the patient to lie supine.

    D. Assess the oxygen saturation level.

106. The renin-angiotensin-aldosterone cascade is initiated by:

    A. Hyponatremia.

    B. Fall in mean arterial pressure/renal artery hypotension.

    C. Fluid retention/overload.

    D. Elevated BUN/creatinine.

107. Symptoms of hypothyroidism include all of the following **except:**

    A. Paresthesia of the fingers.

    B. Sensitivity to cold.

    C. Dry, scaly skin.

    D. Nervousness.

108. A 63-year-old male is recovering from a Whipple procedure and the abdominal wound is healing by secondary intention. Wound care is complex and the son is having difficulty successfully demonstrating the skill. Which intervention would be the most appropriate next step for the nurse?

    A. Provide written step-by-step instructions for the son

    B. Eliminate dressing changes from the skills the son must perform

    C. Provide coaching and the opportunities to repeat the skill

    D. Consult the wound care specialist

109. A 55-year-old patient in the ICU has been admitted for potential organ rejection after a recent kidney transplant. What is the most like sign/symptom the patient would demonstrate?

    A. Increased urine output

    B. Decreased BUN/creatinine

    C. Elevated creatinine

    D. Elevated platelet count

110. Your patient exhibits the following signs and symptoms—temperature 102.6°, heart rate 136, blood pressure 90/50, urine output of 40 cc over the last hour, white blood cell count 10,000, and negative urine, sputum and blood cultures. You suspect the patient has:

    A. cardiogenic shock.

    B. septic shock.

    C. multiple organ dysfunction syndrome (MODS).

    D. systemic inflammatory response syndrome (SIRS).

111. A patient who has narrow QRS supraventricular tachycardia with heart rate of 188 and hypotension may require:

    A. cardioversion.

    B. defibrillation.

    C. pacing.

    D. automatic implantable cardioverter defibrillator (AICD).

112. A patient with acute metabolic acidosis would present with which of the following arterial blood gases results?

    A. pH 7.55, pCO_2 32, pO_2 75, HCO_3- 24

    B. pH 7.50, pCO_2 45, pO_2 73, HCO_3- 30

    C. pH 7.30, pCO_2 55, pO_2 67, HCO_3- 28

    D. pH 7.31, pCO_2 40, pO_2 75, HCO_3- 14

113. Which of the following groups of patient data support the diagnosis of multiple organ dysfunction syndrome (MODS)?

    A. Urine output of 30 cc/hr, blood urea nitrogen (BUN) of 18 mg/dL and white blood cell count (WBC) or 5,120 white blood cells/mcL

    B. Upper GI bleeding, a Glasgow coma score (GCS) of 15, and a hematocrit (Hct) of 25%

    C. A total bilirubin of 15 mg/dL, a serum creatinine of 8 mg/dL, and a platelet count of 2,300 mm^3.

    D. A respiratory rate of 45/minute, a $PaCO_2$ of 60 mmHg, and a chest x-ray with diffuse bilateral infiltrates.

114. In anaphylactic reactions, the primary chemical mediator is:

A. Histamine.

B. Interferon.

C. Interleukin.

D. Tumor necrosis factor.

115. Which of the following diagnostic findings (electrocardiogram; chest x-ray) is consistent with a diagnosis of patent ductus arteriosus?

A. Mild right ventricular hypertrophy; enlarged right ventricle

B. Right atrial enlargement; pulmonary hypertension

C. Left axis deviation; cardiomegaly

D. Left ventricular hypertrophy; left atrial enlargement

116. A "u" wave is a classical clinical symptom of what electrolyte abnormality?

A. Hyperkalemia

B. Hypokalemia

C. Hyponatremia

D. Hypernatremia

117. A premature infant is admitted to the NICU and found to be in respiratory distress. The infant is intubated and ventilated and receives surfactant for the empiric treatment of respiratory distress syndrome. Which of the following is important to consider as a possible complication of these events?

A. Development of bronchopulmonary dysplasia

B. Development of atrial septal defect

C. Development of pneumothorax

D. Development of intestinal obstruction

118. A patient with a BP of 96/66 mmHg took a sublingual .04 mg nitroglycerin tablet five minutes ago and continues to experience chest pain. Which of these actions should a nurse take?

A. Take the patient's blood pressure.

B. Give another dose of nitroglycerin.

C. Check the patient's ECG rhythm.

D. Advise the patient to lie down with legs elevated.

119. A patient's family expresses concern regarding the meaning of numbers on the patient's monitor and asks the nurse for clarification. Which of the following is the most appropriate response for the nurse to give?

A. "The numbers tell us when the patient is having problems."

B. "Which numbers on the monitor concern you?"

C. "The numbers help us determine the best treatment."

D. "What don't you understand about the monitor?"

120. When inspecting the umbilical cord of the newborn, the nurse notices there are two arteries and one vein. What is the best action by the nurse?

A. Notify the delivering provider of the abnormality.

B. Clamp the umbilical cord.

C. Move the baby to the high risk nursery.

D. Look for other abnormalities.

121. The primary management goal for the patient with spinal cord injury upon arrival at the emergency department is to:

    A. transfer the patient from stretcher to bed.

    B. minimize the extent of spinal cord damage.

    C. reduce cervical swelling.

    D. elevate the head to reduce intracranial hypertension.

122. Appropriate response to treatment of myxedema coma would be illustrated by a change in which parameter?

    A. Increase in $PaCO_2$ levels

    B. Reduction in heart rate

    C. Increase in body temperature

    D. Decrease in pH

123. Before administering Nesiritide (Brand name: Natrecor) to a patient who has congestive heart failure, which of the following should a nurse check?

    A. Blood pressure

    B. Cardiac output

    C. Heart rate

    D. Electrocardiogram

124. A 43-year-old construction worker is admitted to the Neuro ICU after a 40-foot fall. He is intubated but alert and following commands. MRI results are pending. Physical exam finds loss of voluntary movement and proprioception with intact pain sensation of the left arm and leg; intact voluntary movement and proprioception but loss of pain sensation of the right arm and leg; fractured left arm; and suspected spinal cord injury. These findings are most consistent with:

    A. Brown-Sequard syndrome.

    B. Cauda equina syndrome.

    C. Central cord syndrome.

    D. Conus medullaris syndrome.

125. A cardiac surgeon has complained that most of the nurses in the ICU do not know how to care for a temporary pacemaker after open heart surgery and he wants to designate certain nurses to care for his patients. Several of the nurses in the unit have formed a task force to evaluate the problem and develop a workable solution. Which of the following is the best first step for the nurses to take to resolve this problem?

    A. Refer the surgeon to the administrative manager to resolve the issue.

    B. Set up mandatory pacemaker in-services for all of the unit nurses.

    C. Include pacemaker care as part of the annual competency review.

    D. Meet with the surgeon to discuss his specific concerns.

126. A patient with gallbladder disease may experience increased pain after a meal of

    A. noodles and broth.

    B. baked chicken and rice.

    C. pizza.

    D. steak.

127. The local hospital is in the process of upgrading from a Level I NICU to a Level III NICU and has appointed a multidisciplinary task force to oversee the project. The unit representative is concerned because the proposed physical layout does not promote developmentally appropriate neonatal care related to lighting and noise issues. Which of the following actions should the nurse take?

    A. Develop strategies to overcome the effects of light and noise in the current model.

    B. Present research studies that identify the importance of a developmentally focused NICU environment.

    C. Report the problems with the current model to nursing administration.

    D. Speak with the unit medical director to enlist his support for changes to the model.

128. The appropriate blood component which should be administered for thrombocytopenia is:

    A. whole blood.

    B. fresh frozen plasma.

    C. platelets.

    D. RBCs.

129. Your patient has a Glasgow Coma Score (GCS) of 5 about two weeks after sustaining a head injury in a motor vehicle crash. The patient is currently not being sedated. You interpret that score as:

    A. not an appropriate measure of neurologic function in a head injured patient.

    B. a devastating traumatic brain injury.

    C. an injury that will not leave the patient with any limitations.

    D. brain death.

130. Of the following methods of supplemental oxygen delivery, which is more likely to be used in infants/pediatrics and/or neonates, but not in adults?

    A. Non-rebreather face mask

    B. Hood

    C. Nasal cannula

    D. Endotracheal intubation

131. Which part of the endocrine system secretes aldosterone?

    A. Zona glomerulosa of the adrenal cortex

    B. Zona fasssciculata of the adrenal cortex

    C. Adrenal medulla

    D. Zona reticularis of the adrenal cortex

132. The following are examples of prerenal conditions which may lead to renal failure **except**:

    A. dehydration.

    B. hypovolemia.

    C. hemorrhage/blood loss.

    D. ureter obstruction.

133. A premature infant was admitted to the NICU for observation and did well clinically. On discharge the mother tells you that her other child had croup and she is interested in trying to prevent this from occurring in her new child. An appropriate response would be:

    A. croup is not preventable with any measures.

    B. croup can be prevented with prophylactic antiobiotics.

    C. croup is not a concern in this age group.

    D. croup has a variety of causes but keeping immunizations up-to-date is important.

134. A patient who has congestive heart failure is receiving Nesiritide (Brand name: Natrecor). Which of these responses should a nurse expect the patient to have if the medication is achieving the desired therapeutic effect?

    A. Increased SVR

    B. Decreased BNP level

    C. Increased contractility

    D. Decreased SVR

135. Your elderly ICU patient is at risk for developing shock. You know that cyanosis of which of the following indicates decreased perfusion in an elderly patient.

    A. Sclera of the eyes

    B. Oral mucous membranes

    C. Skin of the forehead

    D. Nail beds of the fingers and toes

136. Which technique is recommended for eliciting a response to peripheral pain?

    A. Sternal rub

    B. Trapezius muscle squeeze

    C. Nail bed pressure

    D. Mandibular pressure

137. A 53-year-old male patient is admitted to the ED after three days of nausea and vomiting. Initial blood tests reveal the following: BUN 28.0, Creatinine 1.0, K+ 5.9, and Hct 18.0. The patient is alert and oriented and has been only able to drink small quantities of fluids over the last two days. The patient is showing evidence of

    A. acute renal failure.

    B. chronic renal failure.

    C. dehydration.

    D. acute tubular necrosis.

138. Which of the following labs should be most concerning to the nurse caring for a patient with liver disease receiving possible hepatotoxic drugs.

    A. AST 28 units/L

    B. ALT 32 units/L

    C. ALT 50 units/L

    D. AST 10 units/L

139. Primary adrenal insufficiency is characterized by which of the following?

    A. Hyperpigmentation

    B. Hypertension

    C. Bradycardia

    D. Skeletal tremors

140. The primary precursor for all blood cells is the:

    A. Megakaryocyte.

    B. Reticulocyte.

    C. Pluripotential stem cell.

    D. Granulolyte.

141. The adult daughter of a mechanically ventilated patient has agreed to learn how to suction her mother. What is the first task that the nurse must do when developing a teaching plan?

    A. Obtain written information about the procedure.

    B. Determine a schedule for demonstrating the procedure.

    C. Assess the knowledge and skills the daughter needs to learn.

    D. Encourage the daughter to observe the procedure on other patients.

142. You are caring for a young child on gentamycin (Brand name: Garamycin) to treat an infection. Which of the following lab values would indicate that the patient is developing a common complication of gentamycin therapy?

    A. Decreased hematocrit

    B. Increased prothrombin time (PT)

    C. Elevated serum creatinine

    D. Increased carbon dioxide level

143. A patient has been given instructions about his automated implantable cardioverter defibrillator (AICD). Which of these statements, if made by the patient, would indicate that he needs *FURTHER* instruction?

    A. "I will have my device routinely checked to ensure its battery life."

    B. "I won't need to take Betapace (Brand name: Sotalol), since I have an AICD."

    C. "I will need to alert medical staff if I need an MRI exam."

    D. "I won't need hospitalization since I rarely receive electric shocks."

144. Filtration in the glomerulus of the nephron occurs as a result of what condition?

    A. Pressure gradient variations

    B. Glucose shifts

    C. Ion movement

    D. Concentration of urine

145. Another term for adrenal insufficiency is:

    A. Graves' disease.

    B. Myxedema crisis.

    C. Addison's disease.

    D. Cushing's syndrome.

146. In status epilepticus, seizure activity is best described as:

    A. controlled.

    B. absent for at least one year.

    C. escalating in intensity.

    D. a rapid succession of tonic-clonic activity.

147. Precautions for the neutropenic patient should include all **but** the following:

    A. Each person entering room should thoroughly wash hands.

    B. Patient should be kept in a private room with neutropenic protection sign posted.

    C. Patient should not be exposed to/handle fresh flowers.

    D. Patient should be allowed fresh/uncooked fruit and vegetables.

148. After initial shift report and gathering information on assigned patients, the nurse is most compelled to first check on a patient with

    A. gallbladder disease who exhibits Murphy's sign.

    B. gastrointestinal reflux who has a positive Chvostek's sign.

    C. hepatitis who has blood on rectal exam.

    D. abdominal pain who has Grey-Turner's sign.

149. A patient presents to the ICU after a penetrating trauma to the chest. The object is a tree branch which is still present. The patient appears to be relatively hemodynamically stable with BP 95/45 and heart rate 121. Which of the following would be an appropriate course of action?

    A. Remove the impaled object.

    B. Do not remove the impaled object.

    C. Attempt to trim the impaled branch so it does not appear to "sticking" out of the patient.

    D. Remove the object and hold pressure for at least 45 minutes.

150. A six-month-old infant is seen in the ED with a temperature of 38.8° C and a history of cold and flu symptoms for the last 24 hours. The infant is lethargic; HR 188; RR 52; BP 80/45; has sunken fontanelles; and has not wet a diaper in over 18 hours. Which of the following interventions is the first priority for this patient?

    A. Intubate and start mechanical ventilation.

    B. Obtain vascular access.

    C. Place a Foley catheter.

    D. Obtain blood cultures.

CCRN Answers and Explanations

ANSWER KEY

1. A	26. D	51. A	76. A	101. A	126. C
2. D	27. A	52. A	77. B	102. B	127. B
3. A	28. D	53. A	78. A	103. C	128. C
4. C	29. D	54. A	79. C	104. D	129. B
5. A	30. C	55. D	80. D	105. A	130. B
6. D	31. A	56. A	81. B	106. B	131. A
7. C	32. A	57. A	82. C	107. D	132. D
8. B	33. A	58. D	83. C	108. C	133. D
9. B	34. A	59. B	84. B	109. C	134. D
10. D	35. D	60. A	85. B	110. D	135. B
11. D	36. A	61. B	86. C	111. A	136. C
12. D	37. B	62. D	87. C	112. D	137. C
13. A	38. B	63. C	88. B	113. C	138. C
14. B	39. D	64. C	89. C	114. A	139. A
15. C	40. C	65. D	90. D	115. D	140. C
16. C	41. B	66. D	91. D	116. B	141. C
17. B	42. B	67. C	92. B	117. A	142. C
18. A	43. B	68. B	93. B	118. B	143. B
19. B	44. C	69. A	94. A	119. B	144. A
20. A	45. D	70. D	95. D	120. B	145. C
21. B	46. D	71. B	96. D	121. B	146. D
22. C	47. C	72. A	97. C	122. C	147. D
23. A	48. D	73. D	98. A	123. A	148. D
24. A	49. A	74. D	99. A	124. A	149. B
25. A	50. A	75. C	100. A	125. D	150. B

1. A

Patient education for heart failure is now focused on the patient's ejection fraction. While cholesterol panels remain important, new research from AHA and research centers such as the Cleveland Clinic Kaufman Center for Heart Failure has shown that treating heart failure from the aspect of the patient's ejection fraction has better outcomes than previous clinical pathways. A normal ejection fraction is 50–75 percent or greater and an indirect measurement of contractility. Cardiac output is not as specific as a cardiac index. Coronary atherosclerosis is not a measure or monitoring this condition.

2. D

The patient's respiratory status is worsening and he is not abel to comply with face mask with supplemental oxygen. You need to intubate the patient and oxygenate and ventilate him immediately. There is no time to wait to see if he passes a trial of NPPV. Answers A and B are both NPPV. These should only be used in stable clinical situations, not patients with worsening respiratory distress and/or increasing hypoxemia. Choice C is clearly wrong, because sedation will suppress respiratory drive and likely mandate intubation if not warranted earlier. The correct choice is D.

3. A

A is correct because an elevated hematocrit early in resuscitation indicated that the patient is hemoconcentrated due to under resuscitation and needs additional IV fluid. The goal of fluid resuscitation is to maintain tissue perfusion and to insure hemodynamic stability. The formula used as a starting point for fluid resuscitation is the Parkland formula: 2–4ml × body weight (kg) × % body surface area burned. The first half of this should be administered in the first 8 hours and the remainder over the ensuing 16 hours. It may be necessary to increase or decrease this rate based on the pulmonary/cardiac status of the patient.

4. C

The glomerulus and Bowman's capsule are part of the nephron but not part of the tubule system. The responses in B are backwards. The two components in D are in the renal vasculature, not the tubular system.

5. A

When there is increased hormone concentration, physiological control is increased and a stimulus is received in the hypothalamus. This results in inhibition of the hormone-releasing factors. The hypothalamic-hypophysis axis operates by a negative feedback mechanism. Hence, an increase in the concentration of the end hormone of the axis will result in inhibition of the pathway.

6. D

Ischemic stroke results from low cerebral blood flow, usually due to occlusion of a blood vessel by clots, plaque, etc. Transient ischemic attacks (TIA) are reversible and last less than 24 hours, sometimes only minutes. Etiologies of TIA can include arteritis, thrombus emboli, arterial dissection, drugs (e.g., cocaine), stenosis due to atherosclerosis, etc. Hemorrhagic stroke is bleeding into brain tissue. Myocardial infarction is the interruption of coronary perfusion to the heart muscle.

7. C

The use of SCDs, Ted Hose, and LMWH (e.g., lovenox) can be used for the direct prevention of deep vein thromboses. It is true that a pulmonary embolus may originate from a DVT and that the use of the above measures decreases the incidence of PE, but this is secondary to its prevention of DVTs. Myocardial infarctions and COPD exacerbations have no connection with the use of the above measures.

8. B

Corticosteroids can mask infection by suppressing the immune system. Further, their use causes marginalization of neutrophils, resulting in a mild leukocytosis. Hence, not only is the immune system suppressed, but the WBC may appear slightly elevated and falsely raising the suspicion for infection. There is still research being done regarding the effect herbal remedies have on the immune system. Acetaminophen and NSAIDs may mask fever but they should not change the leukocyte count.

9. B

Direct bilirubin is elevated in obstructive jaundice. Although obstructive jaundice can have a number of causes, the most likely thing is obstructive choestasis, i.e., a gallstone blocking the common bile duct. Gallstones may result in biliary colic and/or abdominal pain, but unless they are located in the CBD, the direct bilirubin should not elevate. The total bilirubin is composed of indirect and direct bilirubin and has many more causes than the direct bilirubin. The other choices are not the most likely cause of direct bilirubin elevation.

10. D

Patients feel safe when nurses exhibit technical competence and meet their needs. Not allowing family to stay at the bedside, asking the charge nurse for help with decision making, and talking about your after-work plans does not demonstrate competence or create synergy with the patient or her family.

11. D

The hormones of the adrenal medulla—epinephrine and norepinephrine—are under the control of the autonomic nervous system. The anterior pituitary controls the adrenal cortex. The hypothalamus controls the anterior pituitary and, indirectly, the adrenal cortex.

12. D

I-Flow Corporation, ON-Q system manufacturer recommends stopping catheter removal if resistance is met. Removal of catheter can be retried within 30–60 minutes after changing the patient's position. An x-ray needs only to be obtained if catheter breakage is suspected. The catheter tip is black in color, thus radiopaqued.

13. A

In overwhelming infections, the body uses of all its available resources to respond to the process. In the event that it is sustained over a long period of time, the availability of leukocytes may be significantly reduced, as the body may not be able to mobilize them quick enough. As we age, the ability to produce and respond to stimulus decreases as well. B is incorrect—this scenario would absolutely need to have the immune system stimulated. The bone marrow responds to stimulus from those mechanisms to increase production and release of WBCs. In this case there would be a need to increase release.

14. B

When family members are confused they may not trust the nurses decisions, or they may feel powerless to help their family member. The nurse needs to advocate for the patient by assessing the family members, empowering them to let their needs be known, and assisting them resolve any ethical issues. Choices A, C, and D do not indicate any ethical issues.

15. C

Metoprolol blocks stimulation of $beta_1$ (myocardial) adrenergic receptors. Major side effects associated with beta-blockers are hypotension and bradycardia. There is no such thing as drug-induced cardiogenic syndrome.

16. C

According to the ethical decision-making process, decisions should be made based on the patient's wishes (autonomy). Wishes of the staff or a court would interfere with the patient's autonomy. The family's wishes, while important, are not the primary factor, when seeking an answer to an ethical dilemma.

17. B

A is inaccurate: No organs individually (not even heart or lungs) receive 40 percent of the cardiac output. C and D are too small. The kidneys filter 180 liters of blood each day. To accomplish this, approximately ¼ of the cardiac output must go to the kidneys.

18. A

Bilirubin is a product of hemoglobin breakdown. The other choices are incorrect.

19. B

Leads V_1–V_2 view the septal region of the heart muscle. The septal wall receives it blood flow from the left anterior descending coronary artery. ST-elevation in leads I and aVL reflects a high lateral wall infarction. ST-elevation present in leads II, III, and aVF reflects an inferior wall infarction. ST-elevation present in leads V2–V4 reflects an anterior wall infarction.

20. A

Epidural hematoma is usually caused by a blow to the head, and is often associated with a skull fracture. The artery involved is the middle meningeal artery. The rough edges of the fracture or skull surface impinge on the blood vessels causing bleeding that accumulates between the skull and the dura mater. Intracerebral hemorrhage is bleeding into the brain tissue. Subarachnoid hemorrhage is bleeding into subarachnoid space, usually from a ruptured aneurysm. Subdural hematoma is usually caused by venous bleeding of bridging veins that occurs below the dura mater.

21. B

The quickest and easiest imaging study to order in an emergent situation is a CT with IV contrast. Although pulmonary angiography is the gold standard, it will not be obtained in time to obtain a diagnosis. A V/Q perfusion scan is useful, but again, is not immediately available. Further, the results are reported vaguely as High, Moderate, or Low probability—making the usefulness of the results marginal as a first line study. Finally, without contrast, you will not be able to visualize the pulmonary vessels.

22. C

.9 percent normal saline is the crystalloid of choice for blood transfusions because it is isotonic. The other answer choices are not isotonic and may cause lysis or distortion of the RBC cell membrane due to hypertonicity (3 percent NS). LR is close to isotonic but not exact in all its electrolytes.

23. A

Communication between the hypothalamus and the anterior pituitary occurs via a network of capillary vessels, referred to as portal circulation. The connection with the posterior pituitary is via nerves.

24. A

The FACES scale can be used by simply having the patient point to the appropriate face. Because of this, it is the easiest to use with children, people with language barriers, and intubated patients. The PQRST method, the pain intensity scale, and the Jacox scale all require verbalization and/or writing to communicate pain level.

25. A

Certain medications like nonsteroidal anti-inflammatory medications can predispose patients to GI bleed. The other choices are not possible risk factors for GI bleed.

26. D

Pericarditis is characterized by global ST elevation due to abnormal repolarization secondary to pericardial inflammation. Pericarditis is often mistaken for an inferior wall MI. However, there is no reciprocal ST depression found with pericarditis.

27. A

Silver sulfadiazine (Silvadene) is commonly used to treat burn wounds and contains silver. The other metals are not found in antiseptic cream.

28. D

This patient is vulnerable and susceptible to potential stressors that could negatively affect her outcome. The best response is to ensure that patient and family needs are met in a caring environment. Answers A, B, and C do not consider the patient characteristics according to the Synergy Model.

29. D

A, B, and C are classes of drugs which can produce leukopenia due to the effect they have on either the production or the destruction of leukocytes. Diuretics typically work within the structure of the renal cortex and do not directly have an impact on the WBC count.

30. C

To calculate the cerebral perfusion pressure, the nurse subtracts the ICP from the MAP. Subtracting the MAP from the ICP will give a negative number. Adding or multiplying the numbers would give inappropriate results.

31. A

The patient has a neurological condition that may likely impair her gag reflex and ability to swallow. Hence, the patient is at risk for aspiration. Results of the tracheal aspirate are consistent with this diagnosis of aspiration pneumonia. As a result, the antibiotic coverage will likely include anaerobic organisms. The patient was just admitted to the hospital and does not meet the timeline criteria for nosocomial pneumonia. Although CAP is possible, the clinical situation highly suggests aspiration pneumonia, especially given the tracheal aspirate. COPD is not mentioned in the case, so there is no reason to suspect it.

32. A

Too much potassium in the serum (hyperkalemia) decreases the rate of ventricular depolarization, shortens repolarization, and depresses AV conduction. Therefore, the EKG changes associated with these phenomena are those in A. Prolonged QT segment is commonly due to drug effects such as quinidine or other electrolyte disturbances. Hypokalemia causes the EKG changes which are specified in C. There are many causes for tachycardia, i.e., fever, stress, etc. and ventricular irritability such as ischemia, hypokalemia, etc.

33. A

A moral dilemma is a choice between alternatives that can be justified by moral rules or principles. Answers B, C, and D are either illegal or immoral.

34. A

The most common symptoms of SIADH include personality changes, headache, decreased mentation, lethargy, nausea, vomiting, diminished DTRs, seizures, and coma. These are attributed to the electrolyte disturbances associated with SIADH.

35. D

Following the rules outlined in chapter 5, the pH is less than normal. This eliminates choices A and C, because we know the patient is acidotic. Next, the $PaCO_2$ is greater than 45 mmHg, hence, we know that this is a respiratory acidosis. Finally, the HCO_3- is within the normal range, so there is no combined disorder or compensation as of yet. This is consistent with the short term/acute nature of the occurrence (immediately post-op).

36. A

The major side effects associated with the medication fenoldopam are the following: headache, reflex tachycardia, and hypokalemia. The other side effects listed are not associated with fenoldopan infusion. It should be noted that nitroprusside is considered the "gold standard" medication in the treatment of hypertensive crisis. Nitroprusside itself causes cyanide toxicity (blurred vision, confusion, tinnitus, and seizures); therefore, thiosulfate is added to these infusions. Thiosulfate converts cyanide into thiocyanate which is then excreted in the urine.

37. B

Administration of a fluid bolus will simply dilute the serum and possibly give a false lowered potassium level. Administering an antiarrhythmic will depress ventricular function which would actually potentially worsen a widened QRS and PR interval causing a life threatening arrhythmia such as cardiac standstill or ventricular fibrillation. Restricting fluid may actually concentrate the blood and increase the potassium level. All of these treatments will assist in either increasing excretion of potassium by the exchange of cations or binding the potassium.

38. B

Fever may indicate that the intestinal obstruction has progressed to necrotic bowel, sepsis, and/or perforation. Vomiting, constipation and sweating are expected with patients having an intestinal obstruction.

39. D

Twisting of a nipple is a peripheral pain stimulus, not a central pain stimulus. Answers A, B, and C are appropriate methods of administering a central painful stimulus.

40. C

This patient is highly complex with impaired resources and decreased ability to participate in self-care. The nurse uses system thinking and collaboration by contacting case management or social work for evaluation of the couple's situation. Answers A and B are not appropriate for meeting the patient's stated needs. Answer D is not an appropriate use of nursing time or skills and case management or social work are better prepared to assist the patient.

41. B

Only about 10 percent of the erythropoietin is manufactured in the liver. Bone marrow is the site of RBC production but not erythropoietin. Lungs play no role in the production of either erythropoietin or RBCs.

42. B

SIRS is widespread inflammation with accompanying tachycardia and fever. When it is accompanied by documented infection it is called sepsis.

43. B

A patient who has undergone post-cardiac catheterization is at risk for a retroperitoneal bleed after a transfemoral percutaneous coronary procedure. Blood loss in the retroperitoneal cavity causes severe back pain and a low hemoglobin and hematocrit. The dizziness is associated with a low blood pressure because of this blood loss into the retroperitoneal cavity. These two clinical manifestations are cardinal signs of a retroperitoneal bleed. A nurse priority is to monitor for potential complications of a transfemoral cannulation, which include bleeding or hematoma, retroperitoneal bleed, AV fistula, and psuedoaneurysm. A patient may experience back pain, especially if there is a history of back injury or pain, due to lying on his back for extended periods of time. However, dizziness should not accompany back pain. Administering an analgesic without further investigation is not safe practice in this scenario. Asking the patient to turn and/or lowering his head-of-bed are not addressing the problem.

44. C

The patient is demonstrating paradoxical chest wall movement after trauma. It is highly likely that he has multiple rib fractures in multiple places and has compromised the connection of the chest wall with the pleura. Hence, the chest wall is "sucked" into the thorax with the air when there is negative pressure generated by the intact chest wall. With pulmonary hemorrhage you would expect hemoptysis. Pneumothorax would be diagnosed by chest radiograph and an absence of breath sounds. There was no mention of the heart rhythm being irregularly irregular, hence atrial fibrillation is wrong.

45. D

Treatment of SIADH includes fluid restriction, administration of 3 percent saline, administration of Lasix, and potassium supplements as needed.

46. D

The nurse addresses the situation by indicating that the coworker does not understand the meaning of the request. Using caring practices, moral advocacy, responses to diversity, and clinical inquiry, the nurse works on behalf of the patient's family. She can also act as a facilitator of learning by educating the coworker regarding specific cultural issues. Answers A, B, and C are inappropriate responses to the coworkers concerns.

47. C

Using the Parkland Formula, 4 cc × %TBSA × weight in kg, one gets $4 \times 65 \times 40 = 10400$ cc over 24 hours. Fifty percent of this infuses over the first 8 hours and the rest is spread evenly over the next 16 hours.

48. D

A patient with congestive heart failure has a high preload and afterload with a decreased cardiac output. The goal of treatment is to decrease both preload and afterload and increase cardiac output. Therefore, all other options are incorrect.

49. A

Decreased urine output alone does not indicate injury to the kidneys. It may simply be the body's attempt to preserve water in a dehydrated state. Intermittent drops in mean blood pressure which are not sustained most likely will not cause ischemia, as the body responds with shifts in electrolytes or fluid to compensate. Systolic blood pressure alone is not a good indicator of ischemia, as the patient's normal BP may have a lower systolic BP. A sustained hypotensive episode greater than 40" will result in a decreased blood flow to the kidney and damage to the tubules. As tubules desecrate, renal damage occurs and the ability to filter successfully will decrease.

50. A

Patients who are experiencing acute rejection demonstrate signs and symptoms of acute liver failure including tachycardia, fever, jaundice, and elevated liver enzymes. The patient typically has dark urine which is indicative of bilirubin.

51. A

This patient is moderately resilient, moderately stable, can actively participate in his care, and needs to understand what "extubation" means. The nurse uses clinical judgment, caring practices, and facilitation of learning to provide needed information to the patient. In B, extubation of an awake and responsive patient without any preparation is not appropriate. Choice C may be appropriate for an agitated patient, but is not appropriate for this patient. Choice D is incorrect, since consent is not required to extubate patients.

52. A

The use of oral contraceptive medications is a known risk factor for the development of a deep vein thrombosis. The other medications listed—ASA, vitamin, and PPI—have not been found to increase the risk of a DVT.

53. A

Nuchal rigidity is a clinical manifestation of meningeal irritation in which rigidity of neck muscles limits movement of the neck, including preventing its flexion. Homan's sign is the dorsiflexion of the foot that elicits pain in posterior calf and is considered positive for DVT. Babinski's reflex indicates pyramidal tract damage, an alteration in the motor tracts of the brain. Flaccid paralysis is a clinical manifestation characterized by weakness or paralysis and reduced muscle tone without other obvious cause.

54. A

Partial thickness or second-degree burns are very painful, as the nerve endings are exposed when the dermis is burned off. Body image would not be the highest priority. Four days post-burn, airway maintenance and fluid volume management are not an issue in a patient with a burn to the hand.

55. D

Patients who evidence DIC will most likely have decreased coagulation factors due to the overuse of the coagulation cascade. Therefore, platelet count and fibrinogen levels will be decreased. D-dimer is an indication of hypercoagulability. Choice D, elevated PT and PTT, is indicative of a bleeding disorder.

56. A

Choice A provides the correct steps in the determination of hepatojugular reflux. This assessment indicates right-sided heart failure.

57. A

The objective of treatment is to prevent dehydration and electrolyte imbalances.

58. D

The patient is presenting with a COPD exacerbation. He should receive bronchodilator therapy via nebulizer or inhaler, steroids for airway inflammation, antibiotics, chest radiograph, and cultures prior to antibiotic administration for an infectious work-up. The wrong answer choices are not complete.

59. B

The most frequent clinical symptoms associated with hypocalcemia are Chvostek's or Trousseau's symptoms which are primarily those of a muscular irritability. Hypercalcemia will result in the opposite symptoms, those of muscular depression or weakness and those of apathy. Obtundation is an advanced clinical symptom of a neurological disorder which includes a decrease in consciousness and mental abilities. Thirst is a symptom initiated by the hypothalamus indicating a dehydrated fluid state in the body.

60. A

Lactulose reduces the pH of the intestine and helps the body decrease ammonia levels. It has no action on bilirubin level or urine output.

61. B

Sleeping at the bedside is a coping mechanism when families feel powerless. Answers A, C, and D are methods of avoiding a situation where families feel helpless and powerless.

62. D

The primary cause of cardiac tamponade is myocardial contusion secondary to chest compressions. Performing a pericardial window or pericardiocentesis is the treatment for cardiac tamponade with hemodynamic compromise. Removal of the extra blood or fluid in the pericardial space is not accomplished by cardiac surgery, cardiac catheterization, or echocardiogram. Normally, the pericardial cavity contains between 15–50 ml pericardial fluids. The medical term for an excess of pericardial fluid in this cavity is called pericardial effusion, which is diagnosed by echocardiogram.

63. C

Cerebrospinal fluid is reabsorbed by the arachnoid villi and drains into the venous sinuses. The lateral ventricle is where the CSF circulates. The dura mater is the fibrous membrane that lines the interior of the skull. The subarachnoid cisterns are expanded areas of the subarachnoid space.

64. C

Calcium in the intravascular space is either protein bound or circulating in the ionized state. If the patient has an elevated or a decreased albumin, the serum calcium may be falsely affected. Therefore it is important to evaluate the albumin level to ascertain the amount of bound calcium. The electrolytes sodium and potassium will not impact calcium level significantly. The hematocrit and hemoglobin levels impact the oxygen-carrying capacity of the blood.

65. D

Uremic syndrome is a condition which results from renal failure where the patient continues to ingest water and inappropriate food intake (e.g., high in salt) and impairment of renal failure is extensive. The three categories of acute renal failure are prerenal, intrarenal and postrenal. Therefore, the answer is D, which is not a category of renal failure but a stage of ATN.

66. D

The nurse is using systems thinking and collaboration by making sure that the patient is safe and by working with the appropriate department to assure that equipment is functioning properly. In choice A, resetting a malfunctioning alarm does not solve the problem and puts patient safety at risk. Choices B and C are incorrect, since the physician cannot repair equipment and the FDA only takes reports but does not repair or replace malfunctioning equipment.

67. C

All three actions are appropriate. Critically ill patients need DVT prophylaxis; to prevent skin breakdown they must be repositioned as tolerated and feeding through a nasoenteral tube is usually well-tolerated. Speech therapy is needed after the patient is extubated to evaluate swallowing; nutrition is an integral part of treatment in septic patients; and vital signs need to be monitored much more frequently than each shift. Physical therapy could be consulted to provide passive range of motion exercises.

68. B

Ascites may cause dyspnea and respiratory depression. All the other choices are to be expected and not potentially life-threatening.

69. A

Choice A describes a pneumothroax that meets the criteria of at least 2 cm of air between the chest wall and lateral border of lung parenchyma. Choice B describes the observation/test for asthma. Choice C describes most likely atrial fibrillation and may indicate initiation of anticoagulation, but not a needle thoracostomy of chest tube. Finally, Choice D describes symptoms that would be consistent with pneumonia, and again, does not require a needle thoracostomy or chest tube.

70. D

Functions of the frontal lobe include thought, reasoning, behavior, memory, smell, and movement. Hearing and sensation are functions of the parietal lobe. Vision is processed in the occipital lobe.

71. B

Lortab® is an opioid and may cause decreased gastric motility. All the other choices are permissible.

72. A

A patient in hemorrhagic shock will experience hypotension, since there is less circulating blood volume resulting from blood loss. Less circulating blood causes a low central venous pressure (CVP). A rapid loss of blood volume leads to sympathetic compensation by peripheral constriction, tachycardia, and increased myocardial contractility. A low cardiac output and blood pressure with a normal heart rate do not indicate compensation. A normal cardiac output with a low blood pressure is indicative of septic shock.

73. D

Calcitonin is manufactured in special thyroid cells called parafollicular cells or C cells.

74. D

All but D are correct with regard to leukemia. Patients are at a higher risk for infection.

75. C

An aortic dissection is a tear in the wall of the aorta that causes blood flow between the layers of the arterial wall (intima, media, and tunica adventitia) and forces the layers apart. A false lumen is created. Some organs are perfused by the true lumen and others are perfused by the false lumen. Hypertension is not only the cause of this condition, but it also contributes to further tearing. Rupture and massive blood loss can occur if the tear occurs through all layers of the aorta. For this reason, the top priority for a patient suffering from this condition is blood pressure control. Distal circulation and absence of neurologic symptoms are other real concerns. For this reason, A and D are incorrect. While it is important to monitor renal laboratory values to ascertain kidney perfusion, it is not a top nursing priority of care.

76. A

Pneumomediatinum is what the patient currently has and is not an emergency. She likely developed air in this space when she suffered the pneumothorax, although you cannot be sure. Either way she is hemodynamically stable and the air collection in the mediastinum in this scenario is benign. Inserting the chest tube further or removing it may compromise the patient's status. Again, the patient is stable and not in respiratory distress, so she does not need BiPAP.

77. B

This patient is highly complex, vulnerable, and has a decreased ability to participate in self-care. The nurse with the most experience will demonstrate to him and his a high level of clinical competence, caring practices, and systems thinking that can win their trust. Choice A may not have ever taken care of a patient with a balloon-pump. Choice C would not have the level of skills to demonstrate clinical competence. Choice D is not appropriate if the only reason is because the patients would be next to each other.

78. A

The most commonly ordered study used to evaluate renal trauma patients is the CT of the abdomen which views the retroperitoneal region as well. A chest x-ray is a simple film which will give only basic information about the lungs and bone structure. A rib fracture may cause injury to the kidney, so the chest x-ray will demonstrate the fracture but will not define the damage to the kidney. IVPs evaluate urine filtration and internal tissues. This exam may be used at a later date to evaluate or stage an injury. A renal arteriogram evaluates the arterial blood flow in the kidneys. This may be premature in the evaluation of a patient with no initial clinical evidence of bleeding.

79. C

Increasing lactic acid is most likely indicative of inadequate tissue oxygenation and perfusion. Lactic acid levels should fall with adequate resuscitation—not rise. Elevations in lactic acid may also be seen in patients with metabolic disorders such as diabetic ketoacidosis.

80. D

The three precipitating factors of deep venous thrombosis are known as Virchow's triad and include venous stasis, injury to the endothelium, and hypercoagulable states. Malignancy can serve as a hypercoagulable state due to a paraneoplastic syndrome that is not specific to any particular malignancy. Hemophilia is a condition where patients are at risk for bleeding due to a deficiency in one of the coagulation factors (Factor VIII), so these patients have the exact opposite problems and are anticoagualted.

81. B

In volume control, the ventilator is set to control the tidal volume of each breath received by the patient. The PEEP and respiratory rate will also be set. The current belief is that this mode of ventilation is beneficial because the physician can set a low tidal volume and prevent large volume from being drawn in by the patient. Referred to as low volume ventilation, it is believed to minimize volutrauma in the lungs of ventilated patients.

82. C

The purpose of the CSF is to absorb shock and cushion the brain and spinal cord. Oxygen is transported in the blood vessels. Neurotransmitters are manufactured and released by the neurons. Cerebral perfusion pressure is maintained by autoregulation, chemo-metabolic factors, and intrinsic/extrinsic neurogenic factors.

83. C

Thyroid storm symptoms include hyperthermia, tachycardia, diarrhea, dehydration, diaphoresis, agitation, tremors, delirium, and stupor/coma. Further, exophtalmos is a sign of hyperthyroidism.

84. B

Treatment of thyroid storm is in support of vital functions and reversal of the peripheral effects, with IV propranolol (Inderal®). This will block the peripheral effects of circulating thyroid hormone.

85. B

Arterial occlusion symptoms include white, color, painful, and pulseless extremity. Venous occlusion symptoms include cyanotic, warm, red, painful, and edematous extremity. You can remember this by recalling the three P's: pale, pulseless, and painful.

86. C

The nurse is using advocacy/moral agency since one parent cannot limit the other parent's visitation rights unless court-ordered. Since it is likely that the baby will have a relatively short lifespan, it is important that the mother be allowed to visit if that is her desire. Choice A is not appropriate. Choice B should be offered to the parents first and if that is their choice, then done. Choice D is not appropriate; a picture should be taken for both parents to have for future viewing.

87. C

Billroth II procedure includes anastomosis of the gastric remnant to the jejunum. The other answer choices are incorrect. When such situations arise, there also may be a moral dilemma, as the patient may not fully understand the operation. Hence, notifying the physician in such cases is also appropriate.

88. B

Sensory input is integrated in the parietal lobe. Hearing is processed in the temporal lobe. Vision is the primary function of the occipital lobe. Voluntary motor control occurs in the frontal lobe.

89. C

Eighty percent of all premature infants develop jaundice. Newborns of women with type O or Rh negative blood should have serum bilirubin levels checked. Urinalysis, hemoglobin, and hematocrit are not checked routinely prior to discharge.

90. D

A toddler's head and neck are 18 percent, and an arm, including the hand, 9 percent. Added together, it comes to 27 percent.

91. D

The intra-aortic radiopaqued tip should be located at the two to three intercostal space on x-ray. The IABP catheter can migrate higher in the aorta and occlude the subclavian artery causing a loss in the left arm pulses. This is the reason it is important to assess and document the left arm pulse presence besides the assessment of the pulse in the affected leg. All of the other options (A–C) are not urgent findings that require immediate intervention.

92. B

The two primary pathways in the coagulation cascade are the intrinsic and extrinsic pathways. The intrinsic pathway is initiated when there is endothelium damage and the collagen released comes in contact with factor XII. The extrinsic pathway is when tissue trauma occurs and factor III is released from the damaged tissues and comes in contact with factor VII circulating in the blood. It is called the common pathway. The erythropoietin mechanism is the cascade which precipitates the production of red blood cells when tissue oxygenation occurs. Hypercoagulability is the condition where the normal mechanisms of hemostasis are disrupted and the blood clots inappropriately.

93. B

In this stage of ATN the patient may excrete up to four liters of fluid per day. If the fluid is not replaced as needed, the patient may become dehydrated and electrolyte levels may increase. Restricting fluid intake would only further compound the problem. In addition, administering hypertonic solution may cause a shift from the intracellular space to the intravascular space for a temporary period of time, though as a long-term treatment would worsen the condition. Diuretic therapy is not indicated, as the kidneys are appropriately filtering.

94. A

Gastroesophageal reflux has been associated with AOP, despite the fact that the exact etiology behind AOP is not fully known. Since the question stem does not indicate respiratory distress, invasive ventilation and NPPV are not indicated. As a matter of fact, the treatment that has found to be instrumental is simply supplemental oxygen delivery.

95. D

Initial treatment of patient should be administration of Vitamin K to attempt to reverse the effect of the Coumadin®. The patient's lab studies do not justify administration of RBCs or FFP, since he is not supratherapeutic or actively bleeding—at least that you know of. Cryoprecipitate is not indicated in this situation. It is important that the lab values, such as hemoglobin, in these patients always be compared to previous admissions to determine how far off their baseline is to their current value. It is NOT uncommon for such patients to have anemia, possibly from hemolysis or chronic disease, etc.

96. D

Anaphylactic shock, chronic renal failure and gram-negative sepsis are not common in patients with isolated inhalation injuries. Patients with inhalation injuries are at increased risk of developing bronchopneumonia.

97. C

Treat the problem. Continued assessment of blood pressure or oxygen level will not help the patient. Giving pain medication may decrease respirations more.

98. A

Parathormone stimulation occurs in response to a decreased serum calcium level.

99. A

Quite some time ago, the most common cause of chronic renal failure was glomerulonephritis due to undetected infections which caused renal damage. In more recent times, diabetes has overtaken this condition as the primary cause of chronic renal failure. Thrombosis is not common, but does occur. Sepsis is often the cause of acute renal failure.

100. A

A stroke in the left hemisphere causes aphasia, intellectual impairment, right visual field defects, and slow/cautious behavior. Right hemisphere stroke symptoms include spatial-perceptual deficits, left side neglect, impulsive behavior, and left visual deficits. Stroke in the pons impairs respiratory control. Lesions of the cerebellum cause an inability to coordinate voluntary muscle movement, altered equilibrium, and trunk instability.

101. A

When patients and families are unable speak English, they are considered fragile in terms of vulnerability and can have limited resources available to them. The nurse needs to respond to diversity and systems-think to develop proactive strategies for the patient and family. The most effective method of communicating is by using a translation service. Relying on a family member, ancillary staff, or a communication board are not the most effective methods of communicating. Note also that the patient's family is not English-speaking in this scenario.

102. B

Decorticate posture is flexion of the elbows, extension of the knees, and plantar flexion of the feet. Decerebrate posture is extension of elbows and knees, plantar flexion of feet, and flexion of the wrists. Flexion of both upper and lower extremity position and the extension of upper extremities and flexion of lower extremity positions are used by physical therapists in rehabilitation of injuries.

103. C

Abrupt onset of shortness of breath, chest pain, murmur, and acute development of signs and symptoms of congestive heart failure (due to mitral valve insufficiency) are associated with the development of a papillary muscle rupture. Chest pain and holosystolic murmur manifestations are associated with the development of a perforated ventricular septum, which is another major complication post-myocardial infarction.

104. D

The patient needs to receive supplemental oxygen as the initial treatment for AOP. If this fails, then CPAP can be considered. Further, since gastroesophageal reflux is strongly associated with AOP, it is prudent to treat for this condition as well. It could be argued that you should monitor for this prior to treatment, but the reality is that infants are unable to communicate the subjective complaints of GER, so empiric treatment is acceptable.

105. A

The Fowler's position allows the patient to relax the abdominal muscles and breathe more easily. Rest with the head in the upright position after meals. Coughing or lying supine (flat) will increase indigestion following meals. Checking the oxygen saturation should be done after positioning the patient upright.

106. B

The initiation of the renin-angiotensin-aldosterone cascade stimulates the sympathetic nerve activation. This must be stimulated by the reduction of arterial blood flow to the kidneys and may be the result of prerenal conditions such as hypovolemia. Electrolyte abnormalities do not stimulate this cascade. Initiation of the renin-angiotensin-aldosterone cascade actually causes the release of aldosterone, which further retains water and sodium.

107. D

Symptoms of hypothyroidism includes edema of face, puffiness of eyes, thickened lips, dry and scaly skin, hair loss, altered mentation, weakness, sensitivity to cold, and paresthesia of fingers.

108. C

Since the son desires to participate in his father's care, it is important for the nurse to act as a facilitator of learning and provide adequate opportunities to successfully demonstrate the skill. The best intervention is choice C. Choices A, B, and D will not provide this opportunity and are not appropriate.

109. C

The patient who is evidencing organ rejection would have lab values demonstrating potential renal insufficiency. A or B would be indicative of appropriate renal function. In organ rejection scenarios, the platelet count would most likely decrease; therefore, D is also incorrect.

110. D

The string of data does not support cardiogenic or septic shock or MODS. SIRS is characterized by an increased temperature and heart rate with no documented signs of infection.

111. A

Cardioversion is performed in hopes of converting the abnormal supraventricular rhythm back to normal by delivering low energy joules. Defibrillation and an AICD are not necessary, since the heart is not fibrillating and has narrow QRS complexes. Pacing is not required, because the rhythm is not bradycardic.

112. D

In metabolic acidosis, the pH and bicarbonate should both be low. If it is acute then the carbon dioxide will be about normal since there has not been any time for compensation. The other answers are wrong because:

A. pH 7.55, pCO_2 32, pO_2 75, HCO_3- 24
   Respiratory Alkalosis

B. pH 7.50, pCO_2 45, pO_2 73, HCO_3- 30
   Metabolic Alkalosis

C. pH 7.30, pCO_2 55, pO_2 67, HCO_3- 28
   Respiratory Acidosis

113. C

The string of data shows the liver, kidneys, and bone marrow failing. The values in answer A are all within normal limits. Answer B has a normal Glasgow coma score, and answer D is related to the pulmonary system.

114. A

Histamine is one of the clinical mediators which is stimulated in allergic reactions. Interleukin and tumor necrosis factors are cytokines unrelated to the allergic response. Interferon is a natural protein released when viral exposure occurs.

115. D

This child has moderate levels of vulnerability and susceptibility, given the cardiac condition described. By understanding the pathophysiology of patent ductus arteriosus, the nurse can determine the correct diagnostic findings associated with this disorder. The nurse uses a moderate level of clinical judgment by collecting and interpreting patient data and then making appropriate clinical decisions. Choice A's findings are consistent with an atrial septal defect. Choice B's findings are consistent with a ventricular septal defect. Choice C's findings are consistent with endocardial cushion defect.

116. B

This ECG change is associated with hypokalemia. Hyperkalemia produces peaked ST segments. No specific ECG changes are associated with sodium disturbances.

117. A

The development of bronchopulmonary dysplasia is associated with RDS of infancy and mechanical ventilation. The other conditions have not been associated with bronchopulmonary dysplasia.

118. B

Patients should be instructed to lie down and use this medication at first sign of chest discomfort. However, simply lying down and elevating the patient's legs is not enough. Chest pain relief usually occurs within five minutes of taking sublingual nitroglycerin. Patients can take up to three sublingual tablets every 5 minutes over 15 minutes. Because this patient's chest discomfort is unrelieved and continues to have an acceptable blood pressure, the administration of another sublingual nitrate may resolve the chest discomfort. If the chest discomfort continues after three sublingual tablets, then the patient should go immediately to an emergency room. Although, knowing the ECG would be helpful, more important is that the patient continues to have chest pain with an acceptable blood pressure.

119. B

This family is vulnerable and feeling powerless. The nurse uses compassion to assess the family's concerns and then act as a facilitator of learning by teaching them about the monitor and what the numbers of concern mean. Choices A and C are vague and do not address the family's concerns. Choice D is not appropriate.

120. B

This is an expected finding and should be assessed prior to applying the umbilical clamp.

121. B

The primary goal in the early management of SCI is to minimize the extent of spinal cord damage and prevent secondary injury with the administration of high-dose intravenous (IV) methylprednisolone. Patient-transfer stretcher to bed is part of care, not a management goal. Reduction of cervical swelling does not treat the entire spine. The patient is kept flat and the head is not elevated.

122. C

Presenting signs and symptoms of myxedema coma include: hypothermia, hypoventilation, hypotension, bradycardia, hyporeflexia, hyponatremia, and generalized interstitial edema. Normalization of body temperature is the treatment goal and occurs in response to pharmacologic treatment. Hypoventilation increases $PaCO_2$ levels and the treatment goal is to decrease $PaCO_2$ levels. The treatment goal for bradycardia is to increase the heart rate not reduce it. Alterations in pH are not a component of myxedema coma.

123. A

A major side effect of Natrecor® is hypotension. Oftentimes, a fluid bolus is given before starting this medication. If hypotension occurs after the start of this medication, Trendelenburg or an IV fluid bolus may be ordered. The half-life of Natrecor® is 18 minutes; therefore, hypotension may last for hours.

124. A

Brown-Sequard syndrome is transection of half of the spinal cord with motor paralysis and loss of vibration and position sense on the ipsilateral (same) side of the injury and contralateral (opposite) side loss of pain and temperature sense. Cauda equina syndrome results from injuries below L1–L2 with compression of the cauda equina. Motor, sensory, bowel/bladder and sexual dysfunction may vary. Central cord syndrome presents with upper extremity weakness greater than lower extremity weakness. Conus medullaris syndrome is sometimes used to describe a condition similar to cauda equina syndrome.

125. D

Before setting up mandatory in-services or competency review changes, the best first step should be to meet with the surgeon and identify all of the issues. Meeting with the surgeon shows a high level of collaboration.

126. C

High fat meals stimulate bile to be excreted from the gallbladder into the duodenum.

127. B

The task force may not be aware of the importance of the NICU environment on developmental care and may be using other criteria to determine the layout. By presenting research studies to the group, the nurse is demonstrating a high level of collaboration. This action allows the task force to collaborate and take all logistical, cost, and clinical issues into consideration. Choice A bypasses the task force completely. Choices C and D may alienate the task force and are not appropriate.

128. C

Thrombocytopenia is a low platelet count. The patient should be transfused for platelet counts <50,000 when there is evidence of bleeding. Whole blood does contain platelets, however for simple thrombocytopenia it is not recommended. The indication for FFP is a need for clotting factors. RBCs are given for anemia.

129. B

Glasgow Coma Score was developed to assess brain injury. A GCS less than 8 indicates a significant brain injury. A patient who is brain dead would have a GCS of 3.

130. B

A hood is more likely to be used to deliver oxygen in infants, neonate, and pediatric patients because they may have trouble with the face mask or face tent. Where the latter can easily be used in adults with appropriate instruction, a hood is not necessary in adults. However, the patient population in the question is more amenable to a hood when high levels of FiO_2 are necessary.

131. A

Aldosterone is secreted in the zona glomerulosa.

132. D

Any condition that results in reduced blood flow to the kidneys may be considered prerenal. All of the responses except ureter obstruction could potentially reduce blood flow to the kidneys. That would be a postrenal condition.

133. D

Croup has a variety of causes. The most common are viral. However, there are rare but serious and preventable causes such as diphtheria, Haemophilus influenzae type B (Hib), and measles. Thus, keeping immunizations up-to-date will help. So Croup is preventable, and antibiotics have no role as prophylaxis. Obviously, infants are the age group in whom croup occurs.

134. D

Natrecor® causes venous and arterial dilation. A false increase in BNP is normal for a patient receiving the medication Natrecor®. This is an important consideration if asked to obtain a BNP level on a patient who is receiving this medication for congestive heart failure. Natrecor® has no effect on contractility.

135. B

Cyanosis is most evident in the mucous membranes of older adults. The color of the sclera does not indicate decreased perfusion; skin color is difficult to assess, especially if the patient has dark skin; nail beds may have ridges, fungal infections and yellowing in older patients—therefore they are not good choices.

136. C

Nail bed pressure elicits a peripheral response. Sternal rub, trapezius muscle squeeze, and mandibular pressure elicit a central response.

137. C

The normal BUN to creatinine ratio is less than 20:1. In this situation, the ratio is 28:1 which is strongly indicative of dehydration consistent with his history of nausea and vomiting and the normal creatinine level. The elevated potassium and hematocrit could also result from a dehydration state. It is unlikely that he developed acute renal failure as a result of dehydration over a few days, although a prerenal condition leading to ATN and acute renal failure is hypovolemia.

138. C

Normal ALT and AST should be below 40 units/L.

139. A

Hyperpigmentation occurs in 92 percent of patients with adrenal insufficiency.

140. C

The precursor for all blood cells is the pluripotential stem cell. The other cells listed are the final formations of either white blood cells or red blood cells.

141. C

The nurse is demonstrating facilitation of learning by assessing the daughter's overall level of knowledge and skills prior to planning for teaching sessions. Choices A, B, and D may be used after identifying the daughter's learning needs.

142. C

Nephrotoxicity is a common complication of therapy with aminoglycocides like gentamycin. Hematocrit, prothrombin time and carbon dioxide levels are not affected by gentamycin.

143. B

Concurrent use of antiarrhythmic agents is necessary to decrease the frequency of events. All the other statement choices are evidence that the patient understands information that was taught pertaining to his device.

144. A

The glomerulus serves as the first structure within the nephron as a high pressure capillary bed to filter the blood. The afferent arteriole brings the blood to the glomerulus at a higher pressure than the exiting efferent arteriole. Ions are involved in absorption, secretion and excretion in the proximal and distal tubules and loop of Henle. Glucose is regulated by insulin production in the pancreas not the kidneys. Specific gravity of the urine is indicative of concentration of urine which is collected in the bladder. This filtrate is the final product of kidney functions, not initial filtration.

145. C

Addison's disease is chronic dysfunction of the adrenal glands, resulting in adrenal insufficiency.

146. D

Status epilepticus is either continuous seizures lasting more than five minutes or two or more different seizures with incomplete recovery of consciousness between them. They are not controlled. There is no time-frame in duration or occurrence of status epilepticus. There is no escalation of seizure intensity.

147. D

A, B, and C are all appropriate protective processes for the patient. There is a potential for bacterial infestation in uncooked fruits and vegetables, which the patient should not be exposed to.

148. D

Grey-Turner's sign (bruising in the lower abdomen and flank) indicates retroperitoneal hemorrhage. This patient is most at risk for shock or early changes. Murphy's sign is expected in gallbladder disease. Many normal people exhibit Chvostek's sign (contraction of the facial muscles with light tapping on the facial nerve). Blood on rectal exam is not an emergent condition in a patient with hepatitis with no other indicators of a problem.

149. B

At no cost should an impaled object from a penetrating trauma be removed unless the patient has received indicated diagnostic imaging and is in the operating room where emergent surgical exploration can be conducted. Hence, choices A and D are clearly wrong. Choice C should never be considered. Manipulating an impaled object in any way can result in increased damage to internal organs, as well as acute decomposition. Further, choice C is simply not reasonable or logical.

150. B

This infant is highly vulnerable and has low levels of stability and resiliency. The infant is highly susceptible, fragile, and labile due to severe dehydration. The nurse is using clinical judgment to prioritize the infant's care. Obtaining vascular access and starting fluid replacement is the most important intervention at this time. Choice A is not required for this infant since breathing and airway are adequate at this time. Choices C and D may be required later, but rehydration is the most important goal at this time.

Resources

Chapter 4

Alspach, J. *Core Curriculum for Critical Care Nursing, Chapter 2, The Cardiovascular System.* 5th Edition, Philadelphia: W.B. Saunders, 137–338, 1998.

Furukawa, K., Motomura, T., & Nose, Y. Right ventricular failure left ventricular assist device implantation: The need for an implantable right ventricular assist device. *Artificial Organs.* 29(5), 369–377, 2005.

Guyton, A. & Hall, J. *Textbook of Medical Physiology,* 11th Edition.Philadelphia: Elsevier Saunders, 1998.

Hailey, L. Theraputic Hypothermia after Cardiac Arrest. Retrieved 4/12/08 from *http://www.cardiology.utmb.edu/slides/sec-2-clinical/theraputic%20hypothermia%20after%20cardiac%20arrest_03.pdf.*

Lewis, R., & Mabie, W., Biventricular assist device as a bridge to cardiac transplantation in the treatment of peripartum cardiomyopathy. *Southern Medical Journal.* 90(9), 1997.

Shinn, J. Implantable left ventricular assist devices. *Journal of Cardiovascular Nursing.* 20(55), 522–530, 2005.

Thelan, L., Lough, M., Urden, L., & Stacey, K. *Critical Care Nursing: Diagnosis and Management, Unit 3, Cardiovascular Alterations,* 3rd Edition. St. Louis: Mosby, 1998.

TMR (Transmyocardial Laser Revascularization). Cleveland Clinic–Heart & Vascular Institute. Retrieved 4/12/08 from *http://www.clevlandclinic.org/heartcenter/pub/guide/disease/cad/TMR.htm.*

Walkes, J., Smythe, W. & Reardon, M. *Cardiac Surgery in the Adult, Chapter 63: Cardiac Neoplasms.* New York: McGraw Hill, 1479–1510, 2008.

Chapter 6

Alspach, J. (Ed.). (2006). *AACN core curriculum for critical care nursing.* (6th ed.). St. Louis: Saunders.

American Diabetes Association. (2007). Standards for medical care in diabetes—2007. *Diabetes Care.* 30[Supp 1]: S4–S41.

Benner, Z. (2006). Management of hyperglycemic emergencies. *AACN Clinical Issues.* 17(1): 56–65.

Chulay, M. & Burns, S. (2006). *AACN essentials of critical care nursing.* New York: McGraw-Hill.

Ganong, W. (2005). *Review of medical physiology.* (22nd ed.). New York: McGraw-Hill.

Gearhart, M. & Parbhoo, S. (2006). Hyperglycemia in the critically ill patient. *AACN Clinical Issues.* 17(1): 50–55.

Guller, U., Turek, J., Eubanks, S., DeLong, E., Oertli, D. & Feldman, J. (2006). Detecting pheochromocytoma: Defining the most sensitive test. *Annals of Surgery.* 243(1): 102–107.

Kaplow, R. & Hardin, S. (2007). *Critical care nursing: Synergy for optimal outcomes.* Boston: Jones & Bartlett.

Kitabchi, A. & Nyenwe, E. (2006). Hyperglycemic crises in diabetes mellitus: diabetic ketoacidosis and hyperglycemic hyperosmolar state. *Endocrinology and Metabolism Clinics of North America.* 35: 725–751.

Johnson, K. & Renn, C. (2006). The hypothalamic-pituitary-adrenal axis in critical illness. *AACN Clinical Issues.* 17(1): 39–49.

Singer, P. & Sevilla, L. (2003). Postoperative endocrine management of pituitary tumors. *Neurosurgery Clinics of North America.* 14: 123–138.

Sole, M., Klein, D., & Moseley, M. (2005). *Introduction to critical care nursing.* (4th ed.). St. Louis: Saunders.

Urden, L., Stacy, K., & Lough, M. (2003). *Priorities in critical care nursing.* (4th ed.). St. Louis: Mosby.

Utz, A., Swearingen, B., & Biller, B. (2005). Pituitary surgery and postoperative management in Cushing's disease. *Endocrinology and Metabolism Clinics of North America.* 34: 459–478.

Wartofsky, L. (2006). Myxedema coma. *Endocrinology and Metabolism Clinics of North America.* 35: 687–698.

Weeks, B. (2005). Graves' disease: The importance of early diagnosis. *The Nurse Practitioner.* 30(11): 34–47.

Chapter 7

AACN Core Curriculum for Critical Care Nursing, 5th Edition. Philadelphia: W.B. Saunders Company, 1998.

Guyton, A. C. & Hall, J.E. Renal physiology. In A.C. Guyton and J.E. Hill. Unit VI: Blood Cells, Immunity and Blood Clotting. In A.C. Guyton & J.E. Hill, Textbook of Medical Physiology, 11th Edition. Philadelphia: W.B. Saunders, 419–467, 2006.

Chapter 8

Albano, C., Commandante, L., & Nolan, S. (2005). Innovations in the management of cerebral injury. *Critical Care Nursing Quarterly*. 28(2): 135–149.

Alspach, J. (Ed.). (2006). *AACN core curriculum for critical care nursing*. (6th ed.). St. Louis: Saunders.

Atkinson, S., Carr, R., Maybee, P., & Haynes, D. (2006). The challenges of managing and treating Guillain-Barré syndrome during the acute phase. *Dimensions of Critical Care Nursing*. 25: 256–263.

Bader, M. & Littlejohns, L. (2004). *AANN core curriculum for neuroscience nursing*. (4th ed.). St. Louis: Saunders.

Choi, J & Mohr, J. (2005). Brain arteriovenous malformations in adults. *Lancet Neurology*, 4: 299–308.

Chulay, M. & Burns, S. (2006). *AACN essentials of critical care nursing*. New York: McGraw-Hill.

Estep, M. (2005). Meningococcal meningitis in critical care: An overview. *Critical Care Nursing Quarterly*. 28(2): 111–121.

Fowler, S. & Mancini, B. (2007). Predictive value of biochemical markers of stroke. *Journal of Neuroscience Nursing*. 39: 58–60.

Freeborn, K. (2005). The importance of maintaining spinal precautions. *Critical Care Nursing Quarterly*. 28(2): 195–199.

Ganong, W. (2005). *Review of medical physiology*. (22nd ed.). New York: McGraw-Hill.

Haines, D. (2004). *Neuroanatomy: An atlas of structures, sections, and systems*. Philadelphia: Lippincott Williams & Wilkins.

Hanel, R., Demetrius, K. & Wehman, J. (2005). Endovascular treatment of intracranial aneurysms and vasospasm after aneurysmal subarachnoid hemorrhage. *Neurosurgical Clinics of North America*. 16:317–353.

Hickey, J. (2008). *The clinical practice of neurological and neurosurgical nursing*. (6th ed.). Philadelphia: Lippincott Williams & Wilkins.

Kaplow, R. & Hardin, S. (2007). *Critical care nursing: Synergy for optimal outcomes*. Boston: Jones & Bartlett.

Kosty, T. (2005). Cerebral vasospasm after subarachnoid hemorrhage. *Critical Care Nursing Quarterly.* 28(2): 122–134.

Mortimer, D. & Jancik, J. (2006). Administering hypertonic saline to patients with severe traumatic brain injury. *Journal of Neuroscience Nursing.* 38: 142–146.

Oyama, K. & Criddle, L. (2004). Vasospasm after aneurismal subarachnoid hemorrhage. *Critical Care Nurse.* 24(5):58–67.

Presciutti, M. (2006). Nursing priorities in caring for patients with intracerebral hemorrhage. *Journal of Neuroscience Nursing.* 38 [Supp 4]: 296–299, 315.

Rossetti, A., Logroscino, G., Liaudet, L., Ruffieux, C. et al. (2007). Status epilepticus. *Neurology.* 69: 255–260.

Sheerin, F. (2005). Spinal cord injury: Acute care management. *Emergency Nurse.* 12 (10): 26–34.

Sole, M., Klein, D., & Moseley, M. (2005). *Introduction to critical care nursing.* (4th ed.). St. Louis: Saunders.

Urden, L., Stacy, K., & Lough, M. (2003). *Priorities in critical care nursing.* (4th ed.). St. Louis: Mosby.

Chapter 9

Bickley, L. S. (1999). *Bates Guide to Physical Examination and History Taking.* 7th ed. Philadelphia: Lippincott.

Black, J. M., Hawks, J. H., & Keene, A. M. (2001). *Medical-Surgical Nursing.* 6th ed. Philadelphia: Saunders.

Brozenec, S. A. & Russell, S. S. (1999). *Core Curriculum for Medical-Surgical Nursing.* 2nd ed. New Jersey: Academy of Medical-Surgical Nurses.

Bucher, L. & Melander, S. (1999). *Critical Care Nursing.* Philadelphia: W. B. Saunders.

Fischbach, F. & Dunning, M. B. (2004). *A Manual of Laboratory and Diagnostic Tests.* 7th ed. Philadelphia: Lippincott Williams & Wilkins.

Ignatavicius, D. D. & Workman, M. L. (2002). *Medical-Surgical Nursing.* 4th ed. Philadelphia: W. B. Saunders.

Kidd, P. S. & Wagner, K. D. (2001). *High Acuity Nursing.* 3rd. ed. New Jersey: Prentice Hall.

Lilley, L. L., Harrington, S., & Snyder, J. S. (2005). *Pharmacology and the Nursing Process.* 4th ed. St. Louis, MO: Mosby/Elsevier.

London, M. L., Ladewig, P. W., Ball, J. W., & Bindler, R. C. (2007). *Maternal & Child Nursing Care.* 2nd ed. New Jersey: Pearson/Prentice Hall.

Mims, B. C., Toto, K. H. & Luecke, L. E. (1996). *Critical Care Skills: A Clinical Handbook.* Philadelphia: Saunders.

McNally, P. (2001). *GI/Liver Secrets.* 2nd ed. Philadelphia: Hanley & Belfus/Elsevier.

Pagana, K. & Pagana, T. (2005). *Mosby's Manual of Diagnostic and Laboratory Tests.* 3rd ed. St. Louis, MO: Mosby/Elsevier.

Skidmore-Roth, L. (2004). *Mosby's 2004 Nursing Drug Reference.* St. Louis, MO: Mosby/Elsevier.

Smeltzer, S. & Bare, B. G. (2003). *Brunner and Suddarth's Textbook of Medical-Surgical Nursing.* 10th ed. Philadelphia: Lippincott Williams & Wilkins.

Sole, M. L., Hartshorn, J., & Lamborne, M. L. (2001). *Introduction to Critical Care Nursing.* 3rd ed. Philadelphia: W. B. Saunders/Elsevier.

Sommers, M. S., Johnson, S. A., & Berry, T. A. (2007). *Diseases and Disorders.* 3rd. ed. Philadelphia: F. A. Davis.

Stillwell, S. (2002). *Mosby's Critical Care Nursing References.* 3rd ed. St. Louis, MO: Mosby/Elsevier.

Tucker, S. M., Canobbio, M. M., Paquette, E. V., & Wells, M. F. (2000). *Patient Care Standards.* 7th ed. St. Louis: Mosby.

Urden, L., Lough, M. E., Stacy, K. L. (2005). *Thelan's Critical Care Nursing: Diagnosis and Management.* 5th ed. St. Louis, MO: Mosby/Elsevier.

Chapter 10

AACN Core Curriculum for Critical Care Nursing, 5th Edition. Philadelphia: W.B. Saunders Company, 1998.

Chmielewski, C. Anatomy and overview of nephron function. *Nephrology Nursing.* 30(2): 185–190, 2003.

Dirkes, S. & Hodge, K. Continuous renal replacement therapy in the adult critical care unit. *Critical Care Nurse,* 27(2): 61–80, 2007.

Edwards, S. Tissue viability: Understanding the mechanisms of injury and repair, *Nursing Standard,* 21(13): 48–56, 2005.

French, S. & Banerjee, D. Diagnosis and care of nephritic syndrome. *General Practitioner,* 30–31, 2007.

Goof, C. & Collin, G. Management of renal trauma at a rural, level 1 trauma center. *American Surgeon.* 64(3): 226. Retrieved 12/8/07 from *http://search.ebscohost.com.*

Guyton, A. C. & Hall, J.E. Renal physiology. In A.C. Guyton and J.E. Hill. Unit V: The body and fluids and kidneys. In A.C. Guyton & J.E. Hill, *Textbook of Medical Physiology,* 11th Edition. Philadelphia: W.B. Saunders, 264–379, 2006.

Henke, K. & Eigsti, J. Renal physiology: Review and practical application in the critically ill patient. *Dimensions of Critical Care Nursing.* 22(3): 125–132, 2003.

Kellum, J. & Palevski, P. Renal support in acute kidney injury. *Lancet.* 368(9533): 344–345, 2006.

Klabunder, R. Cardiovascular physiology concepts: Renin-angiotensin-aldosterone system. Retrieved 2/14/08 from *http://www.cvphysiology.com/Blood%20Pressure/BP015htm.*

Star, R. Treatment of acute renal failure: Perspectives in renal medicine. *Kidney International.* 54: 1817–1829, 1998.

Thelan, L., Urden, L. Lough, M., & Stacy, K. *Critical Care Nursing: Diagnosis and Management,* 3rd Edition, Unit VI: Renal alterations. St. Louis: Mosby, 847–916, 1998.

Weglicki, W., Quamme, G., Tucker, K., Haigney, M. & Resnick, L. Potassium, magnesium, and electrolyte imbalance and complications in disease management. *Clinical and Experimental Hypertension.* 95–112, 2004.

Figure 10.1: This article was published in *TEXTBOOK OF MEDICAL PHYSIOLOGY 11E,* Guyton & Hall, Page 309, Figure 26.3, Copyright Elsevier (2006).

Figure 10.2: This article was published in *TEXTBOOK OF MEDICAL PHYSIOLOGY 11E,* Guyton & Hall, Page 310, Figure 26.4, Copyright Elsevier (2006).

Figure 10.3: This article was published in *TEXTBOOK OF MEDICAL PHYSIOLOGY 11E,* Guyton & Hall, Page 314, Figure 26.8, Copyright Elsevier (2006).

Figure 10.4: This article was published in *TEXTBOOK OF MEDICAL PHYSIOLOGY 11E,* Guyton & Hall, Page 318, Figure 26.12, Copyright Elsevier (2006).

Figure 10.5: This article was published in *TEXTBOOK OF MEDICAL PHYSIOLOGY 11E,* Guyton & Hall, Page 358, Figure 28.8, Copyright Elsevier (2006).

Figure 10.6: This article was published in *TEXTBOOK OF MEDICAL PHYSIOLOGY 11E,* Guyton & Hall, Page 375, Figure 29.12, Copyright Elsevier (2006).

Figure 10.7: This article was published in *TEXTBOOK OF MEDICAL PHYSIOLOGY 11E,* Guyton & Hall, Page 414, Figure 31.8, Copyright Elsevier (2006).

Chapter 11

Black, J & Hawks, J. (2005). *Medical Surgical Nursing: Clinical Management for Positive Outcomes.* St. Louis: Saunders.

Bullock, B. & Henze, R. (2000). *Focus on Pathophysiology.* Philadelphia: Lippincott Williams & Wilkins.

Chai, L. (2005) Bloodstream Infections in Children. *Pediatric Critical Care Medicine:* Volume 6(3.) Supplement, pp 542–44.

Creasy, R & Resnick R. (2003). *Maternal-Fetal Medicine: Principles and Practice.* Philadelphia: WB Saunders.

Hockenberry, M. (2005). *Wong's Essentials of Pediatrics.* St. Louis: Mosby

Morton, P, Fontaine, D, Hudak, C, & Gallo, B. (2005). *Critical Care Nursing: A Holistic Approach.* Philadelphia: Lippincott, Williams, & Wilkins.

Shannon, M. (2000). Ingestion of Toxic Substances by Children. *New England Journal of Medicine* 342 (186–91).

Wilkerson, R, Northington, L, Fisher, W. (2005) Ingestions of Toxic Substances by Infants and Children: What we Don't Know Can't Hurt. *Critical Care Nurse* 25(4).

Websites:
http://kidney.niddk.nih.gov/kudiseases/pubs/childkidneydiseases/hemolytic_ureic_syndrome
http://www.bt.cdc.gov/agent/smallpox/disease/faq.asp
http://www.bt.cdc.gov/agent/agentlist-category.asp
http://www.umm.edu/ency/article 002487.htm
http://www.bcm.edu.oto.grand/9293.html
http://www.postgradmed.com/issues/1999/01-99/tomazewski.htm
http://www.emedicine.com
http://www.aapcc.org/DiseGuidelines/index.htm
http://www.safekids.org
http://www.depts.washington.edu/pccm/2-Pediatric%20Burns%20I.
http://www.ncbi.nlm.nih.gov/pubmed

Chapter 12

Alspach, J. (2006). *Core curriculum for critical care nursing.* (6th ed.).St. Louis: Saunders Elsevier.

American Nurses Association, (2001). *Code of ethics for nurses with interpretive statements.* Washington, DC: American Nurses Association.

Beauchamp, T. & Childress, J. (2001). *Principles of biomedical ethics.* (5th ed.). New York: Oxford University Press.

Benner, P. (1984). *From novice to expert: Excellence and power in clinical nursing practice.* Menlo Park, CA: Addison Wesley.

Curley, M. (2007). *Synergy: The unique relationship between nurses and patients.* Indianapolis, IN: Sigma Theta Tau International.

Curley, M. (1998). Patient-nurse synergy: Optimizing patients' outcomes. *American Journal of Critical Care.* 7: 64–72.

Ethics Resource Center Plus Model. Ethics Resource Center, Arlington, Virginia. retrieved June 3, 2008 from: *http://www.ethics.org/resources/decision-making-process.asp*

Hardin, S. & Kaplow, R. (2005). *Synergy for clinical excellence: The AACN synergy model for patient care.* Sudbury, MA: Jones & Bartlett.

Henderson, V. (1960). *Basic principles of nursing care.* London: International Council of Nurses.

Kaplow, R. (2003). AACN Synergy model for patient care: A framework to optimize outcomes. *Critical Care Nurse.* 23: S27–S30.

Rushton, C, & Scanlon, C. (1998). A road map for negotiating end-of-life care. *Medical Surgical Nursing.* 7: 57–59.

Thompson, J. & Thompson, H. (1985). *Bioethical decision-making for nurses.* Norwalk, CT: Appleton Century Crofts.

Index